The Food-Mood-Body Connection

THE FOOD-MOOD-BODY CONNECTION

Nutrition-Based and Environmental Approaches to Mental Health and Physical Wellbeing

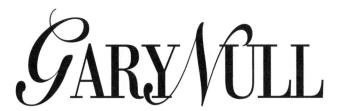

GARY NULL

with Louise Bernikow

SEVEN STORIES PRESS

New York / London / Sydney / Toronto

A Seven Stories Press First Edition

Parts of this book have been adapted from an earlier work by Dr. Null on this topic, *Nutrition and the Mind,* a Seven Stories Press book published in 1995.

This book is not intended to replace the services of a physician. Any application of the information set forth in the following pages is at the reader's discretion. The reader should consult with his or her physician before making any use of the information in this book.

Seven Stories Press
140 Watts Street
New York, NY 10013
http://www.sevenstories.com

In Canada:
Hushion House, 36 Northline Road, Toronto, Ontario M4B 3E2

In the U.K.:
Turnaround Publisher Services Ltd., Unit 3, Olympia Trading Estate, Coburg Road, Wood Green, London N22 6TZ

In Australia: Tower Books, 9/19 Rodborough Road, Frenchs Forest NSW 2086

Library of Congress Cataloging-in-Publication Data

Null, Gary.
    The food-mood-body connection : nutrition-based and environmental approaches to mental health and physical well-being / Gary Null.
        p. cm.
        Includes index.
        ISBN 1-58322-031-3 (cloth) / 1-58322-257-X
        1. Mental health—Nutritional aspects. 2. Health—Nutritional aspects. 3. Mental health—Environmental aspects. 4. Environmental health. 5. Mood (Psychology) I. Title.

RC455.5.N8 N847 2000
613.2—dc21
                                                                    99-461969

9 8 7 6 5 4 3 2 1

College professors may order examination copies of Seven Stories Press titles for a free six-month trial period. To order, visit www.sevenstories.com/textbook, or fax on school letterhead to (212) 226-1411.

Book design by Cindy LaBreacht

Printed in Canada

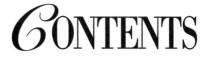ONTENTS

I. Disorders of Mood or Behavior

II. Disorders In Children

III. Organic Conditions Commonly Misdiagnosed As Mental Disease

AUTHOR'S PREFACE

The information in this book represents nearly 30 years of research and clinical experience. In seeking solutions to the complex problems of the food-mood-body connection, I have also interviewed thousands of board-certified clinicians from the fields of immunology, environmental medicine, psychiatry, psychology, as well as other behavioral sciences. From these interviews I have extracted from the clinicians' personal clinical experience the information that is most relevant and easy to understand and utilize. This provides you with the most up-to-date understanding of what may be the answer to the conditions you have or how to prevent unnecessary suffering in the future.

Gary Null, Ph.D.
Naples, Florida
July 2000

ℐNTRODUCTION

At the start of the 21st century, the mental health of the nation and the world is in a state of crisis. In 1999, Dr. David Sacher took the unprecedented step of issuing the first *United States Surgeon General's Report on Mental Health*. Depressive illness, according to the report, affects more than 19 million adults in the United States, not to mention the many millions more who love and care for them. Depressive illness is now the second most common cause of death in the United States, after heart disease. It is a leading cause of death among teens and young adults. Two out of three people who are suffering do not seek treatment.

Like everything else, the epidemic of mental disorders is global. In April, 2000, the World Health Organization examined seven countries and found that almost half the people they studied who experienced at least one disorder in their lifetime came from the United States, but that the rest of the world is not doing very well either. "All predictions are that the future will bring dramatic increase in mental problems," according to Dr. Gro Harlem Brundtland, WHO's General Director, who calls it a "crisis of the 21st century." He blames the "low priority assigned to mental health" for the disaster, as well as "the traditional centralization of mental health services in large, ineffective and often downright harmful psychiatric institutions."

The medical term "depressive illness" only partially describes the problem. We have children so un-balanced they go to school determined to kill, old people so loaded up with prescribed narcotics they can hardly move, and people in between who just feel emotionally lousy. Why?

Dr. Gabriel Cousens believes that what we are really facing is an epidemic of biologically altered brains. "In every generation on a universally poor diet," Dr. Cousens says, "there is a successive increasing degeneration in our mental and physical state. This has been shown in animal studies and we are now finding it in human studies. We have at least 8 million children on Ritalin. At least 10 percent of our children have hyperactivity, where 20 years ago that was not the case at all. We have 500 thousand children on antidepressants, particularly Prozac. One hundred thousand children are active alcoholics. It has to do with the poor nutrition of the parents, which affects the developing brain of the fetus. Then the child is raised on a very poor diet, so the brain, which may be a genetically weakened, becomes even more significantly weakened. Their neurotransmitters have lower amounts, their endorphins are not working quite right and so their brain is actually altered to the point where they need to do something to feel okay. That takes us to the epidemic of addictions which are also mental health diseases."

In spite their usefulness in shedding light on a subject still considered shameful, the *Surgeon General's Report* and the World Health Organization alarm fall far short of what they might have been. Nowhere do they mention the connection between mind and body, which is the starting point of all holistic medicine. Scant attention is paid to the causes of this epidemic of mental trouble—not only "depressive illness," and addictions, but rising numbers of schizophrenics, children who can't sit still long enough to learn anything in school, and ordinary people unable to focus, sleep or think clearly. It's taken for granted that our mental capacities weaken as we get older, but that isn't necessarily true. The environmental poisons and nutritional deficiencies that obviously contribute to mental and physical trouble, disease or deterioration are conspicuously ignored. Even worse, the progress made by orthomolecular doctors and other health professionals still called "alternative," is missing from the picture.

The national and international experts bemoaning a mental health crisis forgot to consider the good news: most mental and emotional conditions can and have been helped, if not cured, by natural means.

As Dr. James D. Gordon, clinical professor at the Georgetown University School of Medicine says, "All aspects of diet can affect all aspects of psychological and emotional functioning" and the fact that the average doctor sees no connection between nutrition and the mind is "staggering. We're not used to understanding the power of food in every healing tradition in the world. Hippocrates said 'Let food be your medicine and medicine your food.' But when we think of putting something in our mouths to affect our health, the reflex is to think of drugs."

Dr. Abram Hoffer, a pioneer in the field of orthomolecular psychiatry, specializing in treating schizophrenia, believes his colleagues in the mental health field are "way behind general medicine, but they're going to have to start budging. We in psychiatry are at least 10 years behind the rest of medicine when it comes to the proper consideration of nutrition, nutrients and other factors in the treatment of mental illness. They're still using treatment that was considered pretty good 30 years ago, and the only treatment today for schizophrenia is one of a variety of tranquilizers. As new ones are produced, they generate tremendous excitement as if a new tranquilizer is gonna do a better job. Some of them are also very dangerous. standard psychiatry merely gives every schizophrenic patient one or more tranquilizers in varying doses and hopes that this will bring the disease under control. if they get well, they start to get side affects, so they cut down the tranquilizer dose, and when they do that, the disease comes back, so the patients are bouncing back an forth between the street and the hospital, between high dose and low dose, between sickness and health. You can see the result. I would guess that half of all the homeless people in North America probably are schizophrenic patients who should have been treated in a hospital and kept there. Most psychiatrists want to put their patients on a tranquilizer on Wednesday, they want to see him better on Thursday, and they want to discharge him on Friday. You simply cannot get a chronic schizophrenic patient well that fast. It takes a lot of time."

Dr. Joseph Debe underlines the time needed for good care: "There are no shortcuts to health, none. You may think it is in a bottle, or a pill, or infommercial, or some other little quick technique but it's not. We deceive ourselves when we think that. You really have to look at it like you are going back to school to learn about yourself, your body, your mind, your spirit—learn all over again because a lot of the lessons you learned weren't your own and didn't apply to you. You took them as your own, you tried to match them, but at some point you woke up and you wore a size six shoe with a size twelve foot. You wonder why you are in such pain and discomfort and all you kept doing is try to make it work, make it fit, well sometimes things aren't meant to work or meant to fit based on upon the misapplication of our energies and our attitude. We've got to realign ourselves with what is essential to us."

In fact, the mainstream health industry has been rushing in the opposite direction. Less time. Less individuality. More and more drugs. Every year, more conditions are "diagnosed" as requiring medication. I recently saw a scientific paper claiming that the disease of "imagined ugliness" should be treated with anti-depressants. The direction is toward more pills, more "quick fixes," and more profit for the pharmaceutical industry.

For many years, the experts on my radio show and I have been protesting the huge and still increasing numbers of Prozac and Ritalin prescriptions written for people suffering from depression or children diagnosed with "Attention Deficit Disorder." In the last decade of the 20th century, Ritalin production increased seven fold. Ninety percent of the Ritalin prescribed in the world is used in the United States. It took the revelation that this Class Two narcotic was being used on children as young as six to alert the public that something was going on. Only now have the dangers and abuses of these drugs begun to provoke an outcry in the mainstream media.

Although generally dismissed as "safe," the huge numbers of prescription drugs, especially those that alter brain chemistry, being consumed by toddlers, adolescents, mature adults and senior citizens does a great deal of proven harm. Dr. Parris Kidd says that up to ten percent of all the people diagnosed with dementia (loss of memory, learning and concentration accompanied by deterioration in mood) are actually suffering from drug-induced brain damage, which is "mimicking dementia. When they are taken off the drug," he says, "they begin to improve." And Dr. Abram Hoffer, who pioneered the whole field of orthomolecular psychiatry, says that anti-psychotic drugs in particular induce "the tranquilizer psychosis, characterized by a decrease in the intensity of the psychotic symptoms but induced in its place are apathy, disinterest, poor judgment, difficulty in thinking and concentration and inability to work."

The more we learn about how the brain and the rest of the body work, the harder it is to believe that disease and deterioration are inevitable as we age. Parris Kidd, a cellular biologist, has, like many others, been insisting that "the modern pattern of brain deterioration is definitely not normal." From simple irritants like forgetting where you put your glasses or keys to forgetting names and faces, brain impairment with aging is, most of all, a product of lifestyle, environment and nutrition. "The brain cells are our largest and most energy demanding and most fragile cells," Dr. Kidd says. "They are particularly vulnerable to toxins like aluminum, mercury fillings, lead from car exhaust, pesticides, even monosodium glutamate and aspartame" in NutraSweet. "As the years go by, cumulative toxic damage will affect function. Although there has been a great shift in emphasis toward looking for genes that cause these problems, there is no aging gene."

What biogenetic company, I wonder, investing millions of dollars in finding a genetic marker for aging and creating a drug of some kind that will affect it, would ever acknowledge the truth of Dr. Kidd's remarks? There is no money in lifestyle change or in a healthy diet. The money is in drug therapy.

In the early 21st century, the money is also in genetic research, based upon the idea that mental illness can be found and treated in the genes. We're told that disorders such as schizophrenia and depression seem to be passed down from generation to generation, therefore it's in your genes. A lot of research talent and money is going into trying to find vaccines so that anyone with a genetic expression of a mental disease will be able to be vaccinated against it. Dr. Ty Colbert, a clinical physiologist and active member of the National Association for Rights, Protection and Advocacy, reminds us that "while there are some true genetic disorders, like Huntington's disease, with which they are making a lot of progress, there has actually been no progress made with any mental illness. No pathophysiological evidence whatsoever exists for mental illness; it's all a series of theories."

The idea that mental illness is in the genes and can, therefore, be inherited, according to Dr. Colbert, "had its roots in the turn of the last century, when there was a strong emphasis on social Darwinism or Eugenics. There was an attempt to prove that defects are passed along, that one race is superior to the other race. So a lot of inheritance studies were developed—with a lot of errors in them—that began to show that mental illness sometimes run in families. They didn't consider other things that run in families—religion, accents, a lot of modeling of behavior. Just because it goes from one generation to the next doesn't mean that it's inherited.

"One of the statistics most quoted by supporters of a genetic theory is that the concordance rate between identical twins with schizophrenia is somewhere between 45 percent and 50 percent. That means if one twin has schizophrenia, the chances of the other one having schizophrenia is 50 percent. That figure is used to substantiate a lot of the biological approach to psychiatry. But more recent, more accurate studies show the concordance rates actually down to something like 17 to 20 percent.

"A psychiatrist was treating a man who was schizophrenic. He also had some unusual abnormalities on his face—his ear lobes were sort of joined together next to his head and he had webs between his fingers. By chance, the psychiatrist happened to be talking to her patient's mother one day and she described an uncle who had some of the same characteristics. This uncle had been diagnosed as schizophrenic too. The psychiatrist concluded that the gene that caused the physical abnormalities in those two people may be the gene that caused the schizophrenia or that the gene that causes physical abnormalities is close to the gene for schizophrenia. If you can find a gene for the abnormalities, maybe you can find a gene for schizophrenia. They were never able to find it. What the doctors didn't consider is that somebody with those weird characteristics is often teased relentlessly by his peers and even maybe rejected by his family, so the problems both individuals had could have been emotionally-based.

"Today, there is an attempt to find a gene for alcoholism. They take a group of alcoholics and a group non-alcoholics and go through the whole genetic code to see if they can't find something different in the genetic codes of the two. If they find something different—it could be blue eyes versus brown eyes—they start to think that gene is close to the gene for alcoholism. That is called a marker. It's not really a defective gene, it's just a marker. They found a marker for alcoholism and then they tried to duplicate it and could not. They found another marker —it hit the newspapers again—that couldn't be duplicated. There have been nearly 100 non-duplications. Those never hit the newspapers."

Nutritional and Environmental Influences on Mental States

Ignoring the nutritional and environmental influences on mental states is a costly and dangerous business. Both are getting worse. Not only are the foods we do eat over-processed, robbed of all nutritional value, but the usual American diet still consists of few fresh fruits and vegetables and inordinate amounts of sugar and caffeine. When I was growing up, we got hot cereal like oatmeal or eggs, whole grain toast and juice for breakfast. Today most children start the day with only a sugared snack, a cola beverage, high levels of caffeine. And we're supposed to believe that there is no connection between that and a child bouncing off the walls an hour later in school? Then the teacher decides that the child has something emotionally wrong with them and shouldn't be in class unless they are under the influence of a medication to control them. We have close to 9 million children taking some form of psychoactive medication each day.

Mid-morning, the kid goes out to a vending machine and gets more sugared, processed foods. By lunch time, there is almost always a toxic reaction—excitotoxins in the food are in the brain. In the afternoon, the kid is bouncing off the walls again. They rarely have a meal with a family where it's really a wholesome meal. It's processed, it's pasteurized, it's salted, it's sugared, it's artificial. No one is going to stop and say, "You know, maybe the child is just having a reaction to the stimulant in the food?" The latest study shows that the average child does not eat one single serving of vegetables and fruits a day. Not one. They gave French fries the benefit of being a half serving of vegetables. So how are these kids supposed to have the biochemistry to allow their bodies and brains to function?

Dr. Gordon tells his patients to start with an experiment: "Cut out the processed food, cut out the sugar, cut out the additives and in some cases, cut out certain foods that may be likely to cause food sensitivities—wheat and milk and milk products, maybe corn. See what happens. In many cases, a kid's behavior has turned around almost 180 degrees. new program.

This needs to be a part of our collective consciousness. Dr. Gordon believes it hasn't been so because "we keep the focus on that magic bullet. The metaphor is a metaphor of attack, an inappropriate metaphor for these kinds of conditions. The question really is—what can we do for ourselves? If we begin to pose the question that way, different kinds of answers come. You can change your diet. You can change your patterns of exercise. You can teach relaxation techniques. You can work with martial arts with kids so they can use their energy in a different way. As long as we keep posing the question—what does the expert have to do to us or for us?—we're in trouble. All we're going to come up with is more drugs.

"I have still not seen a good study that has explored nutrition and the mind. Dean Ornish did that with heart disease—he showed that if you ate a different kind of diet, you could reverse heart disease. The epidemiological evidence is that certain kinds of foods are more likely to predispose you to developing cancer, although they're not the only factor. I think we would find the same kinds of thing with behavior, but there has not been a major push in that direction, partly because there is not a major economic impetus for it. Nobody is going to make money out of basically having a decent diet. You can't patent a decent diet. You can't sell it in a pill. It's something that people have to do for themselves."

What people can do for themselves is laid out very succinctly by Dr. Gordon:

"Eliminate foods that are heavily processed and have been adulterated in any way—with any kind of food additive, preservative, coloring, artificial flavoring, artificial sweetener. Aspartame has been shown to cause serious brain damage in animals.

"If possible, eat food that has been raised organically. That way, you are eliminating the pesticides, herbicides, hormones and antibiotics that go into so much of the food supply, all of which have significant biological effects.

"Eat whole foods. It's crucial. Humans were meant to eat whole foods, not pop tarts. If you eat a whole food diet and then eat a processed food, there are significant effects on intestinal functioning. If the intestine is not functioning well, you are not going to be taking in the nutrients, even if the food is decent.

"Eliminate all of the sugar. A natural honey or rice syrup is fine, but not the nine teaspoons of sugar in every Coke and other sweet carbonated beverages. Cut out the caffeine. Watch for food sensitivities, which are not full-fledged food allergies. The most common culprits are milk and milk products, beef, yeast, wheat, citrus, corn, soy. Eliminate those and then reintroduce them one at a time. See if it clouds your thinking or makes you anxious or depressed.

"As far as supplements go, for anybody living in a society with so much pollution and stress, I recommend a high dose multi-vitamin, multi-mineral with iron if you're a menstruating woman, without iron if you're not menstruating. And at least as a base line, I recommend using some substance with omega three fatty acids—large doses of fish, like salmon, or a couple of tablespoons a day of flax seed. (Flax seed is somewhat better than flax seed oil. You can grind it up and put it on your food.)

"If there are significant psychological problems, check your thyroid. A lot of people are depressed because of low thyroid functioning. Sometimes, those people may show up with normal thyroid functioning on tests. So I suggest that people take their temperature for seven days, early in the morning, putting the thermometer in their armpits for 10 minutes. If the temperature is at 98 or above, that's fine, but many people have temperatures in the 96–97 range. They may be hypothyroid and they may need to go to a nutritionally oriented physician or a naturopath to find out about using supplemental does of thyroid."

Even an extreme mental disease like schizophrenia is linked, according to Dr. Abram Hoffer, to food allergies and nutrient deficiency. "The nutrient deficiencies," Dr. Hoffer says, "are usually some of the B vitamins, especially pyridoxine and niacin or niacinamide, and the chief mineral deficiency is zinc. During World War II in England, when sugar consumption was cut in half, when only a very dark brown flour was available for bread, and when the English were forced to depend more on their own home grown products, the incidence of schizophrenia went down, in spite of the stress of the war and the bombing of London and other cities."

Poor nutrition is one cause of mental health problems. Beyond that, there are several diet-related disorders. Dr. Robert Atkins decries the inaction of conventional physicians treating mental illness when it comes to identifying the root causes of any of these. Depression and anxiety, he says, are both classifiable as diet-related disorders: "I have treated about 45,000 patients in my career. In just about every community around the country, psychiatrists are doing a sort of knee-jerk reaction to the problem of anxiety and depression. They never bother to ask, 'Why is my patient having a problem?' Instead, they immediately ask, 'What is the name of the problem and what's its standard orthodox treatment?' They are bypassing the most important question of all: 'Why is my patient sick?'

"If something is in the diet that is actually contributing enough to this problems like anxiety and depression, we correct the diet, and the problem will disappear. The first question you have to ask is whether the symptoms change from hour to hour. Is the depression worse for an hour, and then it suddenly lifts? Does the anxiety change from hour to hour? That is the cardinal thing to look for because if the depression or anxiety are changeable, then they are almost definitely diet-related.

"There are three major mechanisms of diet-related disorder. The first—and the most important one—is blood-sugar instability. The old name was hypoglycemia, but that really doesn't describe it. It's the condition in which the blood sugar is capable of rapid escalations and rapid falls, so much so that the body is putting out other hormones—particularly adrenaline—to help regulate the blood sugar. Adrenaline is called forth when the blood sugar is on a free fall, which it usually does if something made it go up very fast, like a candy bar or a sugar and caffeine-laden cola drink. You can make your blood sugar go up very fast and if you have this problem, which, I would say, at least half the population has to some extent, then adrenaline is released and you get a panic attack. With blood sugar instability, typically you get your reaction before a meal, if you haven't eaten, or if you have eaten sweets and nothing else, which is the classic way to get it. That is really the basis of most anxiety states. Panic attacks can turn into an absolute phobia. You get a panic attack two or three times, and then become phobic in relation to whatever it was you were doing at the time you got your panic attack.

"The second mechanism is food allergies, which work a little differently. First you eat the offending food—which is often a grain, or milk, or sometimes some of the protein foods. Usually, the foods you are allergic to are whatever you eat most often, and since in our culture so many people eat bread with every meal, you have to suspect wheat. A lot of people drink milk with every meal, so dairy is a prime allergen. After eating foods you are allergic to over a long period of time, you may develop a leaky gut syndrome, and then you will develop the inability to handle the protein complexes that are characteristic of that food. So you get a reaction after you eat it.

"The third mechanism," Dr. Atkins concludes, "is yeast, specifically candida albicans. The yeast itself is capable, through biochemical intermediaries, of making people a little 'flaky' right from the very beginning, but it also makes you more likely to have food intolerances, especially people with sugar imbalances. Very often, people with all three of the above-mentioned conditions are going to a psychiatrist who is not trained to diagnose diet-related disorders. So even though you have psychiatric symptoms, you have a good chance of being incorrectly diagnosed because the doctor you are seeing does not specialize in diet-related disorders."

Food Allergies

There are two definitions of allergies today. The traditional, or classic, definition describes an immunological reaction, and, as Dr. Kendall Gerdes explains, "There are very good data suggesting that food allergies as traditionally defined are a fairly rare phenomenon—maybe three-tenths of one percent in children and even less in adults." Then there is the far more common phenomenon of food intolerance or hypersensitivity, which conventional doctors tend to know very little about. Again, Dr. Gerdes: "People read about food allergies in books they find in health food stores, but then they go to a traditional physician who thinks about allergies in a classic way. So he says, 'Well, this person is talking about something that is really rare.' But in fact, food intolerance or hypersensitivity is much more common. We have to be careful when we talk about allergies, to be sure we know whether we are speaking of the classical definition or the second, more common type.

"Many people do have significant symptoms related to foods, and these are not rare foods. They are not strawberries, or tomatoes, or peanuts that might be involved in the classic, more traditionally described immunological food allergy reactions. They are instead hypersensitivities to the much more commonly eaten everyday foods, such as milk, wheat, and corn. These are the kinds of foods that can get to be problems.

"The immunoglobulin E (IGE) type reaction is really severe. That happens in the person who eats one peanut and has to be taken off to the emergency room. On the other hand, the kind of food sensitivity I am talking about occurs in people who eat fairly large amounts of a particular food, and many times they can't see the cause-and-effect relationship because they are eating that food all the time.

"The first people to do research in the area of food intolerance did so 40 to 50 years ago," Dr. Gerdes continues. "A physician named Herbert Rinkel was the first one to observe that a food a person ate all the time might be causing symptoms, but you couldn't see the relationship. If you took the person off that food for a week and then gave it to them, then you might get a sharp and clear reaction. He called this 'masked food allergy.'

"Dr. Theron Randolph enlarged the concept. He observed that not only did people use these foods often, but they used the foods as if they were addicted to them. They didn't merely have wheat for breakfast, they craved wheat. They loved wheat. They might have it six times a day. They might even, if they had trouble sleeping, eat wheat in the middle of the night to help them get back to sleep. And he found that when people were using certain foods in this kind of pattern, they temporarily felt better after eating the food. By using the same principles that Dr. Rinkel had used, Dr. Randolph would take the person off the food for a week and then challenge them. In that way, many times he could see the reaction that the patient themselves could not see. The critical variable was, once he began to look for the foods that people were addicted to, he found he had a much better basis from which to determine the foods to which people were allergic.

"A person might have a wide array of emotional and mental reactions. He or she might be irritable, depressed, or anxious because of foods that they are eating or because of chemicals in their environment such as perfumes or formaldehyde in particle board or furniture. Research is only beginning to understand how this process works. Dr. Iris Bell, a professor of psychiatry at the University of Arizona, is very interested in this topic and has been exploring it more than anyone else. She is finding that food and chemical sensitivities probably play into the endorphin system—the same system that produces a runner's high. The endorphin system is used as a way for the brain to give a feeling of comfort. For instance, when an infant is crying or upset, the mother gives him some breast milk, and the sugar and fat in the milk probably trigger the endorphin system so that the baby then can go to sleep. That same system can be activated under some circumstances by children and adults in order to make themselves feel good. As a consequence, people find themselves having to use a particular food or a group of foods to make themselves feel better. That is part of the basis of food addiction.

"The simplest approach to use in order to figure out what foods you are sensitive to is to look for the foods that you are using a lot, if you are someone whose symptoms seem to fluctuate over the course of an hour, a day, or a week. This is the same approach that most of the physicians in the Academy of Environmental Medicine use, among others.

"Here's a hypothetical 35-year-old woman. (I say a woman because women go to doctors more frequently than men do, for whatever the reason. Whether this is because men are being more stoic and not coming in, or whether women are more vulnerable, we don't really know.) It would not be uncommon to find a woman who has a fair amount of fatigue, with a low-grade depression that sometimes gets to the point where she almost can't cope with things. When that occurs, and it is a variable type of thing, I will look for the two, or five, or ten foods that she is using a lot and suggest that she take them out of her diet for a week. Then, at the end of that week, many times she will find that she is not so tired and doesn't have that low-grade depression; she has more motivation to do things. Then I get more specific and test one food at a time. I ask her to have a big meal of each of those foods that she has been avoiding. Many times we can find out which food or foods have been causing the low-grade depression and her other symptoms. Though this is a generic example," Dr. Gerdes concludes, "cases just like it are fairly common."

Dr. Abram Hoffer offers another case study: "I treated a young man who was both schizophrenic and alcoholic. He had been working on his Ph.D. when he became so ill that he could not continue. Eventually he came under my care. It turned out that he didn't respond too well to my program—the vitamins and the other things that I was doing—and finally I discovered from his mother, not from him, that he consumed 12 ounces of tomato juice every morning, and had since he was a child. That was one of his basic breakfast foods. And it turned out that he had a tomato allergy. Then his mother told me that she too had been allergic to tomatoes, but she hadn't touched them for at least 60 years.

"When I put the young man on a tomato-free diet, and explained to him why, his depression and his schizophrenia vanished and he became normal. He was my second case in which a food allergy was a major factor in determining the illness of a person. It can be any one food or often a combination of foods—two or even three foods—that people have to learn to avoid, and their mental condition will then improve dramatically."

Dr. Doris Rapp is one of the world's leading experts on food allergies, especially in children. It is no accident that she has focused her energies recently on the so-called "epidemic" of "Attention Deficit Disorder" and the huge numbers of prescriptions for the drug called Ritalin that is being prescribed for it. "There are many studies, here and abroad," she says, "that clearly demonstrate that foods and environmental factors can cause ADD and ADHD. Sixty-six percent of hyperactivity is related to food allergies. Another piece of the puzzle is clearly dust, molds, pollen and chemicals. Mint-flavored Prozac is hardly the answer if a child's depression is due to something eaten, touched or smelled that can be avoided. Environmental medical specialists can turn a child's depression or hyperactivity on and off like a switch with different dilutions of routine allergy extracts. Sure, drugs are helpful, but if the causes can be eliminated, they are not needed."

Heavy Metal Toxicity

Dr. Richard Kunin emphasizes the importance of hair tests, as opposed to the more common blood tests, in the prevention of heavy metal poisoning. To start off, Dr. Kunin offers a personal account of heavy metal toxicity from his own family's experience: "A beautiful son was born to me in October 1971. In about June of 1972, he had enough hair for a hair test and I did one, and found that he had roughly 80 parts per million of lead in his hair. He should have had zero. Eighty parts per million is a toxic load and could only be coming from something he was eating. It was not something that we were putting on his hair; we certainly didn't use hair sprays or dyes. So I knew that my son, before he was a year old, was already poisoned. My heart fell. I almost fainted with grief. We checked things out and found that a toy that he had been given as a gift was tainted with six percent lead in the paint—that's 6,000 parts per million. If we hadn't done a hair test, he would have continued to have been poisoned and would have been mentally retarded.

"Lead poisoning has, first, a bad effect on the brain. The second bad effect is that you get bowel problems and colic. The third thing is you lose your coordination because the hands and feet are weak. Then the immune system is weakened. In other words, you are just not the person you could have been.

"I once had an 18-year-old patient, a beautiful woman, who came to see me who was depressed. She graduated from college with a C average and was disappointed in herself. She had been raised on vitamins and an Adelle Davis diet by a very caring mother. But they had lived overseas, where they had bought native pottery, and as a baby she was already lead-poisoned. I know this because I did a hair analysis of the child's hair samples that her mother had saved at various ages. At one and a half, her hair was 180 parts per million of lead. At five, it was down to 80. At age 12 it was down to practically nothing, and at age 18 we couldn't find it. As she grew, this load of lead that she had picked up as a baby was being absorbed into her tissues and being diluted. But it left behind its damage on her. Her teachers would write on her report card, 'Jennifer could have done so much better if she had really tried.' The teachers couldn't understand it. The girl had an attention deficit based on an early-life toxicity that went undiagnosed because nobody looked.

"In an enlightened society, all children should be tested for lead. But their hair and not their blood should be tested. The government is spending millions of dollars to test children by taking a blood sample for lead, which is absolutely ridiculous. Lead will be filtered out of the blood in a week. If you are exposed to lead this week, by next week it will be gone, but it will remain in your hair for six months. When a hair test is done once a year, you are going to find lead contamination if it is present.

"Hair analysis, for a reasonable price, gives you 30 or more real facts about the levels of mercury, arsenic, cadmium, lead, nickel, aluminum, and fluoride that have built up in your body. Everyone should know what toxic substances and physiologic minerals—chromium, selenium, boron—they're accumulating or are deficient in. We have very few tools that give us this kind of perspective," Dr. Kunin concludes. "The contamination level can be minute and still show up on the test, whose accuracy is quite high."

Dr. Christopher Calapai details some of the sources of our exposure to heavy metal contamination and how the problem can be so damaging to our mental and physical health: "We are exposed to metals from a wide variety of places. They are in our drinking water, in some of our foods, even in our work environment where we breathe in certain toxins. Lead, for example, can come into the body through exposure to metals in paints. We get cadmium from our food, air, and water; mercury from dental fillings and shellfish; and aluminum and excess iron from pots and pans. Many of the metals that are brought into the body are toxic to the brain and to central nervous system tissue. They interfere with normal metabolism by disrupting enzyme systems.

"According to the standard textbook in the field, there have been reports of increased aluminum in the bulk of brain tissue in Alzheimer's patients and, more recently, associations of aluminum with neurofibrillary tangles and neuritic plaques. Aluminum has also been associated with neurofibrillary degeneration in patients with amyotrophic lateral sclerosis and Parkinsonism type dementia. Areas of concern with regard to mercury exposure include kidney dysfunction, neurotoxicity, reduced immune function, hypersensitivity reactions, birth defects and overall changes in general health.

"*The Food Additives Handbook* reports that lead, cadmium, and arsenic are put into animal feed, as are other heavy metals. They are probably placed there intentionally to remove germs. In addition, aluminum is found in baking powder, table salt, and vanilla powder. It's used as an emulsifier, and as an anti-caking agent," Dr. Calapai adds. Testing and treatment protocols for heavy metal poisoning should be holistic and should take into consideration recent refinements in treatment.

"Before treating the condition, we perform a blood test to check vitamin and mineral levels, we examine the person's diet, consider what they do for work, where they work, and what they're exposed to at work, as well as in their home environment. We also do a 24-hour urine test with an intravenous chelation procedure, and test for creatinine clearance (kidney function), as well as testing for heavy metals.

"The latest and best treatment of heavy metal toxicity is a combination of oral vitamins and minerals to maximize immune function, exercise, and intravenous EDTA chelation therapy to remove the metals. Vitamin C is also beneficial. Some people use intravenous vitamin C and alternate that with chelation.

"The vitamins and minerals that we recommend are based upon the individual's particular needs. We check to see if the patient is deficient in different nutrients or if they're not absorbing certain nutrients present in their diet. The ranges are individually different and depend on the result of the physical exam."

Dr. Calapai also discusses chelation therapy, an important modality to treat heavy metal poisoning, as well as certain other illnesses, including heart disease in some cases: "Chelation therapy is a treatment that has been around for many years. It involves using an intravenous application or induction of a protein substance that helps to bind heavy metals, to drag them out and throw them out of the body through the urine. The treatment takes about three hours to perform. It also has been shown to produce significant changes in plaque deposition in the lining of blood vessels, so it can help to open up and improve blood circulation in the body. You can detect how well the metals are being removed by means of a repeat 24-hour urine test. Chelation therapy for people who have heavy metal toxicity may be done once or twice a week for 15 weeks," Dr. Calapai concludes.

Patient story: A single dental filling

A Russian immigrant who had no fillings got a single filling when she was 20. She came to me at 22 with a shopping bag full of medicine. She didn't know what was wrong. She couldn't think. She was nauseated and sick all the time. When I asked her when it started, she said two years before. I looked into her mouth, and saw the single filling. I asked which had come first, the filling or the illness. And she said, "Oh my God. It was three months after the filling was put in that I got sick." She was a very skeptical woman who didn't trust American medicine. I told her she had to have it taken out. She was so desperate that she said, "I don't believe a word you are saying, but I'm going to have it taken out because I'm afraid that I will die if I don't."

She had the filling removed. In 17 days, she was able to start eating some foods that she couldn't eat before. It took about three months before she saw substantial results and she came back and said, "I believe it." Now that was a problem caused by a single filling.

Dr. Alfred Zamm, who convinced the Russian woman to have her dental filling removed, reminds us that "mercury poisoning is like a ghost. You don't know it's there. It comes and goes, wearing masks. Some years ago, I wrote an article listing as many as 50 symptoms associated with mercury poisoning. The top three were fatigue, inappropriate coldness, and sugar intolerance. These patients crave sugar and eat sweet things, and may or may not know that they will get sick. They may eat sweets on Monday and get sick on Tuesday. They may have all sorts of bizarre symptoms—muscle aches and pains, fatigue, headaches, personality changes. You don't have to have all of the symptoms; you can have one, and it may come and go."

Other common symptoms of mercury poisoning are headaches, difficulty concentrating, difficulty with reading comprehension, forgetfulness, depression, and skin changes. "It is very difficult," Dr. Zamm adds, "to prove mercury poisoning, except after the fact, when the mercury is out and the patient feels better. Taking a whole group of fillings out is not a minor matter, so I have devised some tests to assess whether or not it is worth proceeding in this direction.

"If you crave sugar and sugar makes you sick," Dr. Zamm says, "and you are already suspicious about that, then take this test. Try taking selenium, which is a mineral that binds with mercury, cadmium, and arsenic. If you feel better after taking selenium, it is a clue, not a diagnosis. About 20 years ago, when I started to investigate selenium, I realized that there was a paradox. Some people got better right away, some people took about three months, and some people got worse. I finally figured out that the patients who got worse were those who were most sensitive. They were the ones who were really sick—the ones who needed it the most but because of a peculiar intolerance to everything, including the things they needed, couldn't deal with the selenium. To overcome this, I had the very sensitive patients dilute chemically pure selenium down to very small dilutions. By starting with very small dilutions and gradually building up the dosage over a period of three months, these very sick patients started to get better.

"Selenium is an atom that fits into a molecule called glutathionperoxidase, which helps to destroy dangerous, foreign chemicals that just don't belong in our bodies, such as petrochemicals, floor wax, and insecticides. So when you take selenium, you're not only knocking out mercury, cadmium, and arsenic, you are also helping to produce more glutathionperoxidase, which protects you from environmental contaminants. So if you feel better, it is not an absolute diagnosis of mercury poisoning.

"Within pyruvate dehydrogenase complex, there are three enzymes. The first one uses thiamine, vitamin B1. If you are tired all the time, and you take 25 mg of thiamine once or twice a day, which is a low dose, and you notice you feel better, that is another clue you might have mercury poisoning. Now you have the selenium and the thiamine clue.

"The last thing is zinc. Too much cadmium and mercury in the body will replace zinc in the enzymes. Our bodies have 50 to 75 enzymes with zinc in them. So if you have mercury knocking out your zinc, then you know why it is poisoning you. It is inactivating enzymes by knocking out the zinc, which is supposed to be there, and replacing it with mercury which doesn't work. This is cellular poisoning. You are not burning sugar, which is why you are cold and tired, and that's why you are sugar-intolerant.

"Why do some people who have mercury in their bodies not get sick? We are genetically polymorphic, meaning that some people have a lot of enzymes that work very well and some people have less and what they have doesn't work very well. Some of us who have mercury in our bodies are able to deal with it, while others are not able to deal with it. Those who are just getting by, who were born with a slight deficiency, will just get through. But if, at age 12 or 13, people are poisoned by having mercury fillings put in their mouths, those who have strong enzyme systems may not notice much, but those who are less strong start to manifest symptoms, although usually not right away. After a few months, a child can't concentrate at school. Maybe he or she develops allergies, and nobody connects it with the filling that was put in six months earlier.

"I have one patient, a young child, who had a filling the size of a pinhead and I didn't see it because it was in the back. You'd need a special dental mirror. And I said to the mother, 'I don't understand this case. This child can't tolerate sugar, he is hyperkinetic.' (Hyperkinesis, or hyperactivity, is one of the symptoms of mercury poisoning.) I said, 'This has to be a case of mercury poisoning. This child was perfectly well until he was seven. But I don't see any fillings.' She said, 'Doctor, there is a filling there.' So I got a dental mirror from a colleague of mine and looked. Sure enough, there was a filling the size of a pinhead. I couldn't believe it. I had the filling removed, and within three months the child was substantially improved. This child was genetically polymorphic in the sense that he had a very inefficient oxidation process.

"When you talk about genetically polymorphic individuals who are sensitive, such as the Russian emigrant woman, they are going to have many of the symptoms that I have mentioned, including depressions, anxiety, and sleep disturbances. If you are not oxidizing, if you are not burning sugar, you are energy-deficient and you are going to be deficient in many other organ functions. Mercury poisoning from dental fillings is so elusive because it is in effect sabotaging the engine of their lives. Each organ will express itself in its own dysfunction. That is why muscle aches and depression and all those things go together. But some organs are a little stronger than others so they won't manifest symptoms.

"If a patient comes in and says, 'I'm depressed,' one of the causes may be mercury poisoning. I once gave a lecture to a group of graduate students in psychology because the chairman of the department, who was my patient, was so impressed with the fact that you could get the patient better physically and affect the mental illness. The title of the lecture was 'How I Would Like to Be Treated if I Were a Patient.'

"In the case of mercury poisoning, there may be enough oxygen available, but the person's body can't burn it because the burning mechanism has shut down. In every case of depression, physical deficiencies and toxic poisoning should be considered first, before resorting to therapy and psychotropic medications such as antidepressants. I have seen hundreds of these cases respond to diagnosis and treatment of the underlying physical cause.

"How is it possible that, in the new millenium, dentists are continuing to put a toxic substance in our mouths? We need some historical perspective on the issue. In 1826, a Parisian named Taveau discovered that if you took silver coins and filed them into dust and mixed it with mercury, and then squeezed the mercury out, this putty would harden quickly. Then you could take this putty-like material, push it into a cavity in someone's mouth, and it would harden like concrete. Other people realized that this wasn't such a good idea and there were arguments back and forth. Then, in 1833 in New York, two brothers went into the business of doing this process on a mass scale. It's a cheap filling. You don't have to be a good dentist to make a mercury filling.

"The so-called silver amalgam filling is a lie. This 'silver' filling is only 30 percent silver, but it is 50 percent mercury and 20 percent various other metals that can produce hardness. They call it a silver filling when the major ingredient is mercury. So I refer to it as a mercury filling.

"To give you some perspective on just how long ago 1826 was, in terms of the degree of ignorance that was then prevalent, consider that in 1860, 35 years later, a man in Vienna said to doctors, 'If you don't wash your hands before you examine pregnant women, you are going to spread disease.' And this man was thrown out of the medical society because he was impugning the reputation of physicians. They didn't know about germs. It was not until 1875 that Louis Pasteur and others proved that germs were a major cause of disease. And yet dental technology invented back in the medical Dark Ages is what we are still using today, nearly 175 years later.

"How can mercury fillings still be considered to be safe? The answer: If you did it before, it's okay to do it again. For example, lead pipes were the standard for years, so they are still okay now. Luckily, we have finally gotten around to seeing that lead pipes weren't really safe, that the lead leaching into the water causes brain damage. So we've stopped using lead in pipes. We still have tobacco from when the colonists smoked it with the Indians hundreds of years ago. You still can't convince some people that it's not healthy to smoke. We continue to sell tobacco and other poisonous substances out of habit and the profit motive.

"The same is true with mercury fillings. There is no proof that they are safe. Now, if you went out to buy a can of soup in the supermarket, it would be strange to have the clerk behind the counter say to you, 'I'd like you to prove the safety of this can.' You would say, 'What are you talking about? I'm purchasing the can. The fact that you are selling it implies that you are saying that it's safe.' But the clerk says, 'Not when it comes to soup. When it comes to soup, it is the responsibility of the purchaser to prove that it is safe or not safe. We as the sellers don't have to do anything.' That's the situation we're in with mercury fillings. No one has ever proved that mercury fillings are safe in human beings. They should prove it. But instead, the dental industry has turned it around and said, 'No, you have to prove it is unsafe.' Charlemagne said, 'If the populace knew with what idiocy they were ruled, they would revolt.' That goes for some of the things that they do in dentistry, too."

The chemistry of heavy metal poisoning is very important to Dr. tk, who explains that "mercury will decrease about 20 percent of the tubulan, which is a chemical in the brain needed for good brain function, memory, and the transmission of a signal between the memory cells. When they do autopsies on the brains of people with severe memory loss, characteristic of Alzheimer's or Parkinson's disease, they notice that these brains have a definite shortage of tubulan.

"Some people cling to the idea that mercury mixed in an alloy is safe, but the most up to date research shows that while it may not be too harmful when it is mixed, as it stays in your mouth for many years, the acids in your saliva and the digestive juices in your mouth work on those fillings and you begin to off-gas tremendous amounts of mercury.

Most of the mercury getting up into the brain is coming from the off gassing. It goes right up through your nose and gets right in with the oxygen, directly into the brain.

"Mercury passes pretty easily, as does aluminum, through the blood brain barrier. There are four distinct areas in the brain that do not have a blood brain barrier, so when people say, don't worry about it, don't worry about the aluminum lakes and cosmetics, or the mercury in dental amalgams, they're forgetting that even if the blood brain barrier could keep those things out, which it doesn't, there are still four areas of the brain that do not have this protective barrier, and one of the main areas is called the hypothalamus."

Mercury poisoning has other sources and other consequences. Pregnant mothers with this toxicity pass it on to their unborn children, with disturbing results. Scientific studies in 1997 concluded that "millions of children across the world may have been mentally damaged after being exposed to low levels of mercury before they were born." Children whose mothers ate substantial amounts of fish. showed deficits in learning, attention, memory, spatial perception, and motor skills by age 7. The children performed as though they were a few months behind for their age. A U.S. Environmental Protection Agency report estimated that 85,000 U.S. women of childbearing age have excessive exposures to mercury. The mercury in fish comes 60 percent from burning coal and oil, and 36 percent from waste incineration. The Electric Power Research Institute (EPRI) said it would cost up to $10 billion to fit power plant smoke stacks with filters to capture mercury, and that "it's just not worth it."

Dr. Ray Wunderlich offers another example of heavy metal toxicity: "A 30-year-old worker from an orange juice plant in Florida, who was a chemist and had been working there for about three years, came to me because she was depressed, irritable, and anxious; she felt like her brain was in a fog. I did a chemical analysis of this patient: I looked at her blood—her red cells and her plasma—her urine, and her hair. The results showed that she had excesses of five toxic metals: arsenic, cadmium, lead, aluminum, and copper. Now, she had an occupational exposure to heavy metals. Many systems had gone off in the body of this relatively young woman. When she was treated for heavy metal toxicity, she progressively improved and got well. Her case is a very dramatic example of mental dysfunction and emotional problems that cleared up with the elimination of toxins.

"In the U.S.," Dr. Wunderlich continues, "there's a lot of background exposure to heavy metals. Think about all of the auto tires on the road that are spinning off cadmium in their wheels as they wear down, all the 50,000 chemicals in the environment that weren't there 50 years ago. We are all being exposed to toxins. Dr. Davis from England has shown that these gradually and insidiously accumulate in our systems with every decade that we live. So we have to face the strong likelihood that this toxic buildup is interfering with our enzyme function."

Chemicals and Other Environmental Factors Contributing to Mental Conditions

The risk of being exposed to chemicals such as pesticides in our environment is constantly increasing. A variety of common illnesses, including certain types of depression, can be traced to chemical and environmental toxicity as their root cause. Dr. Richard Kunin offers two case histories where exposure to chemicals and other environmental factors were decisive, and where proper diagnosis by a holistic practitioner led to a successful treatment outcome. "Once at a dinner party I met a woman and it turned out that the party was at the home of her psychoanalyst who was a transactional therapist, a psychiatrist, and also an M.D. And she was a victim of a depression that would come and go. The conversation turned to what kind of therapy a doctor like myself—an orthomolecular doctor and a nutrition physician— would use. She decided to come in for a consultation to explain her depressions. In the first two months, as I went through phase one with her, which was the nutrition analysis stage, nothing came of it.

"There was almost a 100-percent probability that we were going to find something chemical because the psychological inputs just didn't explain her depressions. So we went back over the whole case and hit upon something she had forgotten to tell me the first time around, which was that after she had had her third child by Cesarean, she hadn't been able to breathe for a day. Probing further, we found that the anesthesia she was administered was accompanied by a paralysis of her respiratory muscles. It's a short-term muscle relaxant that blocks the neural muscular junction and the transmitter and you are supposed to recover in a matter of minutes. She recovered in a day. If they had not had an automatic pressure respirator there, she would have died.

"She has a potentially fatal disorder. When she was measured they found that her detoxifying enzyme, called cholinesterase, which is supposed to get rid of a chemical like this, was abnormally low on a genetic basis. Now she knew about this but nobody explained to her that it put her at risk for environmental exposure to pesticides that would damage this enzyme further. The common phosphate pesticides were life-threatening to this woman. Nobody told her. Now it turns out that she is a well-to-do woman who could afford to have an exterminator come in and spray her kitchen every month or two. And she would be disabled. The pesticide sprays are supposed to last about a week but it takes about two to three weeks to recover for an ordinary exposure and with her low cholinesterase she would be out for a month.

"She would feel depressed, weak, and shaky. She would have intestinal bloat. She would wheeze a little. She would sleep poorly, have strange dreams. Her saliva would be a little thin. In general, her autonomic nervous system was a wreck.

"When she would visit her family up in Napa Valley, California, which is full of vineyards that are sprayed, everyone else would be playing tennis, and she would be in bed with the covers over her head. Everyone thought that she was neurotic. Nobody measured her cholinesterase until I heard the story, checked, and, sure enough, found she had a genetic deficiency.

"In my own practice, I have come upon four cases like this, about one every two years. But in addition to these four, there have been well over 60 people I've seen in the past six or seven years who don't have the advanced or severe form, but have a milder form of environmental susceptibility. One of these was a nurse who was in the hospital on the psychiatric ward for depression. Although her condition was improving at the hospital, she knew that this wasn't the answer. She wasn't even on medication. Just being in the ward, she was getting better, which already tells us something. She wasn't at home. She was in a new environment, and so the suspicion of environmental factors having an impact goes up.

"This is an important point. If you go on a vacation and feel better, it doesn't necessarily mean that you needed a vacation. Maybe you needed to be out of your home territory where there are environmental factors that make you sick. Now in my practice I always measure cholinesterase levels. This nurse's cholinesterase were also below the normal limit. It turned out that whenever she was visiting her home territory, which was rural, she would be aware that they were spraying by airplane. From a mile away this woman would pick up drifts and her immune system was responding to the solvents and detergents that are used to disperse the sprays over a wide area. But when we measured her cholinesterase, we found that it fluctuated. When it went down—meaning it was inactivated by pesticide exposure—then she would have more symptoms, particularly depressions. When she would recover and be at her high level—meaning she was not impaired—she would feel perfectly healthy and normal and was a vivacious, dynamic person.

"I call this the 'pesticide neurosis.' It's not rare and it's a very significant factor, because people are reacting to common, so-called 'safe' pesticides. These are the same pesticides that California sprayed all over the city of Los Angeles, where there were people who were having all kinds of symptoms, especially when they would spray in two adjacent areas consecutively. If you lived in the cusp between two areas, you got a double dose. In New York in 1999, the entire city was sprayed several days in a row.

"These are the most common pesticide problems that show up as everyday nerve problems. If you eat out in restaurants, they are sprayed every few weeks, and chances are you are going to pick up some of the leftovers of commercial pesticides. They are careful and they do it well, but accidents do happen. If you are having symptoms of environmental susceptibility, you have got to include this in your thinking. Doctors should be including it in their testing."

Dr. Kunin continues: "Judging from the 30 or 40 cases of environmental toxicity that I could refer to from my own clinical experience, it is fairly common for a patient to have a family history. You'll find out that cousin Joe had it or you'll hear that there was a suicide in the family. In fact this may have been the case with the nurse I've been describing. She came to see me looking for nutrition-related answers, and we found instead a toxin-related answer for her. She had a cousin who lived in the San Mateo area, south of San Francisco. When we had the Med Fly scare back in 1983, after the area where her cousin lived was sprayed, he went into a terrible depression and committed suicide. Of course, I can't prove that the depression was brought on by a toxic reaction to the spraying. I didn't get a blood level on him. But when you have one person with a family history of an enzyme weakness and another person with related genes who goes into a deep depression after having been exposed to a bad environmental onslaught, you have to at least consider that the two events are causally related."

These kinds of stories are a wake-up call. Even at this late stage, while we assume everyone is so aware and concerned about pesticides, but that is not the case.

Pesticides: Gary

I'm a good example myself. For 15 years, I didn't eat an orange or an apple because I found I was allergic. Then one day I was up on a farm, a friend of mine had an orchard with great beautiful looking apples. I thought what the heck, I know what's going to happen, I'll get red eyes, raspiness in the throat, my nose is going to run, but it's worth it. What do I care? I want an apple. So I went ahead and ate the apple and nothing happened. I thought, that's strange, maybe my fixed allergy became a cyclic allergy, it only occurs occasionally.

I got back to town and I thought, this is great. I went to the health food store, picked up a beautiful apple and bit into it. Within one block of walking and eating that apple, my nose was running, I had raspiness and itchiness in the back of my throat, my eyelids turned bright red, my eyes turned red. I thought, well, that's a fluke.

The next week, my buddy came to town and brought me some apples. I tried another one. Nothing happened. So then I went back to the store and asked, "Are these certified organic?" The guy said, "Well, we think they are." I went to another store and got some that said certified organic. Nothing happened. I then

I told this story to Dr. Lendon Smith, who educated me further. "It may
not be only the pesticide," he said. "Pesticides are disbursed in the
mist of solvents and detergents, both of which are actually more aller-
genic than the pesticide itself. It may also be, when we say pesticide,
we have to think of the whole picture, you don't get pesticide in pure
form, you get it in the trade forms, whether its kerosene or some other
vehicle, and the vehicle itself may be more noxious and particularly
more sensitizing than the pesticide.

Dr. Alan Pressman recently received a letter from a doctor teaching
in the Department of Anatomy at a college in Illinois who is finding
that the formaldehyde used to preserve the cadavers is actually harm-
ing the students and teachers in their gross anatomy lab. "He has documents going back to the early '80s showing that formaldehyde was
inducing chromosomal changes in medical students who were dissect-
ing cadavers. In fact, anatomists have a higher incidence of brain cancer than populations not exposed to formaldehyde, according to a
number of studies as early as 1984. The formaldehyde is responsible
for additional, toxic mutogentic, and carcinogenic effects, has been
known since the early '80s by the National Cancer Institute. Nothing
gets done. We are not going to be exposed as much to formaldehyde as
we are to certain other chemicals in the environment, perhaps. Look at
dry-cleaning fluid, people that have their clothes dry cleaned and then
wear them are exposed to enormous amounts of chemicals. Plus, we
don't even have to go into the amount of exhaust from automobiles,
exposure to carbon monoxide."

"The government agencies and the higher-ups in the medical political structure are not even half-aware of the complexity of these environmental toxins and their effect on our health," says Dr. Richard Kunin. "The actual interventions that we've seen to date are only partial. As for members of the medical profession generally, they do not really take environmental toxicity seriously. They see it as very rare and therefore don't include hair analysis as part of a routine medical checkup. In fact, doctors have been told not to test for toxins, even though these tests are the best way to screen for poisonous metals as well as to identify how much of various minerals a person is accumulating in the tissues of his or her body."

Dr. Michael Schachter looks for clues in his patients' behavioral habits. Here is one case of a patient with pronounced chemical sensitivities, from his clinical practice: "One woman, whom I have been treating for some time now, becomes very depressed and even has auditory hallucinations when exposed to formaldehyde in department stores. Recently, she was able to improve her condition by using a detoxification program in which she took sauna baths and certain nutrients, such as niacin and vitamin C. It took several weeks of a couple of hours a day of low heat saunas to remove some of the toxic chemicals that were in the fat stores of her body. One possibly relevant factor in her history was that as an adolescent she had engaged in substance abuse, including both marijuana and hallucinogenic drugs like LSD. Though she has improved considerably, she continues to be sensitive to chemicals."

Perfumes have become environmental toxins. Most of the fragrances on the market today do not come from natural flower scents or any natural scents; they're mostly chemicals. Some people can't go into department stores because they get violent headaches. If you're suffering from headaches, that is a sign that your brain is under some kind of attack.

Water has pesticides, heavy metals, and, sometimes, formaldehyde in it because most city water departments only take out bacteria and filter out particles. But heavy metals and products used in unleaded gas get in the air and, when it rains, come down to earth and seep through the ground into the water. Clinicians are urging their patients to drink distilled water, preferably from glass bottles, not plastic ones.

Among household toxins that affect the brain is formaldehyde, used in inexpensive press board furniture as part of the glue. Doctors urge using solid wood furniture and hanging a spider plant, which feeds on formaldehyde. Certainly, a lot of paints are neuro-toxic, as are floor coverings. Many people get the sick carpet syndrome because insecticides have been sprayed on carpets.

A Personal Account of Environmental Toxicity: "Betty"

When I was injured on the job from some paint fumes, my whole life changed. I developed serious food allergies and sensitivities to everything in my environment. I became allergic to everything in my own home, I reacted to plastics of all kinds, and I couldn't breathe outdoor air. The air inside my home had to be filtered especially for me and I had to wear charcoal face masks to breathe. I was literally a captive in my home for the first year.

Also, I had depressions, mood swings, and a lot of confusion and memory loss. I would go into one room and forget why I was there. I know a lot of people have that complaint from time to time, but I had it consistently throughout the day. I couldn't drive myself to the store because I wouldn't be able to find my way. I lost the ability to read normally. Still now, two years later, I have to read things over and over in order to retain the material. I still have that deficit. I have trouble dealing with numbers.

Unfortunately, because my chemical exposure happened to me on the job, I became a workers' compensation patient. This meant that I was often sent to doctors who were unwilling to believe that there was something wrong with me or who didn't understand what the syndrome was all about. So for months at a time, because of their diagnoses, I would go without any treatment at all and I would just get worse.

Luckily I found several doctors who were able to diagnose and treat me. Dr. Wunderlich administered vitamin C drips, a vitamin supplement program, and allergy treatments, because every allergy that you can think of was triggered in my body. To this day, I cannot use any kind of lotions, cosmetics, fragrances, or hair sprays, and I doubt that I ever will be able to use them.

Very slowly, I began to get better. I still have frequent setbacks because of chemical exposures. I can't tolerate anything like gasoline fumes, new plastics, or any kind of new materials in a building. I have very restricted access to public places because of fragrances that are often used in offices, stores, or public restrooms, and because of cleaning solutions and sprays used in public places. After two years, I am still slowly making progress, but I know that I have several more years ahead of me before I can bring my immune system back to where it should be.

I like people and I have always, all my life, been around people. One of my greatest frustrations has been that now I have to dodge people because of the cosmetics, perfumes, and sprays that they use. They set off severe migraine attacks that can put me into bed for two and three days at a time.

I was forced into changing my lifestyle. I had to change my way of eating and a lot of the products that I use in my home. I've gone to a semi-vegetarian diet, mostly organic. I eat very little meat, and no flavorings. I have to be on a completely yeast-free and sugar-free diet. It is extremely restricted. But I have gotten used to it and I realize now that it's an extremely healthy diet.

My experience with doctors has made me see the need for more awareness. So many physicians saw me as a neurotic middle-aged woman because of the symptoms that I had. The symptoms that go with envi-

ronmental illness are numerous and have to be taken
seriously by the medical profession. It is not all in our
heads.

What We're Up Against: The Political and Social Dimensions of Nutrition and Mental Health

With so much expertise available and so many proven solutions, you
have to wonder why Americans still suffer as much as they do and why
the numbers of people afflicted with mental trouble across the spectrum—from mild depression and lack of concentration to schizophrenia and other forms of dementia—continues to increase.

Yet despite the extent of mental disorders, the American medical
establishment has paid little attention to causes, so intent are they on
obtaining the relief of the symptoms of these conditions. Take alcoholism, for instance. There are dozens of studies showing that alcoholics are chronically deficient in certain essential nutrients. Other
studies show that when these nutrients are given at optimal levels, the
chemical imbalances that precipitate the craving for alcohol are
diminished or eliminated, thus biochemically breaking the addictive
response. One would think that the medical establishment would at
least attempt to address the ramifications of these studies. Currently,
many tens of billion dollars are spent yearly on drug and alcohol treatments, of which the vast majority ignore nutrition-based approaches.
Since few of the now-prevalent approaches have been shown to be successful, it is worrisome that nutrition-based approaches continue to be
relegated to the margins. We need to look at the fact that when biochemical imbalances are corrected and chemical sensitivities
addressed, the treatments work, and with a lack of relapse. This is the
kind of cause-and-prevention oriented approach we should be encour-
aging, for alcoholism and other problems. It is in an attempt to help
encourage such an approach that I put together this book.

Thousands of articles in peer-reviewed journals clearly demonstrate that nutrition affects the cause or treatment—or the prevention—of different diseases. It is estimated that up to 90 percent of all
diseases could be eliminated if we understood the role that nutrition,

environment, and lifestyle play. Now that we have the evidence, the question is, why have the medical community, the educational community, and the media not advocated that we implement it?

One of the problems is that once a physician has been trained in a particular area of specialization in a particular way, for that physician to relinquish his or her mind-set and embrace a new paradigm of knowledge is not an easy process. Even with the best of intentions for their patients' well-being, doctors will continue to use modalities that have been outmoded, or that have been shown to be of no benefit, or that are actually harmful, for the simple reason that one uses what one knows.

Dr. Peter Breggin asks, rhetorically, "If the so many drugs prescribed for mental conditions are so dangerous and have such limited usefulness, and if psychosocial approaches are relatively effective, why is the profession so devoted to the drugs? The answer lies in maintaining psychiatric power, prestige, and income. What mainly distinguishes psychiatrists from other mental health professionals, and of course from non-professionals, is their ability to prescribe drugs. To compete against other mental health professionals, psychiatry has wed itself to the medical model, including biological and genetic explanations, and physical treatments. It has no choice: anything else would be professional suicide. In providing psychosocial therapies, psychiatry cannot compete with less expensive, more helpful non-medical therapists, so it must create myths that support the need for medically trained psychiatrists.

"After falling behind economically in competition with psychosocial approaches, psychiatry formed what the American Psychiatric Association admited in 1992 is a 'partnership' with the drug companies. Organized psychiatry has become wholly dependent for financial support on this unholy collaboration with the pharmaceutical industry. To deny the effectiveness of drugs or to admit their dangerousness would result in huge economic losses on every level from the individual psychiatrist who makes his or her living by prescribing medication, to the American Psychiatric Association, which thrives on drug company largesse. If neuroleptics were used to treat anyone other than mental patients, they would have been banned a long time ago. If their use wasn't supported by powerful interest groups, such as the pharmaceutical industry and organized psychiatry, they would be rarely used at all.

"One selling point has been that psychiatric drugs emptied the U.S. mental hospitals. That is a myth. Psychiatric drugs were in widespread use as early as 1954 and 1955, but the hospital population did not decline until nearly ten years later, starting in 1963. That year the federal government first provided disability insurance coverage for mental disorders. The States could at last relieve themselves of the financial burden by refusing admission to new patients and by discharging old ones. The discharged patients, callously abandoned by psychiatry, received a small federal cheque for their support in other facilities, such as nursing or board and care homes. Some patients went home as dependents while others went onto the streets. Follow-up studies in the late 1980s and early 1990s show that very, very few patients became independent or led better lives following these new policies.

"Given that these are exceedingly dangerous drugs, what are their advantages? By suppressing dopamine neurotransmission in the brain, they directly impair the function of the basal ganglia and the emotion-regulating limbic system and frontal lobes. The overall impact is a chemical lobotomy. The patient complains less and becomes more manageable. The neuroleptics mainly suppress aggression, rebelliousness, and spontaneous activity. This is why they are effective whenever and wherever social control is at a premium, such as in mental hospitals, nursing homes, prisons, institutions for persons with developmental disabilities, children's facilities and public clinics, as well as in Russian and Cuban psychiatric political prisons. They are even used in veterinary medicine to bend or subdue the will of animals. When one of our dogs was given a neuroleptic for car sickness, our daughter observed, 'He's behaving himself for the first time in his life.'

"The broader issue is—how are we to understand and to show care for people who undergo emotional pain and anguish? Are we to view them as defective objects or as human beings struggling with emotional and social problems and personal conflict? Are we to drug them into oblivion, or are we to understand and empower them? Giving a drug disempowers the recipient. It says, "You are helpless in the face of your problems. You need less feeling and energy, and less brain function." The true aim of therapy should be to strengthen and to empower the individual. People, not pills, are the only source of real help."

Dr. Peter Braughman, a neurologist, likes to point out that "in 1990, psychiatrist Matthew Dumont suggested that psychiatry give up its coquettish claims to psychotherapy and openly declare itself an arm of the drug industry." He said it need fear no indignant response from a federal government that defines private profit as its reason for being.

"In 1995, the Drug Enforcement Administration learned of financial ties between Ciba-Geigy, the manufacturer of Ritalin, and CHADD, (Children and Adults with Attention Deficit/Hyperactivity Disorder), a supposedly neutral parents' organization that was telling distraught citizens that ADHD is a disease and that Ritalin is essentially not addictive. Ciba-Geigy had given CHADD over a million dollars. The international narcotics control board expressed concern about CHADD's active lobbying for the medical use of Ritalin in children. The financial connection to a pharmaceutical company whose purpose was promoting sales of a controlled addictive substance was considered hidden advertising. Not until the spring of 2000 was a lawsuit on these matters filed. So clearly one just has to follow the money trail.

"In the 1996 elections, Eli Lilly Company, manufacturers of Prozac, made over $770,000 in soft money contributions to prominently placed politicians. By 1996, there were already over 600,000 minors on Prozac and they had a well honed advertising campaign targeting children ready to go. There were plans for candy-coated Prozac as well."

The power and influence of the pharmaceutical industry and of the various medical technology industries are enormous. These would stand to lose a substantial part of the 1.3 trillion dollars, year in and year out, that our national sickness care system costs the American public. Were the public to change its perspective on the nature of acceptable treatment and begin demanding nontoxic therapies, that cash cow would be no more.

"The magic bullet theory"—the idea that a single pill can cure a disease, including a mental or emotional one—not only still dominates medicine, but has become more and more prevalent. In part, this is because of the way managed care works, as Judith Sachs, a Professor at the College of New Jersey in Trenton, recently explained:

"We can no longer sit in a doctor's office. The average managed care visit, whether it is for a cold or a brain tumor, is nine minutes long. In that period of time, you cannot give a full case history, you can't talk about what's going on in your life. You can talk about some symptoms, which may be somatic symptoms that come out of your stress and depression, but you can't get near the root of the problem. It's much easier for doctors to throw a precription at it and say 'take this.'"

In the February 2000 issue of the *Journal of the American Medical Association*, Dr. Joseph T. Coyle of the Harvard Medical School called "the way mental health services are provided to children" one cause of the increasing numbers of prescriptions for psychotropic medications being given to preschoolers. "Many state Medicaid programs now provide quite limited reinbursement for the evaluation of behavioral disorders in children and preclude more than one type of clinical evaluator per day. Thus, the multidisciplinary clinics of the past that brought together pediatric, psychiatric, behavior and family dynamic expertise for difficult cases have largely ceased to exist. As a consequence, it appears that behaviorally disturbed children are now increasingly subjected to quick and inexpensive pharmacologic fixes."

As Dr. Sherry Rogers of Sarasota, Florida so eloquently puts it: "The drug industry clearly owns medicine. That is the bottom line. With the HMOs, medicine has clearly become a business. Every disease has become a drug deficiency. Aspirin has become a Motrin deficiency. Cardiac arrhythmia has become a calcium channel blocker deficiency. Hypertension has become a high blood pressure pill deficiency and depression has become a Prozac deficiency. All of the thought has been removed from medicine. It becomes a no brainer. It's like a little receipt book of computerized flow sheets and the big emphasis is on labels. Label-itis is probably the number one cause of disease or death in the United States. Once you get a label, you are locked into it. Insurance companies cover certain treatments—usually, drugs only—and they penalize or will not pay patients for having looked for the causes, even though they got back to work, got well, got off drugs. They will pay for several $800 MRIs, disability for being unable to work, and at least $100 a month for drugs. There is no rhyme or reason. There is no rationality. We've lost that a long time ago. So people have to take the ball in their court and find out what is wrong with them and then when they get well, to fight for their rights."

Helping people get access to the information that will actually help them get well has been my life's work. I and other people who believe in holistic healing have had to think long and hard about why the information doesn't get through. In part, obviously, it is blocked by vested interests. For example, Dr. Jonathan Zeuss calls the herb St. John's Wort his "first choice for antidepressant treatment for most people," but describes some of the impediments this way: "The synthetic pharmaceutical industry is really scared of St. John's Wort. In Europe, it's bigger than anything like Prozac and it's on its way to becoming like that here. The drug companies know it and they know it's going to take a huge bite out of their profits and I am sure it already has. So it has been really interesting to see how they have responded to it.

"First of all, they know that American doctors have a built-in bias against herbs and especially against herbs that have been studied overseas. There are all kinds of good studies on St. John's Wort from Europe. They have analyzed and analyzed and there is really no question that this stuff works well. But American doctors are still saying, 'well we have to do an American study.' But it was like that with ginkgo too. There were great studies on ginkgo from Europe, but they waited until a study was done here. That study was basically identical to studies already done in Europe. We're using ginkgo now, but doctors are still saying we are waiting for the American study on St. John's Wort. There is a big study going on right now at Duke University, comparing St. John's Wort to Zoloft, a drug basically like Prozac. Most studies on antidepressants take about two months, then they analyze the data and they publish it. A really long study might go three or four months. But the St. John's Wort study will run for four years. I think they wanted to delay getting the results for as long as they could to give the drug companies a few more years of big profits from the synthetic antidepressants. What they should do is publish interim results right now, that would be the ethical thing to do but it remains to be seen if they will do that."

I have been studying and speaking out against the abuses of psychiatry for a long time. One of the most important questions is, who really has the right to determine whether you are normal or not? Once, if a woman was a midwife, she could be considered evil and punished.

Psychiatric terminology has always been used as a form of social control. Until the 1930s, a woman could be given a psychiatric diagnosis for just having her period. For PMS pain, she was considered insane. Before that, women were considered so emotionally imbalanced, they weren't allowed to vote. The "greatest minds" had written scholarly books on it.

In the 1930s, ice pick frontal lobotomies were done frequently and with such brutality that many patients died. But the procedure was widely accepted, there were dozens of "scientific" articles on the importance and rightness of this procedure and who should benefit.

Electro convulsive therapy—shock therapy—is not a scientific procedure and does not cure depression. I have interviewed hundreds of people who have been victimized by it, generally women, and that's still going on. This treatment amounts to the destruction of brain cells by electricity. It is physician-induced brain damage.

In electro convulsive therapy, 180 to 460 volts of electricity are fired through the brain for a 10th of a second to six seconds. The result is a severe convulsion, a seizure of long duration, a grand mal seizure, as in an epileptic fit. As several hundred volts of electricity go through that brain, the brain becomes starved for oxygen and pulls more blood in. This causes blood vessels to break, damaging the brain. Eventually, the brain shrinks as a result of lack of oxygen and the destruction of nerves and neurons. If anyone other than a doctor did this, they would be locked up for cruel and inhumane behavior.

The usual course of treatment involves 10 to 12 shocks over a period of weeks. This extreme treatment is given for depression, and it does work in the short term. A part of the brain damage is memory loss, and the patient just forgets what they were depressed about. Unfortunately, the memory loss is permanent. Permanent learning disability can be another effect of electro convulsive therapy, not to mention emotional problems.

When the patients' underlying problems return, they're even less able to deal with them then they were before the treatment because the brain injury is so severe. The continued use of this type of Medieval therapy would perhaps be understandable if it had been shown to be effective. But studies about the effects of electro convulsive therapy directly contradict the propaganda, put forth by the four manufacturers of electro convulsive therapy devices in the United States—Somatics,

Mecta, Elcot and MedCraft—upon whom physicians and the public rely for information, much as the public relies upon pharmaceutical companies for information on drugs.

The hundreds of thousands of people a year getting electro shocked generate three billions of dollars to the psychiatric industry and the hospitals. Consider this: there has been an ongoing campaign against the health industry in this country for over 50 years. Every day you see advocates of the alternative position challenged as being unscientific and the purveyors of fraud. But what you have here is an industry making about one-fourth the amount of money as all the herbs and organic produce, all of the natural food stores and the vitamins and minerals that are sold, everything that we call the health movement, put all that together. Electro convulsive therapy makes that amount of money, and kills one in 10,000 people.

Fifty-one percent of all senior citizens in nursing homes are given anti-psychotic medication and yet less than one half of one percent have ever been diagnosed as psychotic and the horrors continue.

It's clearly arbitrary to classify someone by a term that makes them seem abnormal. I am very concerned about any group that has the sole power by such nonscientific terminology to say someone has a disease. If you send me someone who is classified with bipolar depression and gee whiz I find out they have low thyroid, reactive hypoglycemia or corrective biological imbalances and—guess what?—they are no longer depressed, maybe they were not depressed to begin with. Someone should be looking at why they had this diagnosis in the first place.

Many of the people I have interviewed confirm my worst fears. Dr. Paula Caplan, Affiliated Scholar at Brown University's Pembroke Center, worked on the *Diagnostic and Statistical Manual* of mental disorders, "the bible of mental health professionals." "The question of who puts this book together and how they do it is of fundamental importance," she says, "because a very small number of people are behind decisions about which of us are crazy and which of us are not. That book is put together by a handful of mostly American psychiatrists, mostly white men.

"According to the manual, there are 374 different kinds of mental illness or mental disorders. The *DSM* is revised periodically; seven years earlier, it had only 297 categories of mental illness. So the whole definition of what are mental illnesses is growing by leaps and bounds. Some of the people who write this "bible" really want to help, and they think the best way is by giving people labels. Other people are very territorial; they think that the more territory this manual covers, the better it is for the mental health professionals. Some people just want to make money—if I can find a way to pathologize anybody who walks through my office door, I am set for life financially.

"I was appalled and amazed when I discovered, on these *DSM* committees, that the people who put this book together ignore what the scientific research shows. We are basically psychologizing, psychiatrizing, pathologizing virtually the entire population. In the current edition, the *DSM* lists Nicotine Dependence Disorder—if you are having trouble quitting smoking, you are mentally ill. There is something called Caffeine-Induced Sleep Disorder—if you drink coffee and it keeps you up at night, you've got a mental disorder.

"Because diagnoses are not drugs, the FDA doesn't regulate them; nobody does. Nobody says 'good heavens we're diagnosing half a million North American women as having premenstrual mental illness, doesn't that seem kind of extreme?'

"It's all the more terrifying when you think about the devastating consequences for people's lives. People are losing custody of their children because they've been given one of these labels and that fact is hauled into court. They can lose their jobs, though legally you are not supposed to be fired for having a diagnosis of metal illness, but in fact, it often happens. They are being declared mentally incompetent. People are being hospitalized against their will. People are being denied various kinds of insurance. If you are given a diagnosis of a mental disorder, you often cannot get disability insurance because you are considered to have a preexisting condition or you are charged exorbitant premiums.

"There should be investigations at every level of government and by private citizen groups of the way psychiatric and mental health diagnosis is done. We need to be challenging it. Like challenges to breast implants and the Dalkon shield, where the people who produced and manufactured them and the individual doctors who used them on their patients have been held liable for the harm that was done. Diagnostic labels are in that same sense products. They are produced by the American Psychiatric Association in the *DSM* and marketed just like the Dalkon Shield, breast implants and cigarettes. The dangers are being covered up. I call the whole process Diagnosisgate because of the parallels with Watergate—the lies, the cover-up. The people who are the most unhappy, in need of help, going to therapists —these are the most vulnerable, the most likely to have these techniques and what is in this book used against them. We need to do something to protect people."

A Personal Account of Psychiatric Abuse: Sandra

When I was a teenager, I had a baby who was born prematurely. He died eleven hours after birth. I had been taught when you are depressed, you put yourself in the hands of your doctor and I did. My mother dropped me off at the hospital on her way to work. I walked in of my own free will. I brought pretty things to dress up in because I thought it was going to be like a vacation. I was told I was going to play games like ping pong and just relax. When the psychiatrist suggested shock treatments, it didn't even cross my mind that it would damage me, so I signed for them. After they started, I had excruciating pain. I could barely remember how I got in the hospital. I was absolutely devastated. I tried to leave and they called the guards, they stopped the elevators, they dragged me down the hall, they shot me full of thorazine, strapped me down in four point restraints—that means having each wrist and each ankle bound securely so that you can't move, you can't bite and you can't get away. To say the very least, it was no way to treat a lady.

It was also the making of an activist. Years later, when Sandra Everett learned that what had happened to her was still happening, even to little children, she "had to start researching and getting involved." She "became a human rights activist, knowing first hand that when an innocent, harmless person gets behind those walls under psychiatric care, nothing they say is taken seriously. Everything is considered an illness."

As founder of Citizens Rescuing Youth, Everett is one of many people organizing against Goal 2000, a law signed into effect by President Clinton in 1994. This law actually mandates that a mental health clinic be established in every school. She is concerned that, "they are labeling everything as a mental illness—oppositional defiance disorder, attention deficit hyperactivity disorder, everything is a disease. If you are bored, that is attention deficit. If you are very active, they call that hyperactivity."

The ones who benefit most greatly from this is the mental health system. In Georgia, where she lives, Everett found that the local school system gets $6,177.33 per year per child labeled with attention deficit hyperactivity disorder and put into special education. If there is a label of mental or emotional disorder on top of that, she says, "they get well over $10,000 per year per child. If that's not putting a bounty on the heads of our children, I don't know what is.

"If a child is labeled as having attention deficit/hyperactivity disorder, they have to carry behavior cards and behavior folders everywhere they go. In one school, the labeled children are not allowed to sit with the other children at lunch. They are being made into outsiders, they are embarrassed about having to go into different classes. They are taunted for taking a pill in order to be able to sit still and concentrate. And it has no scientific validity, because there is no scientific test for this so-called disease. It was invented by the American Psychiatric Association, on the basis of behaviors alone. They did test for alpha waves change in the brain, but alpha waves change in the brain when a person is bored and not paying attention anyway.

"Parents are being told their child could have a chemical imbalance in the brain. They need to send the child in for psychological examination. But there is no scientific test for chemical imbalance in the brain and if there is indeed a chemical imbalance in the brain, it is not an imbalance of Ritalin or Dexedrine or any of the other medications that they use. On one hand, schools are saying just say no to drugs and on the other hand, the school system, infiltrated by psychiatrists and psychologists, is pushing more dangerous drugs than what the child could be getting on the street."

Dr. Braughman says that behind the over-medicating of children lies the fact that "the schools today are in disarray. They confuse psychology and psychiatry with education. While academic achievement and real world preparation for life is declining, the frequency of diagnosis of so called learning disabilities such as dyslexia, specific mathematics disorder and ADHD is on the rise. These things serve as a ready excuse for the fact that educators have failed to educate and that is the lure. It is much more ecstatic and romantic to be a brain diagnostician then it is simply to be one whose job is to impart the skill of reading. So we have teachers all over the country who are deputy diagnosticians, in a diagnostic orgy labeling children as brain diseased and with chemical imbalances of the brain.

"These are troubled children and the adults in their lives, both at home and in schools, are not meeting their emotional needs. They have abdicated and turned instead to colleagues in the greater ADHD industry. So parents are seduced by the educational establishment that has already been totally seduced by mental health as education. Parents tend to believe what they are told by professionals and they're being told that there is a substitute for the real work of tough love. It's a tragic deception, part of the fraud and deception of biologic psychiatry that represents emotional pains as actual diseases when none in fact are."

An ever more egregious abuse of psychiatry is the severe repression of information about the disastrous side effects of commonly prescribed drugs, especially Ritalin and Prozac, not only in their destruction of people's brains, but also the threat to society posed by the propensity to violence people taking these drugs often develop under their influence. Psychiatric drugs, to a large measure, are implicated in the recent school shootings that so horrified the nation. Dennis Clarke of the Citizens Commission on Human Rights observe that "in these incidents, we don't always get the information from the authorities. For example, in the case of Eric Harris in the Littleton, Colorado school murders, toxicology tests reportedly showed that he had no drugs in his body at all. And we're hearing this in case after case after case. The truth is that when they say 'no drugs,' they mean no illegal drugs. They do not report, unless forced to do so, the medical drugs that are in the bodies of these children. That is considered confidential medical information.

"We found out about the drug that Eric Harris was on from Marine Corps recruiters, who are going around this country and finding tremendous numbers of young people ineligible for the military because of their prescription psychiatric drug use. The recruiters had been disappointed by Eric Harris, who they thought they could recruit, because he was on a drug called Luvox. They rejected him three days before the incident.

"But Kip Kinkle, who shot his schoolmates in Oregon, was on Prozac and had previously been on Ritalin. Ritalin causes intense suicidal ideation in children. In fact, on page 136 of the *Diagnostic and Statistical Manual of Mental Disorders* put out by the American Psychiatric Association in 1987, it says that suicide is a major complication of withdrawal from Ritalin.

The Promise of Vitamin Therapy (Orthomolecular) Psychiatry

Despite the forces defending the medical status quo, change is happening. There are some physicians—albeit a relative handful out of the 600,000 in the U.S.—who are using the therapies referred to in this book. These physicians are revolutionizing American health care. There is also a growing segment of the public becoming aware of these nontoxic therapies. But the impact of these new forces is only just beginning to be felt in mainstream America.

Orthomolecular medicine and orthomolecular psychiatry are now over a quarter of a century old, having started with Dr. Linus Pauling's 1968 article in *Science* magazine called "Orthomolecular Psychiatry." As Dr. Philip Hodes explains, "'Orthomolecular' means the right amount of the right nutrients. Thanks to Dr. Roger Williams's concept of 'biochemical individuality,' and Dr. Bernard Rimland's concept of 'toximolecular brains,' we found that many people with so-called mental illnesses, including schizophrenia, autism, depression, and manic-depression, can be helped, in a majority of cases. They must first clean the toxins out of the brain and then provide the brain with the right amounts of the right nutrients.

"Each person is biochemically individual," Dr. Hodes continues, "so the government standards for the minimum daily requirements of various nutrients actually have little if any bearing on the specific needs of any particular human being. What seems to be a mega-amount for one person is the precise amount necessary to keep another person healthy and sane."

Psychiatrist Michael Schachter says that most psychiatrists will consider the possibility of a chemical imbalance in the brain as well as any psychosocial factors. In the former case, they then immediately resort to using some kind of drug to try to right the balance, without looking into the possibility that there could be nutritional factors contributing to the patient's psychological state. "I explore possible imbalances in the body that could be caused by nutritional and other environmental, nonpsychosocial factors that might be playing a role in the development of psychological symptoms. For instance, they don't bother inquiring how much sugar a person is eating, or how much coffee someone is drinking. They do look at alcohol consumption, especially if it's excessive, but most psychiatrists are unaware that sometimes even small amounts can be a problem."

Whenever possible, Dr. Schachter prefers nutrition-based therapies. "I use nutritional substances or substances that are natural to the body, either food substances or accessory food factors—such as vitamins or minerals or amino acids—as the treatment of choice for a person's mental disorder. Sometimes the vitamins may be megadoses because a person may be what we call vitamin-dependent on a particular nutrient. For example, some children who are hyperactive or having learning disorders will respond to one vitamin, for instance vitamin B1 (thiamine), and actually might get worse if you give them large doses of vitamin B6. So treatment really has to be individualized. I try to find what seems to be most effective for that particular child's or adult's condition."

Hand in hand with the nutrition-based approach, Dr. Schachter looks closely at the clinical ecological factors: the foods in the person's current diet, the water he or she drinks, the air he or she breathes, any imbalances in the body, as well as any daily-life habits. "For example, I check for hormonal imbalances or subtle low-thyroid conditions, which are very common in depression. If these are treated, there will often be marked mood improvement. Calcium and magnesium deficiencies are very common as precipitators for anxiety in general or even panic attacks. By correcting some of these nutrient imbalances, you can reduce tremendously the chances of a person having panic attacks. Then, if everything else is not sufficient to bring about improvement, I would use psychotropic drugs if I had to, but I would try to keep them at the lowest possible dose and I would use nutrients and other dietary supplements to minimize their side effects."

In 1955, Dr. Abram Hoffer and several colleagues published a paper in which they showed that nicotinic acid lowered cholesterol levels but that you had to give 3,000 mg per day. This was a major step forward because it proved that you sometimes needed large amounts of a vitamin for a condition not known to be a vitamin deficiency disease. High blood cholesterol was not known to be a vitamin deficiency disease. The term "orthomolecular"—first used by Dr. Linus Pauling in his paper in *Science* in 1968—was based upon his recognition that certain vitamins are effective when they are used in large quantities.

At that time, the conventional wisdom was still that you used vitamins only in tiny amounts and you only needed them for the prevention of deficiency diseases, like scurvy or beriberi. A nutritionist accepted the fact that if you had scurvy you would eat oranges or you would take small quantities of vitamin C. As Dr. Hoffer puts it, "It was unheard of to give someone 1000 mg of vitamin C. If you suggested this they would throw up their hands in horror. The idea that you could use large quantities of vitamins to treat conditions, not just to prevent them, was a major step forward. In fact, it is considered a major paradigm change. So we are now in a paradigm in which we use vitamins as treatment, not just as prevention."

Dr. Hoffer emphasizes this development in his clinical approach. "Orthomolecular psychiatry and medicine was the first major movement to adopt this treatment paradigm. What it means is that when we have a sick patient, we correct their diet. This is vital. I don't talk to any patient until we have spent some time on their diet. We also use any drugs that have to be used. If I have a schizophrenic patient I will use tranquilizers; if I have a depressed patient I will use antidepressants; if they're epileptic I'll use anticonvulsants; if they're suffering and in a lot of pain, I'll use analgesics. But that's not all. In addition to that we use the appropriate nutrients. It can be any one of the 20 or 30 nutrients currently in use. We combine them all. When the patient begins to respond, we gradually withdraw the drugs until we are able to maintain them on the nutrients alone or on such a tiny amount that it doesn't interfere with their ability to function.

"Orthomolecular medicine is the appropriate use of molecules, nutrients, which are native to the body in the appropriate concentration at the appropriate time.

"I don't like the term 'alternative.' I think, rather, that we are going back to our historical roots. If you go back 100 years we had no treatment except nutritional treatment. For 2000 years the best doctors in the world always emphasized good nutrition, but over the past hundred years nutrition suddenly disappeared from medicine. We're just bringing it back again.

"I consider that we are the mainstream of medicine, even though most doctors don't yet recognize it. My colleagues in psychiatry are still ten years out of date. That's because of the natural conservatism of the profession combined with the fact that they have had the least training in biochemistry and physiology of all physicians and thus they are the least likely to look upon the body as a physiological organism. They look upon psychosocial problems as primary when, in fact, in many cases they are secondary. The American psychiatric establishment—including Canada, and including the National Institute of Mental Health—has taken a very strong position against the use of vitamins in psychiatry and have yet to reverse their position, because they're slow learners."

Dr. Garry Vickar believes that "doctors have a tendency to close their minds to anything other than what they read in their literature." He suggests that there are ways to help your physician be a part of the healing process. "The name of the game is getting better. You can't make people want to treat you if you come at them and say, 'You guys are all wrong. You don't know what you're doing.' Doctors want to be helpful, but how you approach them is important.

"Medicines have not been perfect. But without medicines, things are often worse. So let's assume we have to look at the role of medications up to a point. I think you have to have a framework. I think it's important not to become so radical that you say, 'Medicines are no good; they're dangerous all the time and inherently bad.' That's not true. Medicines are not always bad any more than nutritional supplements are always good, because people can be harmed from inappropriately using nutritional supplements, especially herbs that have pharmacological effects in certain doses.

"I don't oppose the use of medications, but I do think there is a time when you have to look towards reducing medications when you start to see some benefit and perhaps enhancing the benefit of the medicine by the addition of vitamins and other supplements.

"My evaluations include making sure that the patients have thorough physical examinations. There are standard blood tests that are done by every doctor. They involve tests of the ability to produce blood cells, and screens for liver function, kidney function, and so on. I test rather routinely for thyroid functioning because it's not at all uncommon to pick up a low thyroid as a cause of depression.

"I don't do a lot of the fancy allergy testing. I do try to get a six-hour glucose tolerance exam on my patients if they'll cooperate. If they simply refuse to consider that, I do instruct them on proper diet—eliminating sugar, caffeine, and a lot of the empty-calorie foods. And of course I discourage smoking and alcohol, but those are pretty fundamental things that every doctor should be doing.

"People who are mentally ill don't usually eat well. I think it's very difficult to bring anyone to any level of positive well-being when they're not healthy."

According to Dr. Richard Kunin, people tend to have ideas about health habits that are too generalized. "Before Linus Pauling and the word 'orthomolecular,' most people thought they were in the avant-garde if they took a multivitamin. These days most people are still proud of themselves if they cut down on their fat consumption and increase their complex carbohydrates and their intake of high-fiber foods. That seems to be the nutritional prescription that is our current consensus. But the orthomolecular approach that, as a doctor, I have learned to respect, goes beyond a 'one-size-fits-all' prescription and looks instead to a person's individual needs as the basis for treatment.

"I have adapted a strategy that allows people a chance to test themselves where diet is concerned in order to identify their needs," Dr. Kunin continues. "I call that test the 'Listen To Your Body Diet.' The bottom line is that people find their own particular food favorites and their own particular dietary balance, especially relative to carbohydrates. Usually, however, it's a blanket thing, like avoid sugars or increase complex carbohydrates. That leaves a lot unanswered until people go for specific tests.

"Whenever we test vitamin levels, we go a step further and also test the enzymes that the vitamins couple with to ultimately make the body chemistry work. We see marked deficiencies in large numbers of the people who come to see us. Remember, they are coming to the doctor because they feel something is wrong. The odds of something being wrong, therefore, are 100 percent. But we catch only about 70 to 80 percent.

"Regarding toxicology and allergy or immunology, there have been great advances. On the toxicology side, since about 1968 or 1970 I have done a screening test for toxins that we call the hair test. It is possible to screen every patient for mercury, lead, arsenic, aluminum, cadmium, nickel, and get an accurate picture of the environmental input into the individual's overall health. The test was, unfortunately, unfairly criticized by the AMA and is not used nearly as much as it should be. Those who are nickel-afflicted are likely to be more allergic. Nickel is a free-radical generator and a sensitizer of the first rank. People with nickel-tainted hair tend to have nickel in their dental alloys or fillings. Nickel is even more sinister than the more well-publicized mercury, which is also a sensitizer. There is nickel in the braces that kids wear, and they can pick up nickel in their systems that way.

"How do we test today if a person is, for example, sensitive to apples or to the sprays that are used on them, that is, to pesticides or chemicals? Some immunology labs are now offering remarkably helpful testing for chemical sensitivities for a relatively low cost. You can get tested for seven or eight of the major solvents and chemicals, such as benzene and others that people haven't heard too much about. There are also plans to include the dioxins in this screening. These tests are a very helpful marker for environmental exposure. In addition, IGG4 and IGE testing can be done in tandem, in which a person is tested for a sample of food, chemical, and inhalant allergies by identifying antibody responses in the blood tests on an automated basis, thus bringing the price way down. These tests make it possible to get a powerful overview of toxicities and allergic responses inside a particular patient.

"Doctors who don't test their patients for toxicities and allergens are getting a limited view of their patients," Dr. Kunin concludes. "This can lead them to rely on treating symptoms with major tranquilizers, antihistamines, or other nonspecific therapies, rather than treating the source of an individual patient's problems."

I

DISORDERS OF MOOD OR BEHAVIOR

1
ADDICTIONS

A Personal Account of Alcoholism: "Bob"

I am a recovered alcoholic. It's been about seven years that I've been off alcohol. At first, I ate a lot of sugar in cakes and things like that. One of the psychological-emotional components of my behavior was that I always had a very difficult time getting started in the morning. The first thing I would think about when I got up was what I was going to eat, which usually included cereal with sugar, a pastry, and sugar-laden coffee. There has been a slow, progressive bettering of my diet, but there has still always been the sugar craving. Sometimes I would be able to get away from it for a week or two weeks, but it would always creep back in.

Recently, I completed a seven-day fast and a colonic cleansing and I found that after that cleansing process the craving pretty much disappeared. Also, I

> wake up in the morning feeling rather alert, and I don't
> have this compulsion to eat sweets. I think that
> because I am staying away from sugar, I generally am
> having better days psychologically.

We have come a long way from the idea that addicts are morally repre-hensible beings who could stop whatever it is they're doing if they only wanted to enough. The medical community, as well as the homeopathic world, now understands that addictions may be diseases, degenerative ones at that. The wisest practitioners know that addictive substances change brain chemistry in ways that persist long after a person stops taking drugs and that no single "medicine" cures any addiction. They are beginning to tease out the best means of helping all kinds of addicts by addressing the specific chemistry of their addiction and recovery, as well as acknowledging the need for mental and spiritual aid.

While we remain a nation of people where, in the new century, an estimated 4 out of 10 can't get through a day without the "fix" of tobac-co, caffeine, alcohol or cocaine, alternative treatments are becoming increasingly sophisticated. It is now believed, for example, that women's hormonal cycles probably influence the ability to stop smok-ing—those who quit during the first fourteen days following menstrua-tion seem to experience less withdrawal and depression than those who quit after the 15th day. For some addicts, acupuncture helps and a few enlightened medical insurance companies are beginning to cover it. In Oregon, heroin addicts must try acupuncture before getting methadone.

The "last frontier" in recognizing how addictive a society we are comes in the attention being paid to substance abuse among the elder-ly. It is now estimated that 2.5 million older adults have alcohol-relat-ed problems, often missed by physicians who mistake symptoms like falling or gastritis for problems associated with aging. Elderly females have less alcoholism as a group, but more depression and more prob-lems from prescription drugs, as well as high rates of nicotine depen-dence. Since the nutritional situation of most elderly people is far from optimal, I'm convinced that the approaches outlined here could go a long way toward improving the situation.

Drug and Alcohol Addiction

According to Dr. Robert Atkins, alcoholism is so tied in with carbohydrate metabolism that it is fair to say they are "genetically superimposable." In other words, it is possible to understand alcoholism in terms of carbohydrate metabolism alone. This is an extremely radical assertion, but one that lends important insight into a problem that plagues our society. "I have seen families in which half of the members were alcoholics and the other half were sugarholics," says Dr. Atkins. "And you could switch them over. You could probably make alcoholics of the people that were addicted to sugar, and it is well known that when alcoholics go through a psychologically based program, and not a biochemically based program, they have a tendency to become sugar addicts." In fact, it is unusual for ex-alcoholics not to become sugar addicts. More commonly, individuals replace one addiction for the other. As Atkins notes: "Unless people get the clue that there is a connection between alcoholism and sugar addiction, they will just go from one to another and will not feel any better. The phrase 'dry drunks' refers to what happens to alcoholics that start switching to sugar instead of getting on a diet in which all the simple sugars are eliminated."

Clearly, in such situations nutritional awareness can make all the difference and Dr. Atkins considers it a necessary component of any successful alcoholism program: "Of course, nutritional support is also important. Minerals, such as chromium, zinc, and manganese, are all very important in regulating this sort of problem. Dr. Abram Hoffer also believes in the nutritional approach: "The general regimen that orthomolecular medicine uses for alcohol addiction (as with depression, schizophrenia, and a number of other mental disorders) is to pay careful attention to nutrition and the use of the right supplements.

"The first order of business," Dr. Hoffer continues, "is to make sure that the individual's basic diet is optimal. We do that by trying to take away most of the additives in food he or she eats on a daily basis. It is impossible to get them all out, but we try to do the best we can. One of the best simple rules is to put the patient on a sugar-free diet, because almost all foods that contain sugar contain a large variety of other chemicals. By avoiding sugar you will cut out most additives, by about 80 or 90 percent. Since we are all individuals, and many of us have food allergies and can't tolerate large quantities of carbohydrates or protein, for example, each one of us has to develop a diet that is optimal for ourselves.

"Second, we add in the supplements that are right for this particular individual. Many of us have been so deprived of these proper supplements over our lifetime that, even with a very good diet, we cannot regain our health. That's why we need supplements. This is where the treatment differs markedly from person to person (and depending upon whether someone is being treated for alcoholism, or a mental illness such as depression or schizophrenia). So while the dietary regimen is largely the same for all—avoid sugar and any foods that make you sick—supplements are determined on a case-by-case basis.

"For alcoholism the basic treatment starts with Alcoholics Anonymous. Bill W., the cofounder of Alcoholics Anonymous, first showed that when you added niacin to the treatment of alcoholism you got a major response that you did not see before. Today, there are a large number of very good alcoholism treatment programs in the United States, where they depend primarily on a combination of the type of nutrition that I have just referred to, the use of the right supplements, and the use of AA and other social aids to help these patients get well."

If you are taking a substance because you're depressed, you might have some form of brain imbalance or your depression may be physiologically induced—an underactive thyroid or a blood sugar imbalance. High blood sugar or low blood sugar manifests as depression. To get away from the chronic feeling of emptiness that frequently happens with depression, people start to drink, which takes away the feelings and gives them the sense of being in a never-never land. The same is true of many drugs. People take drugs to get a euphoria they wouldn't have achieved on their own or that they may have had but couldn't sustain. Once you get used to that, the quick and easy route is just to stick a needle in your arm or some form of narcotic up your nose or drink it or ingest it.

None of this helps us to resolve the underlying conflict. Is the conflict biological in nature, is it psychological, or a combination? I have found that the best way of approaching this problem is not through exercise, not through deep breathing—if someone is really stressed out, getting them to breathe deeply is not going to work.

It's like asking someone grossly overweight to go on a diet—five percent will comply. But if you get them to get into a systematic cleansing program, where they actually break all physical addictions, not just to sugar, but every other thing they could be allergic to, that seems to make for a major first step. Their energy comes back. Any form of addiction withdrawal creates a lack of energy, so when you substitute the energy they would be getting from the drug, and you give it to them naturally, through the body's own process of metabolism, they feel better.

Then you start to rebuild the brain and the center of the brain with phosphatidyl serine, acelialcarnatine, phosphatidyl choline, and herbs that are known to have an impact, like fever few and green tea. You flood the body with flavonoids. This will not work for everyone, but those who follow this kind of program and juice, juice, juice—from four to six juices of freshly made organic vegetable juice a day—after six months to a year, I've seen about 80 percent of addicts cleared up, staying off it, and not coming back.

I would add that if you have a problem drinker in your family, one of the things you can do is just try to see that they take some vitamins. Hopefully, they will. If not, just try to blend them into juices—orange juice or V-8 juice, whatever they are willing to drink.

Alcohol frequently swells the brain if you have a sensitivity to it. Ever notice how some Asians sometimes manifest symptoms of drop-down drunkenness with just one small glass of wine? Studies show that they are having a cerebral allergy. So you need vitamin B1 and I'm talking about a lot. If you're an alcoholic you are looking at at least one hundred milligrams twice a day. Normally, I suggest ten milligrams of B1, fifteen of B2 and fifteen of B6, but not with an alcoholic. In fact they need the whole B complex at a higher level. Also, the essential fatty acids have been used extensively to help people who have problems with alcohol, generally one capsule of about 100 milligrams with a meal.

There are certain amino acids that are helpful. Glutamine, not glutamic acid. I was in a health food store two days ago—I had stopped off there on my way back from a lecture to get a glass of juice—and I heard someone ask, "What do I give my uncle who's got a problem with alcohol?" The salesperson said, "Give him glutamic acid." I turned around and said, "I'm sorry, it's glutamine and you also want thiamine." If you take glutamine with vitamin B6 on an empty stomach—

and it's best to take it on an empty stomach—along with thiamine and vitamin B6, it will affect the brain.

Magnesium is also important in brain detoxification. I've yet to see a person who drinks regularly, even beer, who is not deficient in magnesium. Very important for the adrenal gland is pantothenic acid, which is vitamin B5. The most important however is vitamin C, taken with quercetin, the bioflavonoid. The flavonoids are very powerful healing agents. They have antiviral properties and anti-yeast properties. They are great for people with candida, they are terrific for people with fatigue, people who have a problem with chronic infections, upper respiratory infections that don't go away, nasal infections. Ninety percent of the Vitamin C you take is not utilized unless you take the bioflavonoids with it. I take issue on this point with Linus Pauling, whom I greatly respect. I've yet to see where vitamin C taken by itself is utilized. You just don't get bio availability, where the tissue actually utilizes it. Generally, about two thousand milligrams of the bioflavonoids would be sufficient, but they are very powerful antioxidants also.

Very important for brain functioning overall and helping the liver is lecithin because of its choline inositol. Generally, people who consume even moderate amounts of alcohol have "lipotropic factors," fat build up in their organs, including the liver. That adversely effects metabolism.

You should also look at niacin or niacinamide, if you want to prevent the flush. Milk thistle weed helps repair damage to the liver and so does valerian root.

So those are a few things I suggest if you have problems with alcohol in your family or if you want to have alcohol yourself, but don't want any of the adverse affects that might come from it.

This disease is a challenge to treat and The Health Recovery Center in Minneapolis, founded by Dr. Joan Matthews Larson, is doing something unique. Dr. Larson realized the need to "shift our focus from alcoholism as a psychological disorder to alcoholism as a physical disease that creates cravings, depression and unstable brain functioning. Otherwise, the alcohol is removed and people take the full brunt of the damage that has been done. No matter how much they talk about their resolve, 80 percent or more have relapsed by the end of the first year. One in four deaths of alcoholics who have had formal treatment is from suicide, usually within the first year after treatment."

Dr. Larson went down a new road because that very thing happened in her family. She had a son in his teens. When her husband's father died of a heart attack, the boy got into a lot of drinking at school. He loved the euphoria. He loved drowning his sorrows in the alcohol and he had a tremendous tolerance, could drink most people under the table. But after three or four years, it was changing his brain's stability. He was becoming very depressed. Dr. Larson sought help for him and "he went into a traditional treatment in a hospital setting. Now this person, a kid, who had reached the stage of real emotional instability from the effects of heavy alcohol and some pot use, sat in groups and talked about the misery of his life. He came home from treatment and was home a very short time, a week or two, when he took his life."

Dr. Larson's need to know what might have made a difference in her son's life lead to further study. Many researchers talked about the damage that alcohol inflicts on the brain and central nervous system—depression, mental confusion, anxiety and real cravings. She began to realize that there was no way that talk could change or repair the damage one iota. There had to be more.

She began to look at the natural chemicals the brain uses that support life and sanity. In the beginning, she concentrated on just the B vitamins, to replace the obvious losses. As she became more sophisticated, she used the amino acids, especially glucosamine, an amino acid that will halt the cravings for alcohol. "If an alcoholic just opens the capsule and lets it dissolve under the tongue," she says, "it goes right across the blood brain barrier and shuts down the cravings for alcohol."

Dr. Larson has evolved a detox formula that includes a number of well researched components, all natural chemicals, no toxic drugs:

Amino acids: glutamine, tyrosine, which reloads the norepinephrine, a natural mood enhancer, an antidepressant neurotransmitter. She used to use tryptophan. ("This is the only country in the world where tryptophan is unavailable and that's a pity because there is a great depletion of serotonin by alcohol.") She uses a group of amino acids designed to reload the brain neurotransmitters, which are low from alcohol. The neurotransmitters are important because they create our moods, memory and our emotions.

She does a lot of lab testing and matching of individuals with treatment. Depression, she believes can run in nationalities, like the Finnish people she sees in Minnesota, many of whom have been depressed since childhood and can't lift the depression no matter what they do. Galmanic acid is particularly useful for Scandinavians, Irish, Scots, and American Indians, all of whom seem to have less availability, less ability to get that across the brain into the prostaglandin. And the prostaglandin you want is such a antidepressant metabolite. It takes about seven days.

A lot of calcium and magnesium. The wipe-out of magnesium in the brain causes delirium tremors in the alcoholic after as little as one drink. The loss leaves the nervous system jumpy and the brain distressed.

A good multi vitamin-mineral supplement. Every one of the substances that we use are capsules because we long ago found out that alcoholics have very little ability to break down hard pressed pills. Their pancreatic enzymes are simply not there anymore. We give them some enzymes that have both the hydrochloric acid and the pancreatic enzymes.

Melatonin, so that they can sleep.

A substance called GABA gamma amino butyric acid, which is how the benzodiazepines like Librium and Valium work. They push GABA into the brain and block the re-uptake. By taking GABA, you can reload those neurotransmitters and the firing mechanism is usually fine because of the wipe-out from the drugs and the alcohol.

People who have high histamine have minds that race, don't sleep well, need a small amount of sleep, are compulsive and driven. A lot of times, they are heavy two fisted drinkers. In order to intercept that raciness, we give them methionine; that will block the histamine. Many marijuana users tend to be more high histamine and they love the interruption of all of that activity. It mellows them out. Marijuana does block histamine. It blocks it so well that a person who has used marijuana a long time can lose their zest for life. Their histamine levels are extremely low. Histamine fires all of the neurotransmitters in the brain. So loading them up is one thing but getting them to fire is another. To reload histamine, to raise those levels you use B3, B12, folic acid and histidine. Within weeks, the marijuana user is back to feeling normal again.

Alcoholics say they have been anxious since childhood. They are really enamored of alcohol because it relieves the anxiety for awhile. If we don't relieve the anxiety, they will go right back to drinking again. Often we find high tryptopyrols that are blocking the B6 and zinc and keeping them anxious. That can be totally reversed once it is identified with a urine sample and a lab test. One way to know if you might be a candidate is look at your fingernails. Are there little white dots on all your fingernails and can you remember the content of your dreams consistently? If the answer is, "Yes I've got white dots and no I don't remember my dreams," you need to be tested for phillyrea and have that corrected.

Cocaine-addicted people and heroin addicts have lost certain key chemicals that we need to replace. The cocaine user and the crack cocaine user are firing off norepinephrine like the fourth of July. That's what creates that feeling they love that is so short- lived. Of course, the neurotransmitter has to be reloaded. That is done by taking large amounts of tyrosine. Also, D-phenylalanine which makes endorphins. Now this is not L-phenylalanine; this is D-phenylalanine and it will help replace what the cocaine user has depleted.

At the Health Recovery Center, they put all of these necessary things into an IV.

Dr. Gabriel Cousens has been trying to find out "why, in the year 2000, we have up to 15 million active alcoholics and why five billion tranquilizers are consumed each year and 450 million cups of coffee drunken each day." The answer is that "people's brains and minds are not working clearly, so they turn to drugs to feel okay. They have what I call addictive brains."

Healing the biologically altered brain is the way to eliminate those addictive pressures that send us into sex addiction, drug addiction, alcohol addiction, violence addiction and over eating. We must get our endorphins and neurotransmitters back to normal levels.

Dr. Cousens begins with a familiar program: "detox people, get them on a live food vegetarian diet, see if there are endocrine imbalances, hypoglycemia, hyperthyroid problems. The drugs they have been on—anti-hypertenses, anti-inflammatories, birth control pills, have altered the brain's physiology.

"I study the pH of a person's blood. The brain seems to work at a certain pH, which is 7.46, where it has optimal function. This research was done by Dr. Watson in the 1950s. He discovered that people could have anxiety, depression, paranoia and even schizophrenia, if their blood pH was not at the right level. In a study of over 300 people, he used proper diet to bring the brain pH back to normal and the symptoms went away. The diet is important, then, not just because it is life-force enhancing, but because it actually alters the pH and brings it back to a normal.

"Once I have corrected all these things, I will give free amino acids and other nutrients and certain B vitamins to enhance the functioning of the brain biochemistry so that all the cells are working at their optimal state. I add meditation to calm the mind.

"Lower neurotransmitters and endorphins are partially the result of drug abuse. More men than women abuse drugs—three times more—and up to 5 times more are alcohol abusers. Chronic alcoholics have about a third fewer endorphins working in their brains. Some of the genetic studies show that up to 69 percent of alcoholics are missing a third of the neurotransmitters in the dopamine center. Since dopamine has to do with the pleasure centers, if you are not feeling pleasure, then you have to do something to feel good, like drink or take drugs.

"Cocaine and amphetamines significantly break down the dopamine receptor centers. Prozac can actually deplete the neuroreceptor centers. In the 1960s they used the phrase "better living through chemistry," but it does not work. In 1884, Freud discovered cocaine. It helped with his depression for three years, but after three years, it became an addictive problem. From the 1930s to the 1960s, up to 23 million people were taking amphetamines, about 80 percent of them women. It is a personality enhancing drug—people say 'I feel better' and 'I have more energy'—because it creates a hyper-manic state.

"Prozac and drugs like it are stimulants; they create a hyper-manic state. People who take them pay a price because the drugs alter the brain even more. They are addicting. At first, everybody thought that this was the new panacea, but within a year or two, we began having

Prozac survival groups. Some people did feel better—a hyper-manic state makes them feel more aggressive and gives them the competitive edge. They call Prozac a "selective serotonin enhancer," but it also stimulates the androgens systems, like amphetamines and cocaine do. It also depresses the dopamine receptive centers, which are connected to the pleasure centers.

"These drugs affect the brain in ways that people do not understand. They affect the frontal lobes, which means impaired reason and impulse control, lack of ability to make future plans and for empathy. It is really important because the lack of empathy is partly connected to all the violence that Prozac seems to stimulate. At Columbine High School, at least one of the killers was on Prozac. When you don't have empathy to connect you to human beings, it's really easy to act out with violence.

"Then it affects the limbic system, which is the emotional system, where it creates apathy and indifference. Also, the basoganglion, which is extremely important because that creates abnormal movements, this internal pressure to move around and be active.

"Then it affects the temporal lobes, causing loss of short and long term memory and then parietal lobes and every part of their brain. There is a decrease in understanding and sensory perception and language and sense of self. In the cerebellum, there is loss of regulation of muscle tone and gate. In the hypothalamus, there is loss of temperature and appetite control. It also affects the pituitary gland, the thyroid, adrenals, and sex hormones and stress reactions.

Dr. John Eades has a 20-year history of working in the field of addictive diseases and chemical dependencies with major hospitals. His concerns are social and spiritual. He defines addiction as having three components: "The first is a compulsion or craving. That is a form of a hunger. The second is loss of control. The alcoholic will try to drink two drinks and go home, but he winds up drinking 15 or 16 drinks. The gambling addict may take $100 and leave a credit card in the trunk of the car, but before the evening is over, she is probably back out to the car, getting the credit card. The third is that the consequences of the behavior are bad or negative and the individual continues doing the behavior. The alcoholic gets a DUI, which might stop a person who is just a social drinker. It doesn't stop the alcoholic. A gambler may write a bad check, have problems from that, but it will not stop the behavior.

"In our culture we have addictions to more than drugs. We have people addicted to work. They are on the airplanes all the time with their computers, working and working and working to the exclusion of having a well-rounded life. People are addicted to sexual activity, alcohol, cigarettes and gambling, a new addiction on the horizon that is going to bring tremendous problems as [local and state] governments continue to finance themselves with the revenue from gambling establishments. Another one is addiction to exercise. I have some patients who, if they cannot run on any particular day, actually go into a form of withdrawal. Even when they get injured, they still go out and exacerbate that injury by continuing to exercise."

Myths about happiness, Dr. Eades says, are at the core of the emptiness that leads to addictions. "One of the greatest and most damaging is, 'I'll be happy if I am successful.' The person is always striving, never truly arriving, always reaching, not resting. When this happens we become externally oriented, looking for things outside us to define us. I've worked with too many patients who are very wealthy, but also very discontented and very disconnected in their lives.

"Another myth that we have is, 'I will be happy if I can make another person happy in a relationship.' This leads again to being focused on others. The addict's life revolves around the drug while the co-dependent's life revolves around the addict. Or, 'I'll be happy when a certain situation occurs—when I graduate from school, when I get that job, when I get married, when we have children, when I get that new house, when the children leave home, when I can retire from that job, if I had more money, if I had planned better for my retirement, if I had more years to live.' This myth of 'I'll be happy when or if' can last an entire life.

"A lot of people need the approval of others in order to feel good about themselves. They become a system of mirrors, reflecting back what people think we should be, want us or expect us to be. I also find a lot of people feel that they have to be perfect. When a person starts to fail, as is the normal way of being human, they blame others and this promotes denial of the reality of their imperfection.

"Addictions fill vacuums and, as human beings, we have three kinds of them. One is for things and only things can fill it up—clothes, food, car, shelter. We have a vacuum for people and only people can fill that up. We also have a spiritual vacuum, which can only be filled up with spirituality. The people I work with try to fill up their spiritual vacuum with things and people and are chronically discontent.

"People change when the pain of where they are becomes greater than the pain to change. The alcoholic reaches a place where he says I can't go on this way. I'm killing myself physically. I've lost my job and so forth, but I can't live without it. In addictive relationships, they see that person when they don't want to, they see them more than they mean to, they call them.

"Psychology is limited in its ability to help the addictive mind. William James, the great Harvard psychologist, said that for human beings to change, they must undergo some type of spiritual transformation. One of the myths that permeates our society is that psychologists have all the answers. I know for sure that I don't and I know that as I listen to other professional psychologists talk, that they don't either. We have overlooked the spiritual aspect of the human psyche. Spirituality is necessary. The people that seem the happiest are well rounded and also have a very active spiritual life. They have been able to reach a state of solitude where they can look inward and have a better understanding of life and what's important. Some people are so addicted that no matter what we do, no matter how we analyze that person, no matter what techniques or gimmicks we use, that person probably is only going to change when they undergo some form of spiritual transformation.

"I have a very simple formula. One way that people get reconnected with themselves is by being responsible in their behavior. The word responsible comes from Latin, and it means to be answerable to. Indeed we are answerable to ourselves as well as to other people. The real problems begin when a person behaves irresponsibly and still feels okay about it. At that point, the person begins to distort the world, developing a whole host of ego defense mechanisms, denying and distorting and essentially losing contact with themselves.

"I tell my patients that if they want self esteem, they have to forgive themselves for the past, realize that their futures are spotless and that they are going to have to start being responsible. I urge them to look for internal validation. Focus inward instead of focusing outward. Stop being a victim.

"I ask them not to lie to anybody about anything they are doing for the next ten days. Well, that is a big task for many people in recovery. When they can go through a day without lying, they are probably starting to behave responsibly. If they are behaving irresponsibly and have someone they can tell, honestly, and then move on, that helps.

"In sum, people with addictions have to start being responsible, start striving to be honest, and find a spiritual life. They need to get connected in some kind of organized way perhaps. There is power in people working together toward trying to get connected spiritually. We have to slow down and say hey where am I going? What am I doing with my life? Nothing changes if nothing changes then nothing changes. People expect to continue their same behaviors with their same attitudes and their same thought patterns, but it doesn't work that way. We find great power in helping other people. In AA, people can stay sober because they are helping other people. People are happiest when they lose themselves in activities that help other people with no expected payback.

"Doing good because we hope we will get something good back becomes a form of manipulation. That sham type of behavior leaves a person feeling empty. We need a relationship with ourselves, a relationship with someone else and a relationship with our higher power or our spiritual essence. People who give up their addictions, but transfer those behaviors onto another addiction or keep manipulating, lying and using other people have a false recovery.

"Recovery for most people is not just ceasing a behavior but making a total change. A total holistic change must occur; otherwise, the person will either go back to that drug or that behavior, find another drug or behavior, or continue behaviors that make them very manipulative in nature."

Food Addiction

As I have said and written for many years, food cravings and food addictions often mask food allergies to the very same foods we crave. (See earlier books of mine, such as *The Complete Guide to Sensible*

Eating and *Good Food, Good Mood.*) For the present discussion, I've found holistic practitioners who include in their practice ways of treating food addiction.

One such physician, Dr. Hyla Cass, describes her experience treating patients suffering from food addiction as follows: "Some time ago, a psychologist who specializes in eating disorders began to send her clients to me because she had heard that antidepressant medications worked for these patients. I had shifted to a more holistic way of looking at things, so I told the psychologist that before I did anything with antidepressants I would try some other things. With certain eating disorders, such as food cravings, the underlying problem is a food allergy. We often crave the very foods to which we are allergic. Typically, it's the very things we want to eat that are the most damaging, that create the symptoms. In fact, it's like an addiction to alcohol: As you abstain from the foods you're addicted to, you begin to have withdrawal symptoms and crave those foods even more.

"In order to break the cycle in cases of food addiction, just as when breaking the cycle with drinking (alcoholics are actually allergic to alcohol), you need to supply the body with the appropriate nutrients. When we correct the deficiencies and restore body balance, the food cravings and allergy symptoms will often be relieved. Rather than having to rely strictly on 'willpower,' it is possible for individuals to break addictive cycles by achieving metabolic balance, through avoiding the offending foods and supporting the body with a balanced nutritional program of vitamins, minerals, and amino acids. Often, the cravings will then simply go away. It's quite remarkable: With a good vitamin and mineral product, you can often put a stop to the food allergy and its accompanying symptoms.

"I may order a plasma amino acid analysis, a blood test to determine which amino acids—especially among the essential ones which the body cannot synthesize by itself—are low. The amino acid glutamine, in a dosage of 500–1,000 mg, is particularly useful for reducing cravings, including alcohol cravings.

"There are other things to do for food allergies as well," Dr. Cass adds. "Addictions and allergies are often related to magnesium deficiency and can be corrected by supplementation. There are also techniques that can actually eliminate food allergies through the use of acupuncture and acupressure. As we can see," Dr. Cass concludes, "there are many ways, other than psychotherapy and medication, to approach what at first seems like a psychological problem."

Dr. Doris Rapp brings us more detail concerning the connection between food cravings and allergies: "In my experience, eating disorders and alcoholism can be related to allergies. Frequently, eating disorders are food addictions. When you have a food sensitivity, there is a certain phase of it that makes you really crave that food. And if you happen to be addicted to wheat or baked goods, for example, you can never get enough of them, with the result that you may become obese. To give another example, men who are addicted to corn may drink a lot of beer and they can become alcoholics. They're sensitive to and addicted to the beer, but it's the corn—or sometimes some other component—in the beer that is causing the problem. Sometimes, for those with an allergy to grains, they may feel 'drunk' after eating cereal or certain types of baked goods."

2

ALZHEIMER'S DISEASE

A Doctor's Story: Patient X

A patient came to my office in the Empire State Building. She could not name the building, she didn't know where she was. She could only say that she was in New York. She went on a program using NADH and I saw her again after six months. She said well this is your office in the Empire State Building and this is a blind and this is a window. A couple of months later, her daughter went to visit her and she found a gold button on the floor. She asked her father to whom the button belonged and her mother, the Alzheimer's patient, said, "that's mine I lost it from it from my jacket yesterday." She showed a constant, significant improvement of her mental activity.

I was told this story by Dr. George Birkmayer, the world's leading expert on NADH, which stands for the coenzyme Nicotinamidedenind-inucleotide. This reduced form contains high energy hydrogen—that's the "H" in NADH—that provides energy to your cells. NADH occurs in all the living cells and plays a central role in the energy production of the cells. When you are exercising—power walking, running, swimming or biking—the muscle cells and brain cells contain about 50 micrograms NADH per gram tissue, the heart cells have 90 micrograms, the red blood cells 4. If you supply NADH to the body, it acts as an energy supplement. Dr. Birkmayer has found that NADH "can not only stop the progression of Alzheimer's, but it leads to subtle and significant improvement of certain symptoms, not overnight, but usually in a couple of months."

Alzheimer's disease is caused by the progressive loss of brain cell function. It currently affects over 4 million Americans at a cost to society of $100 billion dollars annually. The disease usually appears after the age of 60, perhaps tripling in numbers of cases every 10 years over age 65. At age 85, the incidence may be as high as 50 percent. Other conditions sometimes diagnosed as dementia include depression, hypothyroidism, vitamin B12 deficiency, folate deficiency, malnutrition and alcohol or drug abuse. Older people with cardiovascular disease are especially prone to it and women appear to have a higher risk of the disease, although higher rates among women may only reflect that women have longer life spans than men.

As life expectancy of both men and women continues to increase, Alzheimer's disease, an only partially understood illness involving deterioration of brain matter and loss of brain function, has become an issue for increasing numbers of people. Demographic projections estimate that as many as 14 million Americans will have AD by 2040, if a highly effective therapy for prevention and reversal is not found.

And yet, as the work of gerontologist Dr. Roy L. Wolford, among others, has shown, it is possible to age in years while remaining functionally younger through enhanced nutrition and a diet different from the typical Western diet relying heavily on meat, dairy products, processed foods, and heaping servings. His book *The Anti-Aging Plan* takes as its starting point the diet developed inside Biosphere 2 and adapts it to the less rigid daily-life habits of Americans, to come up with a low-calorie life-style that appears manageable and satisfying. In studies in mice, nutrient-rich caloric limitation diets largely eliminated age-related slowdown in rate of learning and in memory utilization.

Dr. Philip Hodes has developed a 14-step checklist of approaches he has found helpful in the treatment of Alzheimer's patients:

1. Avoid or eliminate any sources of aluminum exposure: aluminum cookware, utensils, or foil, underarm deodorants, drinking water and any juices and drinks packaged in aluminum-lined cartons. Cut out those vitamins as well as bottled water packaged in bottles with aluminum across the top.

2. Undergo a brain and body detoxification program, which should include a supervised fast. "Now don't attempt to detoxify on your own," Dr. Hodes warns. "You must have holistic physicians or practitioners who are knowledgeable, competent, and experienced in these practices, because if you attempt it on your own you may come up with some upsetting surprises."

Raw juice therapy helps flush out the toxins and supplies enzymes as well as raw vitamins and minerals. Colonic irrigation will help clean out the colon of years of accumulated putrefaction and helps the body function properly. Drinking distilled water, at least in the beginning or for part of the treatment, is also beneficial, along with the use of herbal noncaffeinated teas.

3. Have a practitioner of biological dentistry remove, in proper sequence, your silver-mercury dental amalgam fillings from your teeth. Tom Warren, who wrote *Beating Alzheimer's*, emphasized the importance of this procedure.

4. Bio-oxidative therapies are very effective in bringing oxygen into the brain to increase the individual's ability to think. We live in an external environment with only 19 percent oxygen, when it should contain more, so we all suffer from oxygen insufficiency. Bio-oxidative therapies include hyperbaric oxygen chamber therapy, ozone therapy, and hydrogen peroxide therapy, among others. Also, superoxide dismutase, dimethylglycine, organic-germanium-132, glutathione peroxidase, homozone, vitamin E, aerobic exercising, and deep breathing in a relatively pure environment can be helpful. The herbs ginkgo biloba and butcher's broom are very beneficial.

5. The antioxidants, which work on the brain, are beneficial also. They include: vitamin A, beta carotene, thiamine hydrochloride, riboflavin, niacinamide, pantothenic acid, pyridoxine, B12, folic acid, para-amino-benzoic acid (PABA), biotin, choline and inositol, vitamin E, vitamin C, vitamin P, the bioflavinoids (such as quercetin, hesperiden and pycnogenol), vitamin N, acetyl cysteine, acetyl carnitine, the sulfur-containing amino acids L-cysteine and L-methionine, and the enzymes such as coenzyme Q10, bromelain, papain and pancreatic enzymes.

6. EDTA chelation therapy, performed intravenously, is very good for removing the heavy toxic metals, which include lead, cadmium, arsenic, nickel, copper, iron, mercury, and aluminum. A special chelating agent, desoxyferramine, works well, specifically as an aluminum-chelating agent.

7. Homeopathic remedies will also remove aluminum from the body and the brain, according to Dr. Hodes. "Then you have to take orthomolecular nutritional therapy, intravenously or with intramuscular shots, along with oral supplements of all the nutrients."

8. Dr. Hodes credits clinical ecologists with having made a major contribution in the treatment of people with Alzheimer's disease when they recognized the importance of four to five day diversified food-rotation diets. In a food-rotation diet, you eat a variety of foods and no one food more than once or twice a week—thus eliminating the food allergens to which you are generally "addicted." The rotation diet also lightens the load on your immune system. You should also eliminate alcohol, caffeine, tobacco, sugar, and foods that are refined, processed, or filled with chemicals and artificial colorings and dyes. Replace them with natural, organically grown, pesticide-free wholesome and whole foods.

9. Biomagnetic and electromagnetic pulse therapies are also valuable. Diapulse, magnatherm, biofeedback, acupuncture, and ear acupuncture (auricular therapy) can also be tried.

10. Dr. Hodes also notes the existence of several other, less widespread approaches that are available, involving nutrient substances that increase brain function: An Israeli egg yolk lecithin substance, AL721, which was originally used to give energy and reduce cholesterol in elderly people, and also was used to combat HIV and AIDS,

also helps the brain. You might try Dr. Ana Aslan's treatment called Gerovital (GH3) and live cell therapy, which are illegal in America but available in certain other countries. There is also something called super-triple-phosphatidylcholine.

"There are supplement companies which manufacture brain formulas, which are composed of various amino acids, enzymes, vitamins, minerals, and herbs. Niacin, or vitamin B3, is helpful because it opens up the blood vessels and brings nutrients, blood, oxygen, and other nutrients to the brain. Mineral baths, consisting of sodium, potassium, and magnesium, which seep into our bodies through the pores of the skin, are also helpful."

11. "Herbal remedies are also beneficial: Schussler cell salts, Bach flower remedies, and homeopathic remedies."

12. "Developmental/behavioral optometric vision therapy for improved visualization, perception, cognition, and memory efficiency."

13. "Cranial, sacro-occipital technic, applied kinesiology, and network chiropractic and osteopathic care will improve the efficiency of the flow of the nerve supply and increase oxygen and blood carrying nutrients to the brain."

14. Finally, Dr. Hodes maintains: "Since the brain of an Alzheimer's patient shrinks, we have to rehydrate it with pure water, eight to ten glasses daily. It takes about six months to compensate for the shrinkage."

Dr. Jay Lombard focuses treatment for Alzheimer's on four areas: reducing excessive inflammation; raising a neurotransmitter called acetylcholine, which is very vital to memory in patients; reducing antioxidant activity (free radicals appear to be very involved in Alzheimer's Disease); and boosting the mitochondria. For raising brain acetylcholine levels, there is a natural product called hooperzene A, which blocks the enzyme that breaks down acetylcholine and therefore raises our brain acetylcholine levels. It seems to be very effective in improving memory and preliminary data in Alzheimer's hopefully will be available soon. For antioxidants, ginkgo biloba has been shown to be effective to retard the progression of the disease. Vitamin E and melatonin are very good antioxidants. And for increasing mitochondrial activity, coenzyme Q10 or an analog of coenzyme Q10, an amino acid called acetylecarnitine are useful. There is some data that NAHD may be effective in treating Alzheimer's.

Finally, the last thing for Alzheimer's is looking at hormones, particularly estrogen and DHEA. Estrogen is very effective in inhibiting an enzyme that is detrimental to Alzheimer's patients. This enzyme is called beta secretinase. Estrogen blocks that enzyme and therefore inhibits the production of these pathological proteins found in the brains of Alzheimer's patients. DHEA, a natural adrenal steroid, may be effective in Alzheimer's Disease.

Dr. Michael Schachter reminds us that in dealing with Alzheimer's patients showing signs of senile dementia, "some people have improved quite a bit on a program in which they received injectable B vitamins and magnesium. Some of these elderly people have difficulty absorbing vitamins and minerals simply because of long-term chronic deficiencies, so an injectable program becomes very helpful." He also uses disodium-magnesium EDTA chelation therapy because by using disodium EDTA with magnesium, we're able to reverse some of the aging processes by removing calcium from soft tissues, where it doesn't belong, and trying to get it back into the bone, where it does belong. The chelation process, which is an intravenous treatment, helps with soft tissue decalcification, in addition to removing heavy metals.

"There is some research relating aluminum toxicity to Alzheimer's disease," Dr. Schachter adds. "Dr. Crapper McClaughlin has done some work in Canada, and we have been doing some work recently too, with patients who suffer from dementia using another chelating agent called Deferroxamine or Desferal, which is primarily useful in removing iron and aluminum—but not calcium—from the body. Usually, dementia is a one-way street; people tend to get worse and worse. By using this chelation process, some patients have at least had their dementia process slowed down or stopped for awhile. Some patients have even improved a little using a combination program of supplements, a good diet, and the removal of some of these heavy metals with chelating agents."

Dr. Dharma Singh Khalsa heads the Alzheimer's Prevention Foundation in Tucson, Arizona. His "mission" for several decades has been to make the idea of preventive medicine for the brain available to health care practitioners. He is convinced that memory loss can be prevented and reversed and his work is critical not only for healthy people, but for those suffering all kinds of brain deterioration, including Alzheimer's.

Dr. Khalsa's Seven Step Program for treating Alzheimer's Disease and associated memory impairment is a "complementary" program, combining coventional medical practices with those of alternative medicine.

1. Nutritional Enhancement. "Improved nutrition, all practitioners, agree, enhances cognitive function. At a bare minimum, the diet should have low fat, moderate protein, high complex carbohydrates and a low caloric intake. Adding breast of chicken, fish and non-animal protein products such as tofu is helpful. Certain fish is especially good for the brain. These fish include salmon, tuna, trout, mackerel, and sardines."

2. Nutrient Supplementation. "The B complex vitamins are essential for optimal neurological health. They are especially critical for neurotransmitter control and carbohydrate energy metabolism. Niacin itself (B3) has been shown to have memory improving benefits. For this reason, a high-potency multiple vitamin/mineral package is included in each patient's program in doses above the US RDA, but not in so-called 'orthomolecular' ranges.

"Recent dynamic research has confirmed the neuro-protective role of vitamin E. Vitamin E protects cell membranes from oxidative damage. The dose utilized in this program is 800 IU.

"Other antioxidants prescribed are vitamin C 3000-6000 mg per day and vitamin A 25,000 IU a day. Selenium and zinc are included in the multivitamin/mineral tablet.

"Additional program supplements included 3 newer neuroactive compounds: phosphatidyl serine (PS), 300 mg/day; coenzyme Q-10 (CoQ10), 100 mg/day; and acetyl L carnitine (ALC), 750mg to 1500 mg/day.

"PS is a negatively charged phospholipid, almost exclusively located in cell membranes. It has a series of unique physiological properties that are important to neuronal functions, including stimulation of neurotransmitter release, activation of ion transport mechanisms and increase in glucose and cyclic AMP levels in the brain. In the aging brain, a decline in these functions is associated with memory impairment and deficits in cognitive abilities. PS has been the subject of 23 studies both in America and abroad; 12 of them double-blind. It has been found to improve short-term memory, mood, concentration and activities of daily living. Although initial studies utilized bovine PS, the concern over the risk of a slow viral infection prompted the search for an alternative plant source. A novel PS product made through byenzymatic conversion of soy lecithin has now been developed, and subsequent research has confirmed its positive effects in patients with memory loss.

"CoQ10 is rapidly gaining notice as a powerful neuroprotective agent. It works as a dynamic antioxidant throughout the brain cell membrane and mitochondria, where it is involved in the production of high energy phosphate compounds

"ALC is a superbly versatile metabolite and plays a pivotal role in facilitating energetic pathways in brain cell mitochondria. It is a source of acetyl groups for acetyl-Co-A and facilitates release of acetylcholine and other neurotransmitters and neuropeptides. ALC also has been reported to decrease cortisol levels.

3. Herbs. "Ginkgo biloba was utilized at a dose of 120 mg/day. This dose increases microvascular circulation, scavenges free radicals, and helps improve concentration and short-term memory."

4. Pharmaceuticals. "L-deprenyl citrate, a MAO-B inhibitor was shown to limit degeneration of patients with AD in a 5-year double-blind study with doses of 10 mg/day. The drug increases the levels of important catecholamines, especially dopamine, which are decreased in AD. It also inhibits oxidative deamination, thereby reducing neuronal damage.

"Hydergine, although not utilized in this project, also shows promise in the protection against brain aging.

"A new drug, Aricept (donepezil HCL), was recently approved by the FDA. It is said to be effective in improving cognition and patient function in patients with AD. Apparently it is no more effective than PS, however, and has a greater risk of side effects."

5. Hormone Replacement Therapy. "Research on the effects of estrogen replacement therapy in the prevention of AD has been very exciting. Hippocampal plasticity and nerve growth factors are apparently estrogen-sensitive. The use of either DHEA or pregnenolone, both neurospecific hormones and precursors to estrogen, makes good clinical sense, because of the lower side effect potential. Both have

proved useful in this program at doses of 50mg/day. A recent animal study demonstrated that DHEA affects excitability in the hippocampus, thereby enhancing memory function at moderate dosages. Because the optimal dose needed to facilitate the induction of neuronal plasticity in humans is not yet certain, the dosage level used was arrived at empirically.

"Another study showed for the first time that DHEA enhances acetylcholine release from hippocampal neurons in the rat brain. DHEA has been found to be consistently low in patients with AD.

"Research in animals has proved pregnenolone to be a very powerful memory enhancer. Pregnenolone was also demonstrated to improve memory in humans. More than 50 years ago, researchers at the University of Massachusetts trained 14 subjects to operate an airplane flight simulator. Subjects who received the hormone improved significantly compared with controls. A recent study has demonstrated improved memory with pregnenolone use in older people.

"The hormone melatonin at doses of 0.3mg to 6mg is given at bedtime, when indicated, to restore circadian rhythm in place of benzodiazepines, which can depress cognitive function."

6. Mental Training. Nowhere more than in the brain is the old adage, "Use it or lose it," more appropriate. In fact, Einstein had a fairly normal brain when it came to his neurons. However, what was extremely unusual was the structure of his brain, rich in supporting glial cells. He was the Michael Jordan of mental athletes. Dr. Khalsa's ninety-one year old mother is a prime-time example of how mental exercise helps maintain clarity throughout life. She has been on his Brain Longevity Program for a number of years and enjoys watching game shows. She gets a big kick out of beating the contestants to the answers.

We know that the risk of developing dementia decreases with the number of years of formal education. The lower the educational level, the greater the risk for AD. This highlights research suggesting that mental activity throughout life is neuroprotective. Based on the enriched environment work of Cotman and Diamond, the program includes cognitive stimulation, such as headline discussion, cross word puzzles, music, art and group therapy. Mental training increases dendritic sprouting and enhances central nervous system plasticity.

7. Mind/Body Exercises. "Stress management. It is crucial because chronic, unbalanced stress causes elevation of the hormone cortisol. Cortisol has a toxic effect on the memory center of the brain and can cause memory loss. The stress management tool of meditation decreases cortisol and enhances many aspects of mental function. Massage and guided mental imagery have also recently been shown to lower cortisol levels in the blood.

"To prevent accelerated brain aging and cognitive dysfunction, it is critical to reduce the negative physiological consequences brought about by chronic stress. For this we turn to a practice that is thousands of years old and the subject of many modern scientific research studies: meditation. Besides the awake state, the sleep state and the dream state, there is the fourth state: the transcendent or meditative. In the past three decades, numerous studies have been completed by researchers exploring the far-reaching effects of transcendental meditation, a simple mental technique. Additionally, Herbert Benson, M.D., of the Harvard Medical School's Mind/Body Medical Institute, has studied a wakeful hypometabolic entity, which has become known as the relaxation response (RR). RR is an innate psychophysiological mechanism first demonstrated by Walter Hess, Ph.D. in 1948, a discovery for which he was awarded the Nobel Prize in physiology. Meditation has been found to decrease serum cortisol levels and promotes normalization of adaptive mechanisms. Practitioners of meditation also display lower levels of lipid peroxidase, a marker of free radical production, as well as higher levels of the hormone dehydroepiandrosterone, important for optimal brain function. Elderly meditators have been shown to enjoy greater life expectancy than nonmeditators. The use of meditation as a tool for preventing memory loss, or for reversing it in its early stages, is an avenue ripe for clinical investigation.

"Major chemico-anatomical changes in AD appear to occur as a result of the degeneration of transmitter producing neurons in circumscribed areas of the brain cortex. Pharmacological approaches to the prevention and reversal of memory loss are likely to continue to be difficult because of the presence of multiple neurotransmitter deficits and the difficulty of replacing lost transmitter function in a way that mimics normal neuronal release. For this reason, patients are instructed in the practice of yogic kriyas: specific exercises that combine breathing, finger movement, and regenerating sound currents. The practice of these kriyas serve a dual purpose: they induce the RR and stimulate the central nervous system. Kriyas have been clinically shown to create cerebral stimulation, mental relaxation, and an increased ability to focus. A PET scan has demonstrated that kriyas enhance regional cerebral blood flow, oxygen delivery and glucose utilization.

"Finally, aerobic conditioning has been shown to improve some aspects of mental function by as much as 20 to 30 percent."

3

ANXIETY DISORDERS AND PANIC ATTACKS

D r. Lynne Freeman, Director of the Open Doors Institute in Los Angeles, considers anxiety the number one health problem in the United States today. One specific anxiety disorder is a panic attack, "a very dramatic episode that involves heart palpitations, sweating, feelings of disorientation, shaky limbs and the feeling that one is about to go insane or die." It feels like a heart attack. While there is "a genetic predisposition" to such attacks, they can also be a side effect of certain medications. "Prozac," she says, "can actually increase anxiety symptoms," All kinds of over the counter remedies and prescription drugs can precipitate a panic attack. So it's important to assess the medications you're taking.

One physical condition that often contributes to anxiety is mitral valve prolapse. This is a small heart valve that isn't functioning well, so when the blood passes through the valve, it rushes. A person can experience the quicker pace as a fluttery feeling or a palpitation. This is a pretty innocuous condition, but if you are predisposed to panic disorder or another form of anxiety, you may interpret this sensation as a heart attack, which would set off an anxiety reaction.

The same is true of gastro esophageal acid reflux, which is basically indigestion. Excess stomach acid can produce heart palpitations, arm pain, a feeling that the chest is closing—so it resembles a heart attack or an anxiety attack. other medical conditions often interpreted as anxiety are hormonal changes involved in menopause and premenstrual syndrome, hypoglycemia, even Crohn's disease, where the person sometimes has periods of dehydration. One of the things you always need to look at if you have anxiety is what is going on with you medically.

Environmental allergies are also linked to or mistaken for panic disorders. A significant part of the population is allergic to aspartame, which we find even in natural vitamins. It could be mistaken for anxiety. Or perhaps you're driving and feeling anxious, not realizing that one of the things you may be responding to are the carbon monoxide fumes coming at you.

Very often, people get confused. When they feel anxious, they will be a little premature in labeling that a panic attack. Actually, a panic attack does have a beginning, middle and end, it's a very dramatic episode that involves heart palpitations, sweating, feelings of disorientation, shaky limbs, and the belief that one is about to go insane or possibly die because it can be construed as a heart attack. Panic disorder is consistent episodes of these panic attacks.

There is clearly a genetic predisposition to these experiences. According to the research, anywhere from 60 to 80 percent of agoraphobics, which is a specific kind of anxiety disorder—fear of leaving your immediate safe environment—are women. There are a number of theories for this, partly hormonal causes, partly conditioning. Men have traditionally been responsible for having to make it in the work place, while women have been home and rearing the children. This is clearly changing in our society, and Dr. Freeman expects these statistics in relation to agoraphobia to change as well.

Some forms of anxiety disorder appear to be growing in the new millennium.

Generalized anxiety disorder describes what we often refer to as a worry wart. This person sits around thinking they have cancer, goes to doctors every day, believes they're about to lose their job. We're seeing a lot of this, particularly in the baby boomer generation, who believed that they would be at least as financially well off as their parents, but that's not happening for a lot of people. They're feeling like failures, like they can't manage their lives, and they are just consumed with anxiety. Generalized anxiety disorder can be treated just like panic disorder can, but it does require a different type of intervention.

"Post Traumatic Stress Disorder" originally described people coming back from war, but now we understand that this can apply to anyone who has experienced or witnessed a traumatic event. Some people who only heard about a recent plane crash are actually suffering from symptoms of post traumatic stress disorder—they're having nightmares about flying, don't want to get on a plane, are feeling some depression, some anxiety. They didn't even have to be close to anyone who experienced the crash. Because the media shows us things and gives us information right in our own living rooms, we are exposed to things we've never been exposed to before. Then there is the reality of increased random violence all over. People are feeling much more hyper-vigilant, much more anxious about their vulnerabilities in the world, and so all of these different kinds of anxieties manifest very differently. The most important thing is to know what kind of anxiety you're suffering from and to have it properly assessed.

The treatments that Dr. Freeman finds effective—without medication—are acupuncture and massage, both of which "essentially find a way to reorganize the body's natural chemistries." An acupuncturist can read your body through your pulses. They understand that different organs hold different emotions. For example, the kidney is known to hold fear, so an acupuncturist, by checking pulses and skin temperature and other things can determine that their kidneys need to be "tonified." That means they can rebalance the kidneys. Since the kidneys produce adrenaline, which in turn produces panic reaction, you can see that acupuncture can be very effective in regulating the bio chemistries.

Certain kinds of homeopathic remedies have had reported success. There's been a lot of work on homeopathy in children reported in the French scientific literature, because they've done more research on homeopathy than anyone else I'm aware of. There was a study of high anxiety children, needing instant gratification, easy to overreact, who had stomach aches from the anxiety and the fears. They were given *nux vomica* and it worked. Another group of children had anxiety because of underlying fears—that they wouldn't succeed, wouldn't be accepted, that their parents couldn't accept them unconditionally. They were given *ignatia* and *ignatia* worked.

Dr. Freeman's knowledge of homeopathic remedies focused on calcalcarea carbonica, essentially derived from oyster shells. Like me, she wanted to underline the fact that "a homeopath takes a lot of things into consideration, not just your physical symptoms, your anxiety reactions, but your personality and how you think and operate in the world. So this is just sort of a very general remedy for a certain type of personality, but a homeopath could better prescribe. If a remedy is not prescribed properly, if the energy is too strong, some people may experience heart palpitations, which can translate into more anxiety reactions, so homeopathic remedies really have to be properly prescribed." That is "very different from getting something off the shelf that has some broad based appeal which may or may not help you." One of the biggest problems is that people go to health food stores and inquire and someone who really doesn't know anything about that individual, or has not been trained will recommend very general remedies. For Example, separation anxiety disorder and generalized anxiety disorder are two very distinct anxiety disorders affecting children and they require two different remedies.

Anxiety disorders, including agoraphobia, claustrophobia, panic attacks, etc., often occur in people with prominent allergies. In many cases there is also a diet-related element relating to poor diet and/or poor absorption in the colon. Programs that address what are otherwise usually considered psychological and/or biochemical problems nutritionally have met with much success, as have treatments relying on naturally occurring substances.

According to Dr. Allan Spreen, anxiety disorders will respond to treatment by certain natural substances. The advantages of treatment with natural substances can be numerous and substantial: by freeing people from having to take more toxic medication, the holistic approach can also spare the patient the medication's side effects, as well as the extra expense. "Some amino acids, when given individually," says Dr. Spreen, "in some cases can be very effective in calming down the symptoms of anxiety disorders and panic attacks. For example, tryptophan, which is no longer available, was used as a sleeping agent, until there was a problem with some batches of it being contaminated, which caused a syndrome that wasn't related to the tryptophan but to the contaminant. Some doctors use tyrosine for depression and anxiety. The 'DL' form of phenylalanine is often used on a short-term basis for depression and can be very effective if given correctly. It can lessen anxiety and depression in people by giving them more of an 'up' mood. Phenylalanine is also an appetite suppressant for many people. If they're given correctly there seems to be no toxicity associated with amino acids and they're much cheaper than antidepressants or anti-anxiety prescription medications."

Dr. Walt Stoll has a different approach: "In my clinical experience, I have found that emotional disorders are often linked to the inability to completely break down proteins, during the digestive process, into their amino acids. Just three or four amino acids still hooked together (peptides), if they get through the intestinal lining, can stimulate the immune system to make antibodies against them. Since our body is also made up of peptides, hooked together to make proteins, these antibodies can attack us. To an antibody, a peptide is a peptide. It frequently doesn't matter whether the peptide came from outside the body or is a part of the body. Many of the chronic diseases, which presently are so baffling to the allopathic disease philosophy of conventional Western medicine, are now being found to be related to auto-immune processes.

"In addition," Dr. Stoll adds, "some of these peptides have been found to be identical to certain brain hormones (endorphins) that are associated with panic attacks, depression, manic depression, schizophrenia, and other conditions. In these cases—with more certain to be discovered—there is no need for the immune system to be involved; the effect is direct. The two first examples to be discovered were peptides from imperfectly digested casein (milk protein) and gluten (wheat protein). Of course, these are two of the most commonly eaten foods in our culture!

"All of the mental states listed above are at least partially caused by brain chemistry abnormalities. Generally, I see patients who have already tried many different therapies. These patients come with stacks and stacks of records documenting that nothing seems to have worked in spite of every imaginable test having been done and every imaginable treatment having been tried. Psychoactive drugs have either worked poorly or have even caused the problem to worsen due to the side effects exceeding the benefits.

"Since every other conceivable cause has been ruled out by the time I get to see them, I am free to look for the things that have not been evaluated. One of the first things I look for is how well the lining of their intestinal tract protects them from their environment. I frequently find that either they don't have the normal bacterial balance in the colon or that they have gone beyond that stage to having candidiasis. Candida can only escape from our control if the normal bacteria are not in control. If candida has converted from the normal yeast form into the disease-causing fungal form, it further damages the lining so that the leakage of peptides is much greater.

"The greater the amount of peptide leakage, the more likely it is that the brain will interpret these protein particles as being identical to the endorphins it produces during panic attacks, depression, etc. This same leakage is responsible for the increasing sensitivities we see in patients who are sensitive to environmental substances other than foods. It is much simpler, in most cases, to correct the leakage than it is to eliminate the substance. But why not do both?

"Once the reason for the leakage is corrected, the patient usually sees dramatic improvement in a very short time. The antibodies involved only last for 72 hours. Once the leakage is stopped completely, symptoms lessen substantially in just a few days; and just reduction of the leakage helps. There are many patients today that have had that kind of experience. Not everyone's mental symptoms are caused by poorly digested food playing tricks on the brain. However, in my experience, it is the most commonly missed diagnosis and one that is relatively easy to resolve."

Dr. Michael Schachter emphasizes the importance of proper diet: "If you suffer from an anxiety disorder, you really need to clean up your diet. Getting off sugar and taking calcium and magnesium works. Also, balancing the stresses in your life, through meditation and other anxiety-reducing disciplines, is important."

One of the most popular herbs for treatment of less severe forms of anxiety—as well as for menopausal depression and insomnia—is kava. According to Chris Kilham, author of *Medicine Hunting in Paradise,* which recounts his work as founder of the Cowboy Medicine Expeditions, specializing in researching and creating plant-based products, kava has an exotic history. It was "brought to the Western world after Captain Cook's first voyage to the South Pacific in the late 1700s. There has been ongoing scientific interest in kava since then. It actually was a registered drug in the United States in 1950 for gonorrhea and nervousness. It was never really popular because you can't patent a plant and so drug companies can't make millions of dollars on it. Kava has been for the past several years very popular in Europe and is finally hitting the U.S."

As Kilham explains it, the Polynesians and the Melanesians pound the root and make a beverage out of it, which they drink on an almost daily basis as a relaxing beverage. For medicinal purposes, use extracts of the root. The root contains a group of naturally occurring compounds known as the kava lactones. They are skeletal muscle relaxants. They work in the limbic system of the brain, that area of the brain that has control over emotions, and homeostatic mechanisms like the waking and sleeping cycle, appetite, and the sexual urge. An area known as the amygdala in the brain is the seat of the emotional responses of fear and anxiety. The kava lactones in kava work in the amygdala to mitigate anxiety and they work centrally in the nervous system to relax skeletal muscles. No matter how much kava you use, there is no diminishment of mental function. Clinical studies—which have included toxicological studies, anxiety studies, studies on depression, and studies on sleeplessness—show that kava does not impair function driving an automobile or operating heavy machinery. Toxicity only occurs with huge consumption, in excess of a gallon of the beverage a day, in conjunction with malnutrition. People who are eating a reasonable diet and taking medicinal doses of kava have no cause for concern. The primary toxicity that kava exhibits when it is taken in huge amounts is a patchy skin condition.

But the form in which you take kava does matter. "There is no benefit to consuming capsules or tablets of ground up kava root," Kilham says, "it simply doesn't do anything. You couldn't swallow enough kava root to get an effect. Kava is one of those wonderful plants that actually imparts something you can feel. In that regard, it's quite rare. Clinical studies are done with standardized kava extracts; the doses needed to produce an anti-anxiety, anti-depression or sleep enhancing effect are in excess of 70 milligrams of kava lactones in one, two or three doses a day. What a customer wants to look for is a standardized kava extract with at least 70 milligrams of kava lactones per dose.

"The ultimate test is, do you feel it? I've walked into stores and seen ground up kava root capsule and I've thought, 'People going to swallow them, nothing's going to happen,' and they'll say, 'Oh, this stuff really doesn't work.' What will work is the right quantity of a standardized extract, and if you feel it, you know you've got a good kava product on your hands."

I would add a caveat. If you're depressed, if you have hyperactive disorders, if your personality is always aggressive, if you have unexpressed anger and keep turning around and burning your own bridges, isolating yourself from people, and being short tempered, then kava kava at about 100 milligrams to 150 milligrams could do you a lot of good. But almost all the companies out there who make it use the leaves. The leaves don't have the power. The bark doesn't have the power. The root is potent, the bark and the leaves are not. And it's best in a plant extract form, as Kris Kilham says, because kava lactones should be standardized, and that way you get a pure amount each time. It's been used for thousands of years and it can create a very calm, smooth and even sense of well being.

Obsessive-Compulsive Disorders

In the movie *As Good As It Gets*, Jack Nicholson's character checks and rechecks the locks on his doors, uses a new bar of soap every time he washes his hands and avoids stepping on sidewalk cracks at all costs. He eats the same food in the same restaurant at the same time every day, served by the same waitress. Like an estimated 4 million other Americans, this character suffers from obsessive-compulsive disorder. When his rituals are interrupted, he is gripped by a heart-palpitating, sweat-dripping anxiety attack. In the movie, love cures him. In life, there are other alternatives.

Obsessive-compulsive disorders affect both men and women and are more common than severe mental illnesses like schizophrenia or manic-depressive disorder. This condition is characterized by repetitive thinking and the inability to control or put a stop to this thinking process, which Dr. José Yaryura-Tobias describes as "very forceful, practically taking over the mind. It doesn't allow you to think about anything else. Compulsions are urges that are so extremely demanding that they appear to have to be carried out." Some of the main compulsions are double-checking and hand washing. If the compulsion isn't carried out, there is anxiety that will cease or diminish if it is. This illness has been described in medical literature for at least 200 years.

Dr. Yaryura-Tobias tells us some of the peculiar characteristics of obsessive-compulsive behavior: "It usually takes about seven years or so for a patient to come in for a consultation, which tells us that the condition tends to occur gradually, becoming a part of the patient's behavioral system in a very, very slow manner. It occurs with equal frequency in males and females. Fifty percent of obsessive-compulsive patients manifest their sickness during childhood or adolescence. Later on—primarily after the age of 40—it fades away, and it becomes very rare after the age of 50.

"As to why this condition exists at all, we don't have a sure answer to that question. The behavior may result from a learning process that takes hold during childhood. There is a theory that is now slowly being accepted about a biochemical process at work related to changes in neurotransmitters—the chemical substances in the brain that build bridges between neurons in the nervous cells so that they can transmit signals from the outside into our system or, in the reverse direction, have us act to affect the outside world. The key neurotransmitter that is being studied in this regard is serotonin.

"To treat obsessive-compulsive disorders, behavioral therapy, and an amino acid approach, such as the use of L-tryptophan, would be the treatment of choice, along with some other medications.

"We basically treat with behavioral therapy. We try to use thought-stopping, exposure (flooding) and response prevention to prevent the brain from repeating the same thought. That is difficult, so we also use cognitive therapy to explain the reasons we think the things we do, and try to modify the thought.

"Compulsions are the area where behavioral therapy is most effective. We expose the patient, either in reality or in his or her imagination, to face what he is afraid of. If you have fears of AIDS or of blood, you are exposed to blood or taken to the hospital where there might be patients with AIDS. Or you will read articles on the condition.

"If it is contamination from dirt the patient is afraid of, we teach the person how to touch objects and not to be afraid of them. Then we prevent the patient from washing their hands; in other words, they must remain unclean for awhile. I'm talking about patients who, when they are seriously ill, might completely use up one or two bars of soap per day. They might engage in rituals of washing for many hours. They may wash their hands sometimes a hundred or more times a day. Some of these patients, in addition, will clean their hands with alcohol or other substances. Sometimes their skin becomes extremely raw. I've seen cases where patients require plastic surgery.

"Overall, the treatment takes about six months. With medication there is improvement up to 60 or 70 percent of the time.

"My colleagues and I were the first to use tryptophan and with it we were able to reduce and almost eliminate completely the use of drugs for this condition, and we obtained very good results. Unfortunately, tryptophan has been banned so we can no longer use it. We were using between 3000 and 9000 mg per day.

"Then we used vitamin B6, 100 mg, three times a day. Vitamin B6, pyridoxine phosphate, is a vitamin that is very important for the breakdown of tryptophan into serotonin. The idea behind this was that either these patients didn't have enough serotonin in their brains, were very dependent on serotonin, or that the normal conversion of tryptophan into serotonin was not occurring.

"When we found by measuring that there was a lack of serotonin, this could be reversed by the administration of L-tryptophan with niacin and vitamin B6. Some medications also accomplish this result, but with medications we face many types of side effects.

"About 30 percent of patients do not respond to any form of therapy. But it is not a closed chapter for these patients either. An investigation has to be conducted. Now that we have brain imaging, we are able to visualize the brain. We can measure, for instance, the metabolism of sugar in the brain. We find, for instance, the frontal and temporal lobes and the basal ganglia, that are related to Parkinson's disease, disrupted. We see the metabolism of the breakdown of sugar and also images of an abnormal brain. The same can be seen with some electrophysiological measurements of brain wave tests and so forth.

"Interestingly," Dr. Yaryura-Tobias concludes, "work has been going on using pure behavioral therapy before and after measuring serotonin. With just behavioral therapy, we were able to modify the levels of serotonin in the body. In other words, we may not need medication to change or challenge the presence of a neurotransmitter such as serotonin. Simply the mere interaction of behavioral technique may have an effect."

According to Dr. Robert Atkins, there is some common ground between conventional Western medicine and more holistic approaches such as orthomolecular psychiatry, or what he refers to as "complementary" medicine. "Both orthodox medicine and complementary medicine, which is the nutrition-based alternative to orthodox medicine, recognize that if a certain neurotransmitter is in short supply, certain syndromes will result. A classic example is that the serotonin-deficient person will often be an obsessive-compulsive. These are the people who can't get out of the house because they've got to make sure the light switches are off or the gas jet isn't on—the people who have to wash their hands 20 times a day, and whose desks have to be perfectly neat. These same people are serotonin-deficient."

The difference between the conventional and the alternative medical communities lies in how they address the problem. Dr. Atkins describes the conventional approach: "Now there are drugs that block the degradation of serotonin and allow the serotonin level to lift, but these drugs do a lot of other things: They poison a lot of enzyme systems and that's why so many people got into trouble with Prozac and drugs like that." And the more enlightened alternative approach: "However, you can increase serotonin with the nutrition precursor, tryptophan, which, unfortunately, the FDA took off the market because of a bad batch.

"Dr. Russell Jaffe has done research to indicate that the best treatment for the bad tryptophan syndrome (the eosinophilia myalgic syndrome) is the use of pure unadulterated tryptophan. People with obsessive-compulsive and anxiety disorders often improve on tryptophan. Since the FDA ban on tryptophan, pure tryptophan has not been available in the United States, even by prescription." Some practitioners recommend getting tryptophan from warm milk or in foods like kiwi fruit, turkey, figs and dates.

Some pharmacies, according to Dr. Atkins, "will compound capsules of 5-hydroxy tryptophan. This compound is an intermediary between tryptophan and 5-hydroxy-tryptamine, which is serotonin, the neurotransmitter you are trying to build up. The whole idea of supplying a precursor to build up a neurotransmitter that is in short supply is a fruitful approach to treating psychiatric disorders and should, in my opinion," concludes Dr. Atkins, "be considered before the use of nonphysiologic psychotropic drugs, which have more potential for toxicity."

Acupuncturists also have had a great deal of success with obsessive compulsive disorder. In some situations, their treatment has proven to be more effective than medication.

4

$\mathcal{E}$ATING DISORDERS

Patient Story: Dr. Y

The woman was 47 years old, a psychotherapist with a doctoral degree in psychology, who had been treating patients with eating disorders for almost 15 years. She herself had bulimia—about five binge-purge episodes per day for the last 34 years. She could hardly recount a single day since she was 12 when she did not engage in bulimic activity. We gave her a small amount, about five or 10 milliliters, less than a tablespoon, of liquid zinc and asked her to swirl it around for a few seconds and tell us what she tasted. (If they can't taste the solution, it's evidence of systemic zinc deficiency. This has to do with a zinc dependent polypeptide known as gustine {sp?}, which helps us to distinguish metallic taste, and zinc has a strong metallic taste. She couldn't taste anything. It tasted like water to her. She thought it was a placebo She was given about 120 milliliters of this solution spaced out throughout the day at about 30, 40 milliliters each time, on an empty stomach. Four days later, she called to say she couldn't explain it, but she had no desire to binge or purge that day. That was the first day she could recall feeling good in 34 years.

This story was told by Dr. Alexander Schauss, who has done a lot of important and original work in treating people with eating disorders. The category includes self-starving, bingeing and purging, over-eating and, recently, exercise disorder, a compulsive behavior affliction in which a person cannot refrain from excessive workouts because she or he is terrified of gaining weight. Particularly among women, disordered body images and destructive eating behavior "came out" of the closet in the late 1980s and the 1990s, spurred in part by the revelation that popular singer Karen Carpenter had died of anorexia. Social critics and psychologists have looked to media pressure—and the more available surgeries for re-shaping the human body—as some causes of the dissatisfaction women often feel about "normal" bodies.

Most experts agree that a full spectrum of factors contribute to these diseases—family dynamics, cultural messages, sexual abuse and links with chemical dependency. Nutrition is being recognized as part of the problem and part of the cure. While the most visible sufferers of these diseases have been young women—in magazines, books, television and school educational programs, recent research indicates that men, too, struggle with them. About 10 percent of the diagnosed bulimics and anorexics are men; 40 percent of those with binge-eating disorder. Males with eating disorders are more likely to have alcohol-related conditions and to have had their illness overlooked by doctors, who see it as a specifically female problem.

Dr. Schauss spearheaded the whole understanding of how liquid zinc helps treat these disorders. The psychologist whose case he described had been referred by a local hospital because a serious risk factor with chronic bulimia is that the esophageal flap can tear, resulting in a person choking themselves and dying. He'd had a case like that just two years before, a 19 year old girl at a local university. The psychotherapist's surgeon was trying to stabilize her and had heard about Dr. Schauss's research.

He and his staff were intrigued as to how a simple nutrient like zinc can cause a major change in the way the brain functions. "When you've done something for 34 years, whether it's cigarette smoking, biting your nails, or you're phobic about something, or engaged in bulimia, you have to wonder how it would be possible that in four or five days, such an obsessive compulsive type behavior would just disappear. Five years later, she had not gone back to binge-purging. More important, she was provided no therapy. I never actually met her; the protocol was given to her by a staff member. We're quite convinced in this case and in hundreds of others that it was the liquid zinc that was effective rather than some tangential treatment, which of course would confound our conclusions."

In fact, five year follow up studies done by Dr. Shouse show a 64.1 percent success rate for bulimics on the liquid zinc treatment and an 85 percent recovery rate in anorexic patients. These are extraordinarily high recovery rates for a condition which is considered quite difficult to treat and quite insidious. The mortality rate based on a 20 year study post diagnosis of patients with eating disorders is that 38 percent of them are dead within 20 years of initial diagnosis. And many times the families have spent enormous amounts of money trying to keep their children alive. The average institutional cost right now is about $650 a day, which adds up to about $28,000 to $29,000 per month. Dr. Schauss has had many patients who've been through numerous programs and, half a million dollars later, still did not recover.

"We've known since at least the 1930s, he says, "that when animals were experimentally placed on diets deficient in zinc, they developed anorexia. By 1958, Professor Kung in China—who became a victim of the cultural revolution and we lost track of him—was the first to recognize that zinc was essential in humans. A paper he wrote in Chinese unfortunately never got published in English. About four years later, an American researcher from Wayne State University, working in Egypt, discovered that zinc was intimately required by the human body to develop secondary sexual characteristics. His research eventually lead to the National Academy of Sciences' establishing zinc as an essential nutrient.

"Zinc is pervasive, found in every tissue cell, organ and fluid in the human body, and involved in over 200 enzyme reactions in the brain. That is why we've taken a great interest in what zinc does in the brain that might be of therapeutic value to people with various kinds of neurological psychiatric conditions. We've learned that when humans are placed on zinc deficient diets, they develop eating disorders.

"In morbid obesity—when people are so significantly overweight that it could shorten their lifespan or increase their risk of disease—there is an inverse relationship between the level of obesity and the level of zinc. The more obese they are, the less zinc they have in their body. We don't know yet whether this is cause and effect, but it's a very important observation because at the other end of the continuum, with anorexia nervosa, self induced starvation, people are always zinc deficient. There is strong evidence today from studies done at the University of Kentucky School of Medicine, at Stanford University, and the University of California at Davis, in addition to our research institute's work, that the lower the zinc status is, the more likely it is that the patient will be able to recover from anorexia.

"Similar facts are true of bulimia nervosa. We estimate that on any college or university campus in this country, somewhere between eight and 15 percent of the females attending school are engaging in bulimia, a binge-purge cycle or an effort to use laxatives, purgatives or diuretics to eliminate the calories consumed during binge episodes. Dr. Doris Rapp also believes that zinc deficiency may be a factor, even though the stated reason for the behavior is avoidance of weight gain. According to Dr. Rapp, "In cases where youngsters or adults are eating and then purging themselves in the bathroom by putting a finger down their throats, these individuals are ostensibly getting rid of the food because they don't want to gain weight. But studies have suggested that zinc can be a helpful form of treatment."

Dr. Schauss explains that "the liquid zinc is absorbed directly in the stomach much like water and alcohol, which then goes into portal blood and into the liver. The treatment doesn't cause any favorable response for three to four days because in order for zinc to get into the brain or any other tissue that requires it, it needs a metal carrier, a type of protein that carries metals. That protein is metallothionein. We need to have enough of the protein carrier to help move the zinc to where it's needed in the body. It usually takes several days for the body's extra levels of zinc to facilitate the production of higher amounts of metallothionein. As you continue the treatment, eventually you have a considerable amount of this protein carrier to help move the zinc to where it is required.

"I've had cases where it's taken almost three weeks before the zinc finally starts to saturate brain tissue, which then influences the person's perception of themselves, and that begins to disturb the underlying mechanism that contributes to the eating disorder.

"I'd worked with eating disorder patients for 15 years, hundreds and hundreds of patients, and until I saw this treatment, I felt as most of my colleagues do, that the best we could expect with either bulimia or anorexia was a 20 to 30 percent recovery. And when it occurred, we were not always sure why.

"The zinc research also gives us a much better idea why therapies that are not zinc related may be working. Under conditions of psychological stress, you lose zinc. You can, in fact, measure a two to three fold increase in the amount of zinc in the urine under conditions of psychological stress. Most nutrients are lost at higher levels under physiological stress, such as wounds, surgery, injury, burns, physical trauma. But we lose more zinc if the person's internal, mental ideations place them under constant stress. They may actually be losing zinc at a higher rate than they can replace it through the diet. Combine that with binge-purge activity, where a person is losing a lot of the calories and nutrients in the purge cycle, or with anorexia, where they don't consume enough calories to sustain a balanced level of minerals and vitamins, you begin to understand this problem.

"One of the things that puzzled us early in our research is why so many females have anorexia and bulimia, why not males? We finally realized that zinc is highly concentrated in the male prostate, providing a mineral essential for sperm development. If a male is under psychological stress, he has storages of zinc in the prostate. Since women don't have prostates, they catabolize the zinc from other tissue. The richest tissue in the human body for zinc is the muscle tissue. In anorexia, a common feature is muscle wasting. They're actually eating their own muscle tissue as a way of releasing nutrients that they need to survive.

"It is very, very important to realize that one of the reasons we use zinc is to stop that muscle wasting because the last muscle, one that only contains about one percent of zinc, is the heart muscle. Twenty-nine percent of the zinc in the human body is in skeletal muscle; only one percent is in heart muscle tissue. But when, unfortunately, the body starts to scavenge zinc out of heart muscle tissue, it starts to damage the heart. A weakened heart can result in bradycardia, tachycardia, arrhythmias and eventual heart failure. It is particularly dangerous in patients who are recovering from anorexia—their muscle tissue in their hearts has been damaged and taking on weight puts extra pressure on the heart. That is how the singer Karen Carpenter died.

"The research evidence is strong. The first demonstrated cases of the efficacy of using a liquid zinc were published in *The Lancet* in August of 1984 by my colleague Professor Derick Bry Smith who has been professor of chemistry at the University of Redding for over 35 years. He reasoned that if we could develop just the right polarity of the liquid zinc solution it should pass through the stomach directly into portal blood and into the liver, rather than trying to be absorbed in the small intestine, primarily in the ilium where most of the zinc is absorbed. Because so many of the patients with zinc deficiency have mal absorption for zinc, it creates kind of a catch-22. They need it, but they have difficulty absorbing it. Using the liquid zinc is far more effective than using a powder or capsule.

"It is extremely important to understand that zinc can only be absorbed in the small intestine in the ionic state. If it is combined with another element—zinc sulfate, zinc gluconate, zinc picolinates, amino chelated zincs, zinc proteinates—all of these have to be broken up in the stomach by hydrochloric acid. So if you have low gastric function due to poor secretion of hydrochloric acid or malabsorption of zinc or both, then a zinc tablet or capsule will rarely be as effective as liquid zinc at the lowest concentration, which the body thinks is just plain ole water and you kind of fool it into pulling it into portal blood, and then suddenly the liver recognizes that zinc is there and starts to synthesize more metallothionein and then in its unique process combine it with metallothionein to get it where it needs to go.

"After the first studies, which were just case reports, showed remarkable rates of recovery for anorexics and bulimics, we started to do control trials. One of the first was to see whether in fact there was a difference in taste perception between those who are deficient in zinc and those who are not. We wrote a paper that was presented at the American College of Nutrition in 1986 and published in *Nutrients and Brain Function* in 1987, demonstrating that in fact patients who have zinc deficiency are unable to taste the zinc solution. So we provided relatively strong evidence, based on double blind placebo controlled studies, that this simple non-invasive procedure could be very effective.

"The National Institutes of Health funded studies at the University of Kentucky medical center, which has a large eating disorders program, and several California universities, that showed most patients with eating disorders were, in fact, zinc deficient. Giving them liquid zinc could be highly therapeutic, they found, confirming our earlier clinical observations. But they also found that a diet rich in zinc actually made the patients worse. We still do not understand why. A few years ago, I heard the head of the eating disorders program at the Gutenberg University in Sweden tell a radio audience that she believed that up to 100 percent of patients with eating disorders, including morbid obesity, were zinc deficient. She felt it was imperative that any program that treated patients with an eating disorder use zinc as an adjunct in treatment.

"Why, then do we sometimes see anorexic, bulimic or obese patients recover in programs where no zinc is being used? Remember, you lose zinc under psychological stress. If you send a patient who is stressed to a supportive, warm, nurturing environment, such as many of the eating residential treatment facilities are, after several weeks much of their stress is alleviated. Suddenly the amount of zinc that the body is losing has been decreased, and we believe that that's partially why various treatment modalities have been helping people.

We have long suspected that zinc might act as a useful antidepressant. In our study, we included evaluations of the affective or mood state of our patients, and we were able to monitor this during treatment for some patients for over five years. One of the first things that improved was the degree of depression that they were experiencing. This suggested to us that we might consider using zinc as an antidepressant, because there's growing concern among many patients and even therapists that using antidepressive drugs, such as Prozac, might not be safe in some patients, and we have been looking at viable alternatives. The fact that we discovered this antidepressive effect and could document it in patients under blind conditions, is probably of even greater value to the field of mental health than simply its use in the treatment of patients with eating disorders.

Liquid zinc has been available in the United States since 1984, and there are several companies that sell it. It is a shocking thing to realize how for about $12 to $15 of treatment per day, people recover. When I first saw this work, I didn't think anybody would believe me, and I thought certainly my colleagues would throw me in the river for suggesting such a simple solution for such a complex problem. So we did it over and over and over again, we waited until colleagues and other centers confirmed our results, and it was only recently that my co-author Carolyn Costin and I finally decided to talk to some of our colleagues at international and national meetings of mental health specialists. It would have been easy 10 years ago to just jump out, get on the Oprah show and say hey, we've got it, but we thought we'd better be cautious. From a scientific standpoint, that's been good, but what really bothers me is I do get phone calls from parents who are angry as hell because then they lost their daughter and if information had been readily available to professionals and physicians and pediatricians, maybe their daughter would be alive today. I've had to deal with the anguish of the cost to human life that has been necessary to provide my colleagues enough convincing evidence that there is really something here.

But I have also had some experiences which have been nothing short of shocking. I might be invited to a hospital that has an eating disorder unit. I present the data to the staff, they are enthusiastic and usually they've tried it out on a few patients and seen the benefits, but then the business manager steps in and talks about how much money the hospital will lose if it engages in what is basically an outpatient treatment program. That happened at a local hospital here in Washington state and I got so mad that money was more important than health that I went to every support group for bulimic and anorexics I could find in the area and showed them how they could use this on their own. Within a year, that eating disorder unit closed down because it didn't have enough patients to sustain it. The trustee who had invited me to the hospital resigned his position. But it didn't really solve the problem, which is how do patients get this information?"

Dr. José Yaryura-Tobias reminds us of the life-threatening severity of a condition like anorexia nervosa, and of his view that any nutritional approach must be preceded by a program of cognitive therapy. "Anorexia nervosa, from our perspective, is an obsessive-compulsive disorder that is related to self-image, the way that we perceive ourselves. Basically, anorexia nervosa is the process by which a human being self-starves. Thirty percent of the population who self-starve eventually die.

"From the biochemical viewpoint, in the vast majority of cases when patients come for a consultation they are already very emaciated. The chemistry we can measure is very altered. We know that there is a groove that is related to an area of the brain called the limbic system. This is the hypothalamic area, which regulates sugar, thirst, appetite, and so forth. This information can help us classify some of these patients, but does not tell us how to manage and eventually cure the problem. The rest of the problem, we feel, has to do with body image perception, the way that these patients see their own bodies. They feel too fat, too slim. They have different perspectives than the rest of us.

"How do we treat this condition? Basically we use a nutritional approach after the patient has undertaken a behavioral program with cognitive therapy. Cognitive therapy is important because the idea is to educate the person about their problems and to discuss with them how many false beliefs they have about who they are, why they think this way, why their body looks the way it does for them, and so forth. So false-belief modification is an important part of treatment."

Psychologist Lynne Freedman approaches treating patients with eating disorders from a different point of view. "People with anorexia," she says, "unlike other people with panic disorders that involve constant reminders of one's mortality, have a real denial about their own mortality. They are highly destructive, depriving their bodies of nutrients and in a lot of denial about the ramifications of that. But there is a medical condition that most anorexics will have to face at some time—they become dehydrated from lack of food and fluids. In a state of dehydration, they experience heart palpitations and shortness of breath. Eventually, many anorexics develop heart problems. Some need pacemakers because their hearts have taken such beatings.

"So there's clearly a relationship between anorexia and anxiety. In fact, 38 percent of anorexics have reported a history of having anxiety. At some point, an anorexic may recognize that if she doesn't eat, she will die. But she has been avoiding food for so long—much as the agoraphobic has been avoiding leaving home—that she has developed an actual food phobia. She can sit there with a plate of food, knowing that she needs to eat and completely unable to eat, no longer in that place of intentionally withholding. She really wants to eat, and can't. This is one of the reasons doctors are using a lot of antidepressant medications on anorexia just as they would for someone with an anxiety disorder, hoping that they can somehow break that food phobia. Unfortunately it hasn't been very successful.

"Bulimia is a slightly different situation because it does involve the compulsion to eat as opposed to the avoidance of eating. Certainly the dehydration and the physical symptoms do eventually erupt in a bulimic, and so they can experience anxiety as well."

Laura Norman is a registered, certified reflexologist and a New York State licensed massage practitioner in private practice for 25 years. She offers specific ways eating disorders can be treated with reflexology, which she defines as "a science and an art that deals with the principle that there are reflex areas in your feet that correspond to all parts of the body. When we stimulate these areas, it helps to bring about homeostasis, balance in the body, without side affects. It deeply relaxes, which helps to reduce vascular constriction, so your blood and nerve supply can flow more freely. Improving circulation can help to eliminate toxins in the body and break up congestion or blockages resulting from the accumulation of excess mucus, uric acid, lactic acid, calcium deposits. It enhances the flow of blood, helps to relieve pain and discomfort, and activates the release of endorphins. It's a natural opiate, like substances normally produced in the brain that alter and regulate moods. Mainly, it helps to promote a sense of inner peace, tranquility and well being.

"There are more than 7,000 nerves in each foot. When we stimulate a reflex area, there is a response to this stimulus, that is why we called it reflexology. A well trained reflexologist can apply specific pressure to reflex areas using their fingers and thumbs. Anorexia and bulimia are mostly stress induced. the main thing the reflexology will do is help the person affected relax. For all eating disorders, anorexia, bulimia, or even people who are just plain overweight, we focus on the same organs and glands to help balance the eating disorder.

"The first and most common technique that we use, mainly on the bottom and sides of the foot is 'thumb walking.' using our thumb, we move in a forward motion inching along like a caterpillar on the entire sole and sides of the foot.

"Next, we do 'finger walking,' which is very similar, using the pointer finger bending the finger at the first joint and moving in a forward motion, on the top of the foot because it is more bony

"The third technique is called rotation on a point; where we want to press a little deeper we place our thumb into the point, using our other hand to grip the foot And rotate. For even deeper, harder to reach points we hook in, press our thumb into that point.

"For eating disorders, the points are these:
➤the pituitary gland (to coordinate activity of all the other glands and to stimulate and regulate the hormonal secretions);
➤the brain (to enhance circulation of blood to the brain and to promote normal brain wave activity);
➤the solar plexus (to orchestrate and increase circulation to the abdominal organs and help relax the person overall);
➤the spine (to soothe the nerves and enhance transmission of impulses to all the parts of the body)
➤the thyroid (to regulate metabolism and to modify activity of the nervous system);
➤the parathyroid (to promote metabolism of calcium And phosphorus, enhance nerve transmission, and for muscle tone);
➤the adrenal gland (to release hormones to regulate metabolism, rejuvenate hyperactivity in response to stress, and to stimulate energy);
➤the kidneys (to maintain water balance, balance blood pressure and filter toxins and waste from the blood);
➤the stomach area (to help soothe the muscles and nerves and increase blood circulation into the stomach);
➤the pancreas (to control balance of blood sugar and aid in digestion of food and nutrient extraction);

➤the liver (to filter toxins from the blood and regulate nutrient absorption);

➤the gallbladder (to release bile to encourage peristalsis and promote absorption of fat and soluble vitamins.

➤the intestines again (to promote peristalsis and increase blood circulation and nutrient absorption, and to stimulate elimination of solid wastes)

"For bulimia, I would also work on the mouth, teeth, gums and the esophagus."

Norman explains how to find the points in the feet corresponding to these organs:

➤For the pituitary gland—in the center of the big toe and deep in the center of each foot.

➤The brain reflexes are on all the tips of the big toes. Work the smaller toes also for fine tuning.

➤The thyroid is found in the base of the big toe.

➤For the mouth, gums and teeth, support the fingers of your right hand behind the fingers of your left hand on the back of the toes and press in the base of the toenails.

➤The reflexes to the esophagus are located mainly on the bottom of the left foot, underneath the big toe. Use the thumb walk in that area.

A lot of these overlap because we are now working on the digestive system, which will overlap for the digestive conditions, so people can remember this for those conditions as well.

➤The pancreas area is under the ball of the foot on the left foot. Just press your thumbs across that area.

➤The liver reflex is on the right foot, and since the liver is the largest organ in the body, the reflex covers the whole section under the ball of the foot down to the middle of the foot.

➤The gallbladder point is embedded in the liver reflex, under the ball of the foot and the middle of the foot, underneath the third and fourth toes. Hook in back up under the fourth toe just a little above the middle of the foot.

The kidneys are a very easy point to locate, right in the center of the foot, underneath your second and third toe, just in the middle of the foot.

Those are the main points to work for eating disorders, which do overlap with the digestive organs, it is mainly working digestive organs and glands to help those other conditions.

5

$\mathscr{D}$EPRESSION
(Unipolar Disorder)

Personal Story: Catherine Carrigan

I can't remember when I first felt depressed—it was always with me. I began seeing psychiatrists at the age of 16, and began taking various medications at age 18. I was hospitalized at the age of 20. At the time, the inference was that I should be very ashamed of myself. I was on lithium and antidepressants for 18 years and I developed chronic fatigue as a result of the side effects of all the medications. The whole time I was on drugs, I was suicidal every other month. When I first got off my drugs, I had to spend a lot of time taking care of myself. After being told all my life that the best I could do was to take drugs, talk about my childhood forever and shut up to the rest of the world about it, I want to offer hope that it is possible to overcome depression.

Depression is a great leveler. It affects one in four Americans and doesn't differentiate between rich and poor, although it does appear to afflict women more than it does men. It is a serious disease, often related to—some even think it is the cause of—other illnesses like heart disease, arthritis, allergies and cancer. To Dr. Sherry Rogers, among others, depression accompanies most diseases—especially those that affect vessels in the brain (arteriosclerosis) or the auto-immune system (lupus) or many hormonal diseases, "because most diseases are not limited to affecting one organ, but have effects throughout the body, including the brain."

On the other hand, I have seen many people who have been diagnosed with depression, medicated, even institutionalized, and when I check them I find physical conditions that can be helped. Recent estimates are that half the people diagnosed as suffering from depression can obtain relief simply by having an underlying physical disease identified and treated. I have found under active thyroid, low blood sugar, cerebral allergy, a nutritionally induced or environmentally induced allergy, a nutrient deficiency or simply a life issue that could have been dealt with in a non toxic way. By changing those things, people who were incapacitated emotionally found completely normal and healthy lives. There are many practitioners within the orthomolecular movement who see things this way, yet most people continue to go right off the psychiatrist or psychologist and get into standard therapeutic models. I have a great deal of concern, as I have said at some length elsewhere, because Prozac is a very dangerous drug.

Catherine Carrigan, whose self-healing from crippling depression and the books she has written about it have inspired many other people, believes the disease has mental, physical and spiritual causes and solutions. She recommends checking for physical health problems first. "Studies show that if you go to a psychiatrist alone, the chances of medical, non-mental factors being discovered are less than one in ten." Physical health problems that may be contributing to depression include: candida or yeast infection, hypoglycemia, thyroid problems or other endocrine disorders, environmental allergies, food sensitivities, amino acid deficiencies, electrolyte imbalances, vitamin or mineral deficiencies, toxic exposure to heavy metals or chemicals, cardiopulmonary obstructive disease, brain tumors, Alzheimer's, stroke, seizure, hypertension, viral infections, diabetes, insulin resistance or difficulty metabolizing carbohydrates, any chronic illness.

There are different degrees of depression, and its treatment has varied considerably according to trends in psychiatry, psychology, and psychopharmacology in recent decades, and depending on the severity of the condition. Some of us call it "depression" when we are struck by feelings of mild sadness, of the kind that affect nearly everyone from time to time, often for no obvious reason we can put our fingers on. Certain times of the year are associated with mood lows, particularly at the beginning and end of winter, for example. Commonly, when someone close to us moves away or dies, or if we lose a job or have some other major disappointment, there's apt to be an even stronger mood reaction in almost everybody. There will be some sadness, perhaps some grief. Usually such periods of sadness or grief are of a limited duration. When they drag on for a longer period of time, or become much more profound, we may begin to speak of clinical depression.

The causes of depression may include genetic factors. As Dr. William Goldwag explains, "These may be related to changes in the brain metabolism and the nervous system. We know about genetic factors through the action of certain drugs. We see what chemical changes take place. Obviously our individual chemistry is to a great extent determined by our genes. There are genes presently under investigation that are believed to be responsible for manic-depression-type illnesses, in which one fluctuates from hyperactivity to depression or limited activity. Every day another gene is being found that is responsible for some of these illnesses. The gene expresses itself through a change in chemistry."

It's common for depressed people to have a family history of depression. In addition to the genetic factor, such family histories may also be due to common environmental factors, shared experiences in depressed families, and poor eating habits that are passed on from one generation to another.

Environmental factors may play multiple roles among the causes of depression. For example, being raised in a family in which one or more people are depressed may often be associated with poor nutrition. As Dr. William Goldwag reminds us, "Just being exposed to depressed people can be an influence, since children learn how to behave by imitation. Also, family members are eating the same food, and if, for instance, the mother is depressed and cooking and serving her family, that food is apt to be sparse in nutrients since she is interested in just getting the meal over with and has difficulty finding enough energy to prepare it."

Being abused physically or verbally can be another factor that inhibits children of depressed parents. As a way of handling abuse the child may withdraw and become depressed and inactive as a defense against very harsh treatment from the parent.

As Dr. Doris Rapp describes it, mood disorders often lead to battering of family members and intimates: "Husbands batter wives, wives batter husbands, they both batter the children, and boyfriends batter their girlfriends. Mother battering, I might add, is very common. Many of the children I treat beat, kick, bruise, bite, and pinch their mothers. When some individuals have typical allergies and environmental illness, if they have a mood problem, they can become nasty and irritable and angry. All I ask is, 'What did you eat, touch, and smell?' To help find the cause I try to discover whether the change in behavior occurs inside or outside, after eating, or after smelling a chemical. It might be a food, dust, mold, pollens, or chemicals, which not only affect the brain, but discrete areas of the brain. As a result, the allergen or food or chemical exposure might make you tired or, if it affects the frontal lobes, it might make you behave in an inappropriate way. It could affect the speech center of the brain so that you speak too rapidly, or unclearly, or stutter, or don't speak intelligently. It's just potluck as to what area of the brain or body will be affected when you are exposed to something to which you are allergic."

Dr. Goldwag names specific characteristic signs of severe depression: reduction in appetite, reduction in sleep ability, fatigue, lack of energy, agitation or retardation in motor activity, loss of interest in usual activities, loss of interest in sex, feelings of worthlessness or guilt, slowed thinking, inability to concentrate to a severe degree, and recurring thoughts of suicide, or suicide attempts."

Everyone from time to time has one or more of these symptoms. "Generally these should be present for at least two weeks and represent a change from a previous state. But when approximately four or five of these are present for a long period of time, and when this represents a departure from a person's usual personality, the possibility of depression should be considered."

In the not-so-distant past, before drug therapy became popular, severe depression was treated through hospitalization, electroshock therapy, and even insulin shock therapy. Dr. Goldwag describes the reasoning behind such extreme measures: "The idea was that somehow or other when you shock the brain it shakes things up. A lot of the disturbed thought processes seemed to almost get blanked out, and you could sort of start all over again with an individual.

"Psychotherapy, of course, has always been popular," adds Dr. Goldwag. "That can range from just the presence of a close, supportive friend or relative to more in-depth treatment with a psychiatrist or psychologist."

Perhaps most importantly, when depression is relatively mild, there is much the individual can do on his or her own. According to Dr. Goldwag: "There are many, many things that individuals can do to help themselves. What we want to ask is, what can we do nutritionally and in other ways? What lifestyle factors are under our own control that we can manipulate in order to alleviate symptoms of depression or prevent them?"

Three of the most important areas where answers to that question can be found by the individual himself or herself are exercise, interaction with others, and nutrition.

Catherine Carrigan says it is important to "do what you can to lower your stress level because when you get stressed out, your cortisol level goes up. Cortisol is a hormone secreted by the adrenal gland. When your cortisol level is high, you get depressed. Stress equals high cortisol, high cortisol equals depression. Cortisol balances in the body with insulin, so to recover from depression, you need to lower your stress level and balance your blood sugar.

"If you tend to be a negative thinker, studies prove that even antidepressants won't help you. Five minutes of pure anger raises your cortisol level for up to six hours. On the other hand, five minutes caring about other people, such as praying, raises your immune system for up to six hours. If you are depressed you need to understand that there is a direct chemical connection between how you choose to think and your body chemistry and how you end up feeling.

"You might need to detoxify your body. There are forty chemicals proven to depress the nervous system. De-toxing could include taking special supplements to remove heavy metals, improve your digestion, clear your liver, etc. Detoxification has been proven to be a short cut to recovery for numerous mental and physical diseases.

"Don't overlook the spiritual connection. What have you learned? Ask yourself what depression has to teach you. For myself, depression was all about learning faith because anyone can have a lot of faith when the sun is shining and everything is going great but it takes a special kind of person who can have faith when they feel terrible."

Dr. Goldwag also emphasizes interaction with others as an important step the depressed individual may attempt on his or her own: "The next step may involve doing some volunteer work, getting out and doing things for other people. This is very important in trying to get the depressed person's mind off himself or herself. Depressed people are continually negative. They have dark thoughts, guilt, sad feelings, grief, regrets. Such negative thoughts are characteristic of depression. You can't talk the depressed individual out of them or try to convince them otherwise, but you can distract them. Physical activity is one distraction. Doing things for other people is another. So getting the person involved in someone else's problems can be a very effective way of dealing with depressed individuals."

Then comes nutrition. It is surprising how often diet and nutrition are factors in depression, and how effective enhanced or improved nutrition can be in helping someone suffering from depression to improve their mood. As Dr. Goldwag says, "Nutrition is important in preventing depression and treating it. Often the quality of the diet suffers in depressed people. If the depression is profound, the individual doesn't even feel like eating. Depressed people who live alone or who are major providers or cooks in the house may not feel like preparing meals or even shopping. They're apt to restrict their nutrition to fast food or just anything to get eating over with." In many cases, weight loss is a symptom of severe depression. In many other cases, there is substantial weight gain.

As Dr. Goldwag notes, significant weight loss is likely to bring about "marked deprivation of the essential nutrients, including the amino acids needed to manufacture the proper proteins, as well as a deficiency in many vitamins and minerals. That in itself can then aggravate the depression."

Dr. Goldwag suggests straightforward solutions to at least some of the challenges associated with depression: "There are some simple ways to prepare food in advance so that the food has to be prepared less often. I recommend preparing a raw salad once a week. Certain fresh vegetables can be stored for quite a period in a refrigerator and will keep quite well. There are a whole variety to choose from: carrots, celery, radishes, cauliflower, broccoli, peppers, red cabbage, green onions, snow peas, string beans. These can all be cut up and mixed together. They can be stored in a plastic bag or sealed container. When mealtime comes, a person can take a handful of these vegetables and then perhaps add some other ones that don't keep as well, such as tomatoes or sprouts. You then have a fresh salad that is already prepared with a lot of important nutrients. This is just one way of having food prepared in advance. It's good for people who are depressed and don't have the energy to make a whole meal."

Dr. Goldwag believes that the B complex vitamins are especially important. "One of the major groups of vitamins to incorporate are from the B complex family. Years and years ago, when people suffered from severe vitamin deficiencies, some of the resultant diseases like pellagra and so forth were characterized by accompanying psychotic reactions. That is, the thinking process was the most obvious one to be affected by the vitamin deficiency. Simply providing the proper vitamin, in this case vitamin B3 or niacin, was the treatment. It cleared up the psychosis.

"There's no doubt that brain function is very dependent upon nutrients like niacin and others, because when they're absent there is apt to be some very disturbed thinking. Depression is one of the symptoms that can occur with this.

"It is important to get all the B complex vitamins, since they work together. Thiamine, B1, is important, as is riboflavin to a lesser extent. Another important one is B6, pyridoxine. B12 is still another one that can affect the mental processes.

"Niacin is often used in much higher doses than the others in order to accomplish some of these changes. Niacin is a ubiquitous vitamin. It is being used greatly to help reduce cholesterol levels, to improve the good cholesterol and reduce the bad. The dosages being used are much greater than those used to simply overcome a deficiency."

The importance of the B vitamins is underscored by researcher Sid Baumel, who says that "the most often studied vitamin connection to depression has been the B vitamins, which are the most closely associated with the normal maintenance of mood and the brain." If you have a really significant B vitamin deficiency, the kind that gives you bleeding gums and obvious skin problems, depression is one of the other symptoms you'd be likely to have. People who are clinically depressed don't routinely get their blood levels of B vitamins measured, but it has been proven that the more depressed a person is, the lower the level of one particular B vitamin, called folic acid, is. There have been a number of studies looking into blood levels of folic acid and the prevention of relapse in people who have recovered from a depression. These studies found that people with high levels of folic acid—whether because of their diets or because they are taking supplement—were less likely to suffer a relapse. People low in folic acid have been given supplements of folic acid and reported a very good clinical response. More recently, there have been studies of a natural derivative of folic acid called methyl folate, showing it to be an antidepressant comparable in effect to the antidepressant drug it was being compared to. And this supports the claim that nutritionally oriented doctors including ortho molecular psychiatrists have been making for many years now that folic acid prescribed in megadoses appears to be a stimulating antidepressant for some of their patients. Folic acid is one of the better researched examples of nutritional deficiencies with a strong connection to depression.

The amino acid tryptophan can be another key substance in the treatment of depression. Tryptophan is a precursor to serotonin and Prozac and other drugs like it, drugs that amplify the activity of serotonin in the brain. Tryptophan, the substance from which the brain manufacturers its own serotonin, does the same kind of thing when it is taken as a supplement. In controlled studies beginning in the 1950s, it was found consistently to be as effective as the antidepressant drugs that were available. It never has been compared directly to Prozac, but Prozac has not been proven significantly more effective than any of the other antidepressant drugs. Five hydroxy tryptophan is another natural compound which is a little bit closer to serotonin. It's an orphan drug and it's available by special request to doctors and it seems to be even more effective than tryptophan.

According to Dr. Goldwag, tryptophan helps to raise the levels of a naturally occurring chemical in the brain called serotonin, which have been found to be abnormally low in depressed people. "We learned about serotonin from experiments in which certain drugs that preserve it from being destroyed in the brain seem to work as antidepressants. The theory is that whatever can supply or aid the serotonin factor will help depression. Some foods that contain tryptophan can act as antidepressants. It is found most abundantly in milk and turkey. Tryptophan used to be obtainable until the FDA took it off the market several years ago because there were some serious blood problems in people who took it. This was later tracked down to a contaminant; the problem was not due to the tryptophan itself. Unfortunately the FDA has been rather lax in not allowing it back on the market again. Increasing the intake of milk and turkey are at least two ways of getting tryptophan."

At the same time, there are plenty of foods that should be avoided. Fast foods can affect mental symptoms by causing blood sugar abnormalities. People who tend to hypoglycemia or low blood sugar patterns should avoid eating too many simple carbohydrates, such as candy bars, which are converted very rapidly to sugar in the blood. As Dr. Goldwag says, "Simple carbohydrate foods temporarily raise the blood sugar, but then they drop it to a very low level several hours later, resulting in depression. This encourages the individual to repeat the cycle of taking sugar or some simple carbohydrate that's converted to sugar in order to feel that high again. This constant seesaw from high to low mood can account for many episodes of depression in individuals."

Dr. Jonathan Zeuss has no doubt that depression is "to a very large degree a nutritionally-caused disease. If you only know one thing about nutrition and depression, it should be about the omega three fatty acids. They are absolutely crucial. There is a huge amount of evidence now in the 1990s linking omega three deficiency and depression. Around a quarter of the dry weight of our brains is made up of omega threes and if you are deficient in them, the cells in your brain malfunction and you are much more likely to become depressed.

"They are essential fatty acids. Your body can't make them itself, so it's essential that you get them in your diet. Omega threes are found in fish and green leafy plants like spinach and in supplements you can buy like flax oil and fish oil. You can't get them any other way. Most Americans do not eat enough fish and greens. If you look at other countries, you can predict the prevalence of depression in the population just by knowing the average annual fish consumption. In Germany, the average person eats just 20 pounds of fish per year and they have a very high rate of depression there. In Japan, fish is a staple of the diet, the average person eats about 150 pounds of it per year and they have an incredibly low rate of depression. The U.S. is about in the middle between those two extremes.

"There are several clinical studies going on right now using omega threes in the form of fish oil to treat depression. We already know that fish oil is quite effective for treating manic depression or bipolar disorder and schizophrenia. Fish oil capsules have two different types of omega threes in them called EPA and DHA. It usually comes in 1000 milligram capsules and you need to take quite a lot of it. I recommend a total of about 10 grams per day of EPA and DHA divided into two doses. That usually works out to about 20 capsules per day. So you should also increase the amount of fish and greens in your diet. If you have a bleeding disorder or if you are on aspirin or Coumadin or other drugs affecting your clotting, you should really only take fish oil under the close monitoring of a physician because fish oils do thin the blood. It takes several weeks to alter the fatty acid composition of the cell membranes in your brain, but some people feel the depression lift before that. Take vitamin E along with the fish oils to protect yourself from any peroxidized oils in the capsules."

"People with mood disorders tend to have very sensitive body chemistry," according to Catherine Carrigan. She recommends investigating amino acid imbalance. "In the past three years, researchers have discovered that the bodies of people with mood disorders have difficulty producing a specific amino acid called GABA, gamma amino butyric acid. In fact, this is the closest thing scientists have ever come to a blood test for predisposition to mood disorders. GABA is supposed to synthesize in the body from other amino acids. Even four years after they are no longer depressed, people with mood disorders still have trouble making GABA. GABA helps you to relax."

Both alcoholics and chronic dieters often have depressive tendencies. Alcoholics often suffer from symptoms of low mood, and although alcohol may appear at first as a stimulant and mood enhancer, it is in fact a depressant and substantially decreases the ability of the body to extract nutrients from the food we eat. Dieters tend to eat very few B-complex-containing foods, and they often suffer from depression as well.

As Dr. Goldwag reminds us, "The first drugs ever used for treating depression were amphetamines. In their time, before they got such a bad reputation, they were considered helpful. In the old days—20, 30, or 40 years ago—amphetamines were used for weight control. They did diminish the appetite, and they also made a person feel good, alert, and more energetic. People who went on diets and took amphetamines felt great.

"Of course, the problem came when you stopped the amphetamines. People would go into a depression. For that reason amphetamines were recognized to be very habit-forming. In order to feel good a person had to keep on taking them. For many people that still seemed okay, at least for a while. For a fair percentage though, the dose became inadequate as the person started feeling like he or she needed more and more of the drug. This created all kinds of problems with the body's chemistry.

"There are still some medications on the market that act a little bit like the amphetamines, although they are not anywhere near as powerful. These are mild sympathetic nervous system stimulants that are sold over the counter, such as those people use to keep awake when they have to drive. In some instances I'm sure there are people who take them as a way of counteracting depression.

"The next group of drugs to come along were the tricyclic antidepressants. They're called tricyclic because of their chemical structure, which is a triple cycle. There are a whole bunch of them now on the market. The newer group are those that inhibit the enzymes that break down serotonin. They are designed to try to raise the serotonin level in the brain. In that way they counteract depression.

"They are all to varying degrees effective, but they all have side effects. Some of the side effects are severe; some are mild. They usually take days or weeks before they are effective, and in this way they are different than the amphetamines used to be, because those would work in a matter of minutes or hours. Of course, in the long run the present-day antidepressants may be more effective.

"As far as nutritional protocols, the ones I know of that are of practical use are the ones that use high doses of B complex, specifically niacin. Those have been used for some time now. You have to be a little bit careful of niacin because over long periods of time, in high doses, there can be some effects on the liver. The doses of niacin that have been used, mostly by Dr. Hoffer, have been in the ranges of 1 to 3 grams a day. That's thousands of milligrams a day, whereas the requirements for avoiding a deficiency are measured in just 10 or 20 mg."

Dr. Robert Atkins distinguishes between two types of depression, each with its respective type of therapeutic approach. "Clinically, you can divide depressions into two different categories: the apathetic depression where you just can't get interested in or enjoy anything, and the agitated or anxious depression, where basically you are depressed and nervous. The latter is responsive to increasing serotonin levels and is best treated with tryptophan. Tryptophan is extremely valuable in cases of agitated depression. Apathetic depression is best treated with tyrosine or what we now call acetyltyrosine, and a product called Noraval."

Dr. Doris Rapp, like many other doctors we interviewed, discerned environmental and nutritional causes of depression. "There is no doubt that certain people become sad when they eat certain foods. One youngster became depressed and nearly suicidal when she was on fluoride tablets. Then she was put on imipramine and she could barely walk. All we did was make an allergy extract of the fluoride and we could change her drawings from happy faces to tear-stained faces and she would start to cry. For two years, the fluoride had been causing her trouble, but none of her doctors would believe that a fluoride tablet could cause this problem. Now fluoride isn't necessarily bad for everybody, but it is certainly not a good preparation for certain individuals.

"I see patients who don't have asthma and hay fever during the pollen season, but they become suicidal and depressed every year at the same time when a certain tree pollinates, when the grass pollinates, on moldy days, and when the ragweed pollinates. So if you can see a pattern to your depression, it is worth trying to figure out what might be the reason for that pattern."

Dr. Richard Kunin believes that "most of the problems that we would identify as fatigue and depression up to the moderate level—depression that makes life an effort but not impossible—are environmental problems based on nutrition, environmental pollution, toxins in the environment, sensitization due to chemicals that stick to our cell membranes and alter them and make them allergy causing. These are the things that cause people to feel miserable, and to feel miserable for long enough so that when you add to it the slings and arrows part of life, it's not hard to understand this thing called depression. Psychotic depression is different; it's a distinct minority of cases."

Dr. Lendon Smith agrees. "A poor immune system as the result of bad diet and pesticides on top of some genetic deficiency are leading to a lot of sickness now. A balanced chemistry will lead to a reasonably normal life. We are just bags of chemicals. People who have allergies are usually too alkaline and they need some vinegar, ammonium chloride or some acidifier and that will balance their chemistry, so their allergies are under control. We can balance their chemistry to handle the ordinary pesticides. Why doesn't everybody who is exposed to pesticides get sick? Well, maybe they don't have enough of some nutrients, but there are other ways to improve this and we know that naturopathic methods work. We've got to get people to be more aware of the alternate methods of care."

Dr. Michael Schachter reports that "Sometimes depression is caused by a deficiency of the neurotransmitter for norepinephrine. In such a case the amino acid L-tyrosine, or the amino acid DL-phenylalanine may be helpful. DL-phenylalanine consists of two forms of phenylalanine, namely D-phenylalanine and L-phenylalanine. L-phenylalanine is used by the body to make proteins. D-phenylalanine is a precursor of the brain substance D-phenylethylamine, which is frequently deficient in people who are suffering from depression. I also recommend the mineral magnesium, and vitamin B1 (thiamine) for depression. But the course of treatment really has to be individualized."

Dr. Lendon Smith addresses some of the more baffling aspects of depression in today's society. "The more we hear about the rising tide of suicides in adolescents and even in children as young as eight, nine, and ten, it seems astounding that such a thing should overwhelm substantial numbers of children in what is supposed to be the happiest time of life. I evaluate children and adults who are depressed. For some of them there is no apparent reason for their overwhelming sadness. They've got good relationships with other people. Their social organization is intact. They've had a good upbringing. They have a good self-image. They have good school or work performance and they're getting nice accolades from relatives and friends. Why are they depressed? It just doesn't seem right.

"When we do blood tests on these people we find, in general, that there are two things wrong. One is that they're nutrient deficient. In the particular program I'm doing, we go by the deviation from the mean. If, for instance, calcium's range is 8.5 to 10.5, then 9.5 is the mean. If they're down to 9 or 8.6, the doctor will say, 'Everything is okay.' Still, if there are enough of those scores below the mean, these people don't have enough wherewithal, enough nutrients, to satisfy all their enzyme requirements.

"Fifteen years ago, for example, a 20-year-old woman came to see me who was depressed for no apparent reason. She came from a good family, and had a nice boyfriend and a good job. Everything seemed fine but she would still get depressed every once in a while. At that time I was experimenting with vitamins. I thought it would be quite safe to give her a shot of the mixed B complex vitamins. I included a cc of everything from B1 to folic acid and B12. I would give about 50 mg of each one of these vitamins and 50 mcg of the B12 intramuscularly every day. "After two or three of these shots this patient told me that the treatment wasn't working very well for her. She asked, 'Couldn't you give them as separate vitamins?' I started giving her injections of isolated vitamins. I gave her a shot of 100 mg of B1 on Monday and B2 on Tuesday. I gave her separate shots of B3, B6, B12, and folic acid.

"She reported feeling terrible after receiving B1, thiamine. She asked me never to do that again. I thought that seemed odd. After the B2 she came back and said that it was okay but nothing special. She said the same thing after receiving the B3. But after B6 she came back and said, 'I think you're onto something.' She also really liked the B12 and the folic acid.

"These three vitamins were the important ones for her. I mixed them up and gave them to her every week or two. With that combination, she was apparently satisfied.

"About five or six years ago, I started a new program where we have people smell vitamins to see what they need. If it's a good smell or no smell, they need it. If it's a bad smell, they don't.

"I had her open up thiamine and smell it. She said, 'Good lord. Somebody must have done something awful to this.' I explained to her that nothing was wrong with the vitamin but that she didn't need it. She had some bacteria in her intestinal tract that helped her make her own thiamine. Her body was therefore rejecting it. B3 had no smell; she needed that. B6 had a good smell; she needed that. B12 and folic acid had no smell so she needed that. Her body told her what she needed, and she could satisfy its requirements. Apparently this method of using the sense of smell and taste is highly accurate in determining people's needs. It should be used rather than just taking multivitamins willy-nilly.

"Craving chocolate is also a sign of depression. It usually means that people need magnesium, because there's magnesium in chocolate. Women, the day before their menstrual period, often find themselves searching through the cupboards for chocolate. They find a big canister of Hershey's and drink it down before feeling better from the magnesium. I often had the delightful experience of giving an intravenous mixture of vitamin C, calcium, magnesium, and B vitamins. Usually it has more magnesium than calcium. Afterwards I asked patients whether they would like some chocolate and they told me they didn't need it. It really is connected.

"Women in the sixth month of pregnancy will often send their husbands out for ice cream because the baby is starting to grow fast. The woman has a conscious need for dairy products because she knows they will bring her the calcium she needs, but she also says, 'Don't forget the pickles.' She knows, somehow, that she needs to acidify that calcium source for the baby. She will not get much out of it and she will suffer from leg cramps.

"The chemist I work with in Spokane discovered something about GGT, a liver and gallbladder enzyme called gamma glutamil transpeptidase. The mean level would be about 20. Someone with a level below

20 is more likely to have magnesium deficiency symptoms—short attention span, trouble relaxing or sleeping, little muscle cramps in the feet and legs, and a craving for chocolate. Most of these people don't like to be touched. They may be a little crabby. Those symptoms go with low magnesium.

"Magnesium is one of the first minerals to disappear from food when it's been processed. Magnesium is also one of the first minerals to leave the body when there is stress, which accounts for how many women behave a day or so before their periods. They feel stressed because they're losing their magnesium.

"We need to supply magnesium to these people. We can determine who needs it by the blood test and by the sense of smell. If people smell a bottle of pure magnesium salt—magnesium chloride is a good one—if it smells good or if there's no smell, then the person needs it. The blood test we usually use is the 24 chem. screen, the standard blood test.

"Many symptoms of depression, hyperactivity, headaches, loss of weight, and other conditions are related to genetic tendencies. If there is a tendency to be depressed in the family, a magnesium deficiency will allow that tendency to show up. If there's alcoholism, diabetes, obesity in the family, then low magnesium may allow those things to show up in a person. There are reasons to explain all these things and nutrition is basic to this. The patients don't have an antidepressant pill deficiency; they usually have a magnesium deficiency."

Dr. Sherry Rogers is even more emphatic. "In 27 years of medical practice, the one nutrient I have been very impressed with is magnesium. In treating people with panic disorders, anxiety, insomnia, fatigue and depression, just by merely correcting their magnesium—something so simple, so inexpensive, so relatively harmless—has made a dramatic difference."

The first thing Dr. Smith does is ask people what they're eating. "If I find that they're eating a lot of dairy products, and that as a child they had their tonsils taken out, and that they had a lot of strep throat and ear infections, then I know they're allergic to milk and they're looking for calcium. Sure enough, the blood tests will show this. That's the first thing they have to stop. Whatever they love is probably causing the trouble because food sensitivities can cause low blood sugar."

Summing up, Dr. Smith cites low blood sugar and magnesium deficiency as two key hidden causes of depression. "As we know—those of us who have worked with nutrition at all—low blood sugar, not just eating sugar, can do that, but also eating foods to which a person is sensitive, will make the blood sugar fall and that can lead to depression. So lack of magnesium and falling blood sugar, for whatever reason, are the two most significant things responsible for a susceptibility to depression."

Recent years have seen remarkable breakthroughs in the use of natural substances to fight depression. For Dr. Rogers, "phosphatidyl choline in its pure form has made a dramatic difference for many people with severe depression. It should, because the cell membranes are where the "happy hormones" or the neurotransmitters have to hook into the cell. In order for them to insert into these cell membranes, the receptors have to be healthy. Healthy receptors in the membrane are made out of the constituents that make up cell membrane. Phosphatidyl choline is one of those. People just don't get enough of it any more because they don't eat beans, which are rich in phosphatidyl choline. It is considered a peasant food because you have to soak them and cook them a long time and people are into fast foods. They don't eat eggs because they are trying to lower their cholesterol—but you do need cholesterol for the brain. In fact, one of the reasons many people on certain cholesterol lowering drugs have high suicide rates is because they got depressed when their cholesterol got too low. They didn't have enough cholesterol in the hormone receptors in the brain and died by suicide."

Syd Baumel reports that norepinephrine, a brain chemical called PEA, tyrosine and L-phenylalanine and DL-phenylalanine all have a body of evidence of controlled studies supporting their effectiveness as antidepressants.

The most popular natural treatments for depression in the new century are St. John's Wort and SAM-e. Dr. Jonathan Zeuss calls St. John's Wort his "first choice for antidepressant treatment for most people," although he is emphatically against using even natural supplements as "magic bullets" for a disease as complex as depression. "Rather than just recommending a different kind of pill for them to take," his holistic approach includes treatment for "the levels of thought and the spiritual level, which might encompass psychotherapy, spiritual practices like prayer and meditation, and lifestyle interventions like light therapy and exercise.

"St. John's Wort "works as well as conventional antidepressants like Prozac, but it has only a fraction of the side effects and it's dirt cheap. The raw material of St. John's Wort is very inexpensive. It's basically a weed that grows everywhere. Manufacturers are less likely to try to thin it out by using fillers. It is pretty unique among antidepressants because it appears to work in many different ways at once. It works on reuptake of serotonin, norepinephrine and dopamine and also through a few other types of receptors. It also has immune-enhancing effects, which probably add to the overall antidepressant effect. The side effects are minimal. Don't mix St. John's Wort with any other kind of antidepressant medication, except fish oils, which should be safe.

"St. John's Wort comes in a number of different forms, mostly tablets and liquid extracts. The liquid is the least processed form. There are probably more than a dozen active ingredients in St. John's Wort and they all contribute to its effect. Sustained released tablets have recently come out, naturally, they're more expensive, but it's really just a marketing gimmick. There is no need for sustained released form because St. John's Wort has a long enough half-life in your body. Virtually everyone I've prescribed St. John's Wort for takes a non-sustained released form twice a day and there is no problem with that at all."

Letha Hadady, herbalist and certified acupuncturist, has a different approach. She uses certain Asian herbs because "when we take serotonin drugs, we lose our connection with our own body and our own healing powers. Simply breathing in the light and sending out love opens up all our possibilities for self healing. There are other sources of serotonin—sunshine, bananas, the ions from the seashore—but herbs also can give us the natural warmth and grounding and centering that we get from anti-depression herbs.

She starts by focusing on digestion "because when we have better metabolism and better digestion we have fewer toxins in the body that can interfere with our processing; our emotional center is also our digestive center. By clearing the problems of digestion, we can also digest our thoughts and our problems better. There is a very good Chinese remedy for this called Xiao Yao Wan. Several very important herbs that you can find easily are in that remedy to balance and strengthen our digestive center. This morning for breakfast, I had ginger, which is one of them. I had green tea, which I drink all day. Radish has anti congestion energy that clears our senses and helps us think better and I wanted to add a sour taste to balance the hot, pungent and bitter. Lately I have been eating a lot of star fruit, which is slightly sour, but other people might want to have lemon. So we have green tea, ginger, radish, and something sour, like lemon. This helps balance and strengthen the digestion.

"The link between digestion and depression is very clear. When our digestion is weak, we can't process our foods, but neither can we process our emotions and our sadness. We feel overcome; everything is too heavy for us to deal with and we give in to an addiction, like ice cream—milk and cheese and cream—which makes it all worse, which makes our digestion weaker and sets us up for major problems. Barley soup helps clear away the kind of congestion that makes us feel heavy. Sometimes feeling loaded down with problems is really water retention and excess phlegm. Barley soup helps. You might want to chop in some garlic and ginger and cardamom. Cardamom is very spicy and delicious and it speeds and strengthens the heart and strengthens the heart, but it is also sharp and piercing and cuts through phlegm. Another herb that is good for that too is hawthorn.

"Don't have it every day, because hawthorn every day might give you stomach burn. But when you need it, when you need to clarify your senses and you need to speed your digestion, a bit of cardamom, a bit of hawthorn is very, very good.

"Sometimes we get depressed because we don't have good circulation from our hearts. When our energy cannot nourish the brain, we have problems like speediness and heart palpitations. There are remedies in the Chinese medical tradition, such as cerebral tonic pills, which help ease the heart action so we don't wake up with panic attacks at night or become so maniac because we are depressed, we cannot sleep. Asian remedies do not sedate our brain in the hopes of trying to rid us of our problems. We don't put our brains to sleep, but we clarify our thinking and clarify our senses so that we can actually deal with our problems better.

"Some people just don't have the energy to get up out of their chair and do what they need to do. Or they have abused their energy with stimulants like coffee and cocaine so they don't have the energy for strong sexuality or for concentration. They need a tonic, something to pick their energy up. One that is used a lot is ginseng tonic pills. It's ginseng with other ingredients that help nourish the brain. A number of good stimulants use ginseng and fo-ti. Fo-ti nourishes the brain and the brain cells and the moisture in the body and ginseng balances and speeds our metabolism. So we need both, the hot and the cold, the yin and yang.

"People sometimes feel chilled and weak and have sexual weakness, which can lead to depression. They also have frequent urination. They feel weak from the waist down. This kind of depression happens after jet lag, after child birth, with chronic asthma or chronic diarrhea. There are a couple of wonderful things you can take for that. One is a Chinese remedy called sexoton, it comes in pills, you can take ten pills three times a day if you need it. Clove can have the same effect, giving you a deeper breath and more courage. When we breathe in deeply and our adrenal glands are strong, we have the fortitude and the vitality to go out there and do our work and get it done. Clove clears our congestion and strengthens the adrenal glands in our lungs so that we can take in that deep breath."

Depression and Tobacco

Dr. Abram Hoffer tells the story of a classic case of a misdiagnosis corrected, enabling one man to start anew after his previous life had already been ruined. "A high school teacher and principal of about 45 developed a severe depression. In fact, I believe he was misdiagnosed as a schizophrenic. He exhibited what we call a straightforward, deep-seated, endogenous depression. He was in a mental hospital for about a year or two, and then discharged. He was so depressed that no one could live with him. His wife divorced him and eventually he was living with his aunt, who looked after him as if he were a child. As a last resort, he was referred to me.

"When he came to see me, which was many years ago, I had just started looking into the question of allergies. At that time, I wasn't very familiar with food allergies, but I thought he was a very interesting case and I said to myself, 'He is a classic case of a depression, maybe schizophrenic. He'd be the last person in the world who would respond to this anti-allergy approach.' At that time I was using—and I still do—a four-day water fast. This is a way of determining whether or not these allergies are present. He agreed that he would do the fast, which also involved refraining from any smoking or consuming of alcohol; he had to drink about eight glasses of water a day and nothing else. His aunt said she would help make sure he complied. When he came back to see me two weeks later, he and his aunt explained that, at the end of the four-day fast, he was normal. All of the depression was gone.

"This same man then began to get tested for food allergies and he found that not a single food made him sick. But now he began to smoke again. Within a day after he resumed smoking, he was back in his deep depression. The ironic thing was that he had a brother who was a tobacco company executive, who kept sending him free cartons of cigarettes. Now when we made the connection to his cigarette smoking, he stopped smoking. Thirty days later, after he had been depressed for four years and hadn't been able to work, he was back in school teaching. And I remember this clearly because the insurance company that was then paying his monthly pension was so astounded at this dramatic response that they sent one of their agents to see me, to find out what the magic wand was that I had waved to get this patient off their rolls. This is a classic case of an allergy to tobacco that was causing this man's depression."

Effect of Exercise, Nutrition, and Lifestyle on Depression

Dr. William Goldwag insists on the importance of those changes which can be made by the patient himself or herself. "When we have patients who are depressed and we can get them moving, the depression is greatly alleviated. Of course, drugs have changed the whole treatment of depression greatly, but the impact exercise can have on depression has often been overlooked, and it needs to be re-emphasized. People who are on antidepressants may improve, but the way for them to really get back to functioning well—back in touch with their environment, back to work, back in relationships with their family—is to get them moving. And there's no better way to get people moving than through exercise, whose healing potential has no limits."

Exercise is one of the most profound aids in the treatment of depression, according to Dr. Goldwag: "One of the major errors in the thinking of patients and therapists is the notion that in order to be active you have to feel better. This is exactly contrary to what we are recommending.

"We recommend that you do first, and then the feeling comes later. In other words, you must do what you have to do regardless of how you feel. This aids in feeling better. You can't wait until you feel good and then do something, because in depression that may take days, weeks, months, or even years. You want to accelerate the process.

"Those of us who exercise regularly have had days when we just didn't feel like it. That's the way depressed people feel about everything. They just don't feel like it. They don't have the energy, the motivation, the stimulation to go and do even the ordinary things. When it's severe, the person may not even have the will or desire to get out of bed in the morning.

"The exercise may consist of very, very simple things, like just getting out and walking, getting up and doing some simple movements, some mild calisthenics, any kind of physical movement that gets the body in action. For some people just getting out of bed and getting dressed is a big accomplishment. That may be the first step.

"It is important for depressed people to get up and get dressed. They should not walk around in the pajamas or nightgowns because this maintains that connection to the bed and the bed means inactivity. That's the thing you're trying to overcome. Exercise may take the form of walking, walking the dog perhaps, or going outside to do some simple gardening. These are all very important for overcoming that feeling of lassitude that is so characteristic of depression.

"Another benefit of exercise is a feeling of accomplishment. Even doing a little bit of exercise will make you feel more energized later on. Finishing an exercise routine, even one that's fatiguing, after a brief period of rest, will give you a feeling of revitalization, of energy, and a psychological feeling of accomplishment. It gives a feeling of, 'I've done it. It's completed.' For the depressed individual, the boost to self-esteem that this can give is important.

"The individual is the important thing to take into account when I recommend exercise. There is no one exercise that is good for everybody. Some people can just do a little bit; some can push themselves much further. Ask anybody who has gone from a relatively sedentary life to an exercise program and they will all report the same thing: more energy, more interest in what is going on, a clearer mind, and less stress. Being active, therefore, is an integral part of any kind of medical program, particularly for people who are having mental disturbances.

"I have many patients who have had very stressful medical histories or emotional histories. Today, as more and more people are revealing the difficulties they had as children—the abuse, both sexual and nonsexual—their history, and the stress it causes based on these early childhood experiences continues to have an impact on their lives. Even though their lives may be relatively serene now, psychically they are still dealing with a lot of these issues.

"At the same time, they have to be made to realize that nutrition plays an integral role in their feeling well. They have to supply their bodies with proper nutrients and eliminate excesses or chronic addictions to alcohol, drugs, or food (including sweets and sugar). Inevitably, I find that if someone gets away from an addiction to sugar, they function much better. The old term hypoglycemia is very appropriate for their condition, particularly for people with chronic depression, chronic fatigue syndrome, and chronic immune system dysfunction. These people find that when they modify their diets and get off sugars, their mental functioning improves considerably.

"This is the first step: switching to a healthy diet containing lots of vegetables, fruits, and whole grains, and minimizing the amount of meat in the diet. Now some people will feel better once they modify their diet, and they'll be able to move right into more activity. Some people need to start off with some kind of moderate exercise program and almost automatically they will start to look for a more nutritious diet. The two seem to go hand in hand. Nowadays, so many athletes are paying a lot more attention to what they eat, in addition to their workouts. Similarly, many people who are paying attention to their diets now find that exercise almost becomes an inevitable consequence of paying attention to promoting good health."

Dr. Judith Sachs agrees that exercise "triggers all of these brain stimulants that make us feel good, these natural opiates. This is another system we have in the brain that takes away pain and gives us pleasure. A lot of people who run say, 'well it feels so good when I stop,' but even people who are not crazy about that kind of exercise are finding that they feel better in their body. They feel efficient, like the body is not just this house that they happen to live in, but has actually become an integral part of their mind, their spirit, the whole way that they approach themselves and other people. That can really turn around a lack of self confidence, a lack of self esteem. When you've said 'all I could do was to walk down to the mailbox to get my mail' and suddenly you are able to run up five flights of stairs or run a mini-marathon—that can make you feel very effective as a person. I suggest to people who are feeling kind of low and blue that they set themselves some kind of exercise goal. Something that they enjoy doing, whether it is roller blading, dancing (maybe they enter a dance competition with a partner) or taking a class in something they have never done before, like boxing which has become popular and also alleviates some of those aggressive tendencies. It can make you feel effective and part of things, especially if you do a team sport that involves a group where people rely on you, you count. It's not whether you have made that home run but how you have helped other people to get to that home run. Exercise actually works the body, but it also revitalizes our sense of spirit and I think that is really important. It can also help to motivate us to stick with a good diet, a good helpful diet. I don't mean a weight loss diet.

"After paying attention to exercise and nutrition, you need to be aware of the stresses of your own lifestyle, your own patterns of behavior, how they are manifested, and how they may be altered by more healthy ways of thinking. For example, if you frequently get upset by dwelling on the past, then you need to try not to think so much about what took place in the past or what is going to happen in the future. Your emotional work is to learn how to focus on the present reality, what's going on now, by putting the body in a mode where it is accepting what's happening now, so you're ready for anything that may happen, instead of reliving crises over and over again."

6
MANIC DEPRESSION
(Bipolar Disorder)

D r. Garry Vickar describes bipolar disease as an illness that has a manic component and a depressed component. If we want to look at mood disorders as a distinct group, which he describes as useful, we're talking about "diseases of unknown etiology characterized by recurrences of disturbed mood."

"If the mood is one of either agitation or elevated mood," Dr. Vickar continues, "one calls that hypomanic or, at the most extreme, manic. Manic individuals are those whose moods are elevated, with, typically, accompanying disorders of energy, both physical and emotional.

"The opposite pole, which is where this term of polarity comes in, is that of depressed mood. Here, there's slowness of thinking, a low-ness of mood, a slowness of motor activity. Of course, there are people whose mood disorders consist of simply one pole, that is, they have recurrent depression.

"The primary problem associated with mood disorders is exactly what it says: There is a problem with mood. Along with that come other features: e.g., people who have depressed moods will also very often end up having slowdowns in body functions, such as disturbances in sleep and reduced appetite for food, sex, and pleasurable pursuits. Depressed people often find that food doesn't taste as good as it once did. They lose their ability to enjoy pleasurable activities, whether these are sports, hobbies, or sexual activity.

"With depression there's an overwhelmingly painful, heavy, loss of one's sense of having the ability to function in the world, a sense of one's uselessness. The danger, of course, is that people may become so overwhelmed by their own subjective experience of loss and uselessness that they think their lives are not worth living or they come to believe that others think that their lives are not worth living. In the worst case, someone will lose perspective and think that the world is so terrible that their loved ones shouldn't live. Then you have the specter of the potential of homicidal/suicidal activities.

"There are illnesses that fall under the rubric of mood disorders that don't have a manic component. These are recurrent depressions. Generally, the incidence of mood disorders, especially depressive disorders, is substantially greater, that is, more common, than schizophrenic disorders. Recurrent depressions certainly occur frequently. Depression is a very serious illness and a very insidious one in which people lose their perspective on themselves and their views of where they fit into the world.

"At the opposite pole of the depression is what I consider a hypomanic state. Today it is uncommon to see people whose illness is so out of control that they become truly manic. More often you will see individuals who are manic-depressive becoming excessively elevated in their moods. They become more expansive. They might go on spending sprees and spend money they don't have, or get involved in activities that they truly are not qualified for. They may run up charge cards, or get involved in gambling, financial affairs, extramarital affairs, alcohol, or possibly drug abuse that they would not otherwise be doing. It becomes almost the reverse of the depression spectrum—they need less sleep, they need less food, and everything is very intense. It can become rather horrific because people can become exhausted. They're sleeping two or three hours a day, if that. They may be getting by on a cup of coffee and a soda and cigarettes. At the same time they have this overwhelming sense of omnipotence about themselves and their abilities. So it can be a very, very dangerous period of time."

As Dr. Vickar reminds us, a manic episode may also take forms very different from the euphoria described above: "It can also be a period when, instead of being overly expansive, people become overly suspicious. They become paranoid. The opposite side of persecutory paranoia is grandiosity. Sometimes the grandiose patient grows irritable, angry, and upset at other people who are getting in the way of the wonderful achievements he or she has to offer the world.

"When treating patients suffering from manic-depression, also known as bipolar disorder, we have certain advantages if we accept that the mood disorders are related to possibly disturbed serotonin metabolism. In Canada they have tryptophan; we used to have it here.

"I don't use other amino acids but I certainly use lithium. Now we're discovering that some of the other anti-seizure medications may work in patients with lithium intolerance. Lithium is a naturally occurring substance so I prefer it over the other anti-seizure medications which are, of course, man-made. In fact, lithium is a perfect example of a naturally occurring substance being used by traditional psychiatrists to treat biochemical diseases. Sometimes you use lithium in schizophrenic patients who also have secondary depressions of their moods. You want to be cautious, however.

"If a patient is manic and having psychotic symptoms, I tend to use a formulation similar to that given to psychotic patients. Lithium is certainly added in large part. If the patient's mood is low and he or she is depressed, lithium is sometimes of value, but not always. In addition to traditional antidepressants, I make sure they have enough B complex vitamins.

"Before tryptophan was taken off the market, I used a fair amount of it. There are some people who use phenylalanine or tyrosine, and these substances can be purchased, but it is often difficult for patients to get them. Not every hospital will stock them for you either. Also, sometimes the quality of the product is hard to verify."

Dr. Vickar describes a case history involving manic depression: "I treated a patient who had, for 40 years, exhibited a history that was very clearly that of a manic depressive: He was erratic, impulsive, had marital problems, and was in and out of jobs. His response came when

I added lithium to the vitamins, and nothing else. In over 40 years of his marriage, nobody had ever taken a look at the possibility that he had a biochemical abnormality. They just thought he was immature, or impulsive, or perhaps a bit antisocial. I see him once a year, and he takes lithium and vitamins and nothing else. Lithium is a naturally occurring substance that manic-depressives need in higher doses than the rest of us. So here is a case of somebody who, for the better part of a lifetime of illness, hadn't been diagnosed at all."

7
$\mathcal{S}$CHIZOPHRENIA

A Personal Account of Schizophrenia:
"Howard"

My illness started around 1977, when I developed a persecution complex and delusions of grandeur. I was seeing about three different psychiatrists and they were unable to help me. One psychiatrist thought I was manic-depressive. I wasn't being treated for schizophrenia, which is what I have. The orthomolecular approach made me well again. Now I am on a regimen of vitamins and antipsychotic drugs. The vitamins, I am told, enhance the good effects of the drugs so that I don't have to take high doses of the drugs in order to remain normal or stable. Before I got on this regimen I had not been taking any vitamins. Using the orthomolecular approach to help treat my schizophrenia, I basically feel normal and have my life back again.

Schizophrenia is a group of illnesses of unknown cause that have as their common features disorders of perception and emotion. Schizophrenic illnesses are classified, according to common terminology, as paranoid or nonparanoid, and they are termed either chronic or acute. According to Dr. Garry Vickar, "The new research that's being done suggests that there are, in fact, differences in prognosis"—in other words the likely outcome for patients suffering from schizophrenia—"in part related to the shape of the brain itself, the age at onset, and complicating factors relating to any co-existing drug abuse or other concurrent conditions.

"Clearly," Dr. Vickar continues, "schizophrenic illnesses as a group are among the most serious biochemical disorders there are; it can be said that schizophrenia is to psychiatry what cancers are to general medicine. The bulk of the lost revenue to society, the bulk of psychiatric expense, and the sheer horror to the families, which is not easily quantifiable, are unfortunately all consequences associated with the diagnosis of schizophrenia.

"The most disturbing part of schizophrenia is the disturbance of thought. These are patients who may have vague symptoms, who go through periods of what German psychiatrists used to call 'stage fright,' and then something happens and they start to believe that their disordered perceptions represent true events. Their strong belief in these disordered perceptions transforms them into delusions, which are simply fixed, false beliefs. Patients will start to believe their delusions and then start to believe their misinterpretation of a perceptual nature. They may hear a voice and believe that the voice is real and represents some real event or real person. They'll act on that. An example would be, if I hear somebody calling my name, if I don't think it's my thought anymore but that there really is somebody calling my name, I will act accordingly. If I think that people are looking at me and making faces, I might think there is something very wrong with me and feel bad or upset about it. If I'm eating my meal and there's a piece of moldy cheese, I might think I've been poisoned and that someone did it to me purposefully. The process starts to escalate and snowball.

"The most diabolical part of the illness is the loss of insight, loss of the ability to reality-test. For instance, if you're driving down the street at night and it's dark and hard to see, and you see something at the side

of the road, you might slow down to be cautious, thinking that somebody is going to cross the street. Then you get close enough and see
that it's really just shrubs or a mailbox or just part of the normal land-
scape, and you say, I'm glad I was cautious. If instead, however, you
start to distort the original perception and really believe that there's
someone who might jump out on the road or that somebody is trying to
hurt you and can get in the way of your vehicle, you might take evasive
action. In the process, you could have an accident or cause somebody
else to have one. You start to distort things without realizing that you
are distorting them. That's similar to what happens when the really disastrous part of the illness takes over.

"When you become paranoid and don't know why, you begin to
wonder, 'What is it about me that's so bad? Why are people saying bad
things about me?' It can become very serious. I had a patient who
believed that then-President Reagan was making comments about
him—about this individual—and he felt compelled to call the White
House and protest to the FBI that he was being hounded by President
Reagan. He firmly believed it. When he recovered he didn't believe it,
but when he was delusional he firmly believed that the President was,
in fact, personally interfering with his life. Such paranoid delusions
can become all-consuming and unfortunately very painful."

Dr. Philip Hodes sketches the history of the treatment of schizophrenia in orthomolecular psychiatry as follows: "In the field of schizophrenia, in the 1950s there were three pioneers in orthomolecular
psychiatry: Dr. Abram Hoffer, Dr. Humphry Osmond, and Dr. John
Smythies, who used large amounts of niacinamide, vitamin C, and
some of the other B vitamins, to help their schizophrenic patients
recover. In the 1970s, Dr. Alan Cott went to Russia and brought back
the practice of fasting, and helped to detoxify many of the brains of
schizophrenics who had not responded to any other kind of treatment.
He helped them clear their brains so that they became rational and
normal.

"Today we live in a state of environmental pollution. There are
over 90,000 chemicals in the external environment that we ingest
through what we eat, drink, and breathe. Contaminants are in the soil,
water, air, and food supply. The particles which are toxic penetrate
and leak through the blood brain barrier over time and get into the

brain. This process also happens with several of the heavy toxic metals, such as lead, cadmium, copper, iron, arsenic, mercury, and aluminum. These chemicals and heavy metals, by affecting brain chemistry, affect the mind and behavior, so they must be removed. They need to be chelated out.

"In the Science Section of *The New York Times*, on April 27, 1993, an article stated, 'New suspect in bacterial resistance, amalgam. The mercury in dental fillings may spur resistance to antibiotics.' Dr. Hal Huggins has shown that the silver mercury dental amalgams are very harmful; when you chew, the mercury is released, causing immune suppression and brain poisoning. Many of the people who have developed so-called 'mental illnesses' are suffering from things like mercury, lead, copper, iron, and aluminum poisonings. These toxic metals affect one's thinking and behavior. People can develop bizarre behavior and distorted thinking, along with warped perceptions, as a result of these toxic metals. Add to this toxic stew all the insecticides, pesticides, and herbicides that we ingest daily.

"The orthomolecular approach to schizophrenics is to detoxify them, change their diets, and remove foods that are chemically treated, or that contain a lot of sugar and refined carbohydrates, or that have been laced with pesticides. Then these patients are placed on the optimal doses of nutrients for their individual bodies. The nutrients used include vitamin B complex—especially thiamine, niacin, pyridoxine (B6), and B12.

"The late Dr. Henry (Hank) Newbold demonstrated that many of his schizophrenic psychiatric patients were suffering from a vitamin B12 'dependency' and that they needed large amounts in order to feel well and sane again. Then as the years went by, orthomolecular doctors discovered that the essential minerals—macro minerals such as calcium and magnesium, as well as the trace mineral elements zinc, manganese, chromium, and selenium—also helped balance the cerebral chemistry of schizophrenics. Dr. Priscilla Slagle published her research in a book, *Up From Depression*, showing the important role of amino acids in the brain, and in the treatment of manic depressives and schizophrenics.

"You also have to look at the water supply. Many water supplies contain chemicals, such as iron, silicone, aluminum, fluoride, and chlorine.

We ingest all of these things and once they hit the blood stream, they are rushed to all of the 64 to 67 trillion cells in the body. These toxins block out the opportunity for the vital nutrients to be absorbed.

"The basic constituents of the human body are proteins, amino acids (the building blocks of proteins), carbohydrates, fats, vitamins, minerals, oxygen, enzymes, nucleic acids, water, and electromagnetic and biomagnetic energy forms. If any of these are unbalanced or deficient, and there are nutritional deficiencies, different conditions and diseases can arise. Our diet is not really a healthy diet: the soil our food is grown in has been overworked; there have been artificial fertilizers put in; and the foods are refined, processed, and sprayed with all kinds of chemicals and inundated with all kinds of food coloring and dyes.

"When we eat these foods we become both malnourished and toxic. In answer to those who say, 'Oh, you don't need vitamins. Just eat a well-balanced diet,' I say you can't get a well-balanced diet and you do need extra nutrients to help stave off the deleterious effects of all the chemical pollutants in the environment. With orthomolecular therapy," Dr. Hodes concludes, "many people feel a lot better when they get more nutrients than their diet gives them."

Researcher Eva Edelman adds that a low state of histamine is sometimes associated with schizophrenia and that this, too, can be environmentally related. "Perhaps 40 to 50 percent of individuals diagnosed as schizophrenic are low histamines. They typically have a pear shaped body, low metabolism, and a tendency to dental cavities. They may have upper body pain, and tend to be young looking and resistant to shock—because histamine plays an important role in producing shock reactions in the body. They also tend to have food and chemical sensitivity.

"This condition produces the most typical mental symptoms of schizophrenia, the kind conventional psychiatry would readily identify. Low histamine is often caused by an excess of copper in the body. While copper is a very important nutrient for most people, it's very easy to get an excess because copper is prevalent in our diets and in good herbs; it's often in the pipes that conduct water to our houses. Also in vitamin pills—a lot of companies provide what would be a maximum dose for many people. Blood type A can create a tendency to accumulate copper. Copper depletes histamine levels and it also depletes vitamin B3 and C, which are needed to support mental functioning in low histamine individuals."

Dr. Abram Hoffer reminds us that very early treatment efforts involving orthomolecular psychiatry existed and were critical to the field's current resurgence: "The orthomolecular treatment of schizophrenia was started in Saskatchewan in 1951 when we ran the first double-blind controlled experiments in North American medicine and also the first in worldwide psychiatry. On the basis of these experiments, where we compared the effect of vitamin B3 against a placebo, we found that the addition of the vitamin to the standard treatment of that day, which was only electroconvulsant therapy, doubled the two-year recovery rate from 35 percent to 70 percent. That was the beginning.

"After that we ran another three double-blind controlled experiments. Since that time we have accumulated massive clinical experience; I myself have seen many thousands of schizophrenic patients. The treatment for the schizophrenic patient is really relatively simple. It's a combination of the best of modern psychiatry, which includes the proper use of tranquilizers, antidepressants, or other drugs, with proper attention to diet and the use of nutrients.

"The main nutrient is vitamin B3, which has to be given in large quantities. It's not enough to give the tiny amount present in food. One will have to give many thousands of times as much in the standard dose. For the patients I work with, I give 3000 mg per day of either nicotinic acid or nicotinamide, which are both forms of vitamin B3.

"I also use vitamin C at the same dose level and sometimes a lot more because vitamin C is a very good water-soluble antioxidant. It is considered the foremost, the most active water-soluble antioxidant present in the human body. That's extremely important.

"In many cases," Dr. Hoffer continues, "we use vitamin B6 as well for a particular group of schizophrenic patients. This is combined with an overall nutritional approach that may also include the use of a very important mineral, zinc. Zinc and B6 function together and are extremely important.

"Finally, we use manganese to protect our patients against developing tardive dyskinesia. This is a condition which afflicts chronic schizophrenic patients who are placed upon large quantities of tranquilizers.

According to Dr. Richard Kunin from San Francisco, when you take tranquilizers for a long period of time you take manganese out of the body, which is the reason patients develop tardive dyskinesia. When you give them back the manganese this condition may go away in a few cases.

"I put my patients on a diet that is junk-free. I exclude any of the prepared foods that contain additives, including sugar. I also pay attention to patients' allergies, because 50 or 60 percent of all schizophrenics have major food allergies. If these are not detected and eliminated, the patients are not going to get any better.

"This is essentially the treatment for schizophrenia, although there is one more important variable—the patients themselves. You have to take a lot of time dealing with schizophrenic patients. I will just briefly review what I have done recently. I have re-examined 27 of my chronic schizophrenic patients who have been working with me for at least ten years. They had been sick an average of seven years before they came to see me. They had all failed to respond to any of the standard treatments—drugs, tranquilizers, or shock treatments. They had not been given any vitamins.

"I did a survey of what happened to them after being with me for ten years. Of the 27 really chronic patients, 17 today are normal. They really are well. They're paying taxes."

Patient Story: Mister Y

A man from eastern Canada was a very paranoid schizophrenic. He was in and out of the Ontario mental hospital system. He was so sick that his wife divorced him and his family disowned him. He moved out west to Victoria and was living as a homeless person there for awhile. He came under Dr. Hoffer's care and remained on the vitamins, to the doctor's surprise. Three or four years ago he got his degree at the local university in Toronto and the last time Dr. Hoffer saw him he was looking for a job. He thinks this is quite an accomplishment for someone who had been a very sick patient.

"Another patient," Dr. Hoffer says, was a woman who, in a psychotic frenzy, burned down her house. She now runs her own business and supervises 12 people. These are examples of some of the recoveries we've had.

"The other ten are not well yet. Some may never be well because they've been sick for too long, but they're certainly an awful lot better than they were when we found them. They're now comfortable. They're able to live with any hallucinations or delusions they still have.

"This is a very chronic group of patients, the kind that normally don't respond. The important thing—going back to the view that you have to expect slow, progressive improvement rather than any sudden cure—is that it took five to seven years of continuous treatment before they reached their current stage of improvement.

"Acute patients, patients who have only been sick for a year, do a lot better, of course," Dr. Hoffer reminds us. "I fully expect that if I see 100 schizophrenic patients who have been sick a year or two or less, after two years of this kind of treatment, 95 percent of them will be well. In fact, the 17 young men and women I mentioned above who made complete recoveries had all become schizophrenic in their teens. They were placed upon vitamin treatment in various parts of Canada and the United States. These 17 young men and women all went into medicine. Today they are practicing psychiatry. One went to Harvard Medical School and is now a doctor in Boston. One became a president of a major psychiatric association in North America. The other members of that association did not know that he had a history of having been psychotic at one time. That's a pretty good record."

Dr. Garry Vickar emphasizes the holistic foundation of the treatment approach he prefers. "I think in any chronic illness, such as schizophrenia, you have to maximize the person's whole functioning. You want to make them as healthy as possible. You don't want to have an imbalance where your left arm is really maximally in shape because you're a pitcher but the rest of you is flab. You have to have the whole organism as healthy as possible.

"If, in fact, people have abnormal thinking because of deficiencies of B12, maybe they have a lack of an enzyme in their stomach that doesn't carry out the necessary conversion of B12 into what the body needs. These people have a disease called pernicious anemia that can result in their becoming paranoid. Once in awhile you'll find a person who lacks this thing called intrinsic factor. You have to give B12 supplements to prevent them from becoming paranoid and from developing nervous system signs and symptoms and gait disturbances. With B12 they get better. So there are simple things like that which can be done and which, in this modern age, can get overlooked by conventional physicians.

"I check for magnesium levels in all my patients, especially adolescents who drink a lot of soda pop. I also do zinc, copper, and manganese levels because there is some evidence that low manganese is implicated in tardive dyskinesia. A low magnesium level is implicated in irritability, nervousness, even nerve conduction problems and seizures. The worst-case scenario is a premenopausal woman who just had a baby, was on birth control pills prior to her pregnancy, is on prenatal vitamins, and goes back on the pill after the baby is born. She'll have sky-high copper levels, almost toxic relative to zinc.

"With the schizophrenic patient I use niacinamide or niacin (more frequently niacinamide because most patients won't tolerate niacin). I tend to use much of what Abram Hoffer has come up with. I look for a minimum of 3000 mg of niacinamide a day with an equal amount of vitamin C. I recommend a B complex with 50 to 150 mg of the entire B complex, mineral balance, depending upon zinc and copper levels. We try to titrate a dose until we reach a level of improvement with the least amount of medicine and the amount of vitamin and mineral supplements that the patient can tolerate."

Dr. Vickar continues, expressing the broad philosophy of his treatment of schizophrenic patients: "I have patients who have been diagnosed as having schizophrenia, and while I don't argue with the diagnosis, it hasn't captured the whole essence of what is going on with that patient. I prefer to see it as an incomplete diagnosis, rather than as a misdiagnosis. Very often the goal, in the schizophrenic diagnosis, is just to subdue behavior. When people are in such states of distress that their behavior is inappropriate, or agitated, or out of control, the goal is primarily to treat that behavior. I think that there is more we can do. We have to try to understand why the patient is doing what he or she is doing—not necessarily psychologically, but in some way biochemically.

"We don't know what the ultimate causes of schizophrenia are. Each new drug that comes along throws the current theory into such disarray that it doesn't apply anymore, because the new drug doesn't work the way that those preceding it did. So I don't think that anybody knows the causes, but there is one thing that we are sure of: We can make a big difference in how a schizophrenic is doing by applying two basic principles, as Dr. Hoffer has indicated: good sound nutrition and vitamin supplements.

"These are not synonymous. Nutrition has to be the floor upon which the treatment is built. Then, after that, you have to start looking at other factors—whether it be smoking, co-existing alcohol-related problems, dietary disturbances, or absorption difficulties. Also, the patient may not be doing well because what they have been given is, in fact, creating more problems. So we have to be sensitive to such reactions to treatment and continue to modify the treatment all the way along. And again, the approach I find to be most useful is that schizophrenia is not so much a missed diagnosis as it is an incomplete one."

Dr. Peter Breggin, an expert of the side effects of anti-psychotic drugs, points out that while "the neuroleptics are supposedly most effective in treating the acute phase of schizophrenia, a definitive review of controlled studies in 1989 showed that they perform no better than sedatives or narcotics and even no better than placebo. On the other hand, studies have shown that patients diagnosed with acute schizophrenia improve better without medication in small home-like settings run by non-professional staff who know how to listen and to care. The patients become more independent, and do so at no greater financial cost, because non-professional salaries are so much lower. As an enormous added benefit, the drug-free patients do not get tardive dyskinesia or tardive dementia, as well as other drug-induced and sometimes life-threatening disorders.

"But isn't schizophrenia a biochemical and genetic disease? In reality, there's no convincing evidence that schizophrenia is a biochemical disorder. While there are a host of conjectures about biochemical imbalances, the only ones we know of in the brains of mental patients are those produced by the drugs. Similarly, no substantial evidence exists for a genetic basis of schizophrenia. The frequently cited

Scandinavian genetic studies of the mid-1970s actually confirm an environmental factor while disproving a genetic one. But even if schizophrenia were a brain disease, it would not make sense to add further brain damage and dysfunction by administering neuroleptics."

Schizophrenia and Alcoholism

Dr. Abram Hoffer estimates that about ten percent of all schizophrenic patients are also alcoholic. "It's not a big figure," he adds, "if you remember that ten percent of all adults in North America are probably alcoholic. In other words, the same proportion is present in schizophrenics. If you start the other way, a certain percentage of alcoholics are, in fact, also schizophrenic. There is an overlap.

"It has been acknowledged for many years that this particular group that have both problems is very tough to treat. The first person to really show that you can help them was Dr. David Hawkins, who was then practicing on Long Island. He found that when he placed his alcoholic schizophrenic patients on the proper vitamin treatment, including mostly niacin and vitamin C, he began to see a fantastic number of recoveries. I have seen some recoveries, but not as many as he has.

"I can attest to the fact that patients do a lot better if they are treated for both conditions. This treatment includes niacin or niacinic acid and the other vitamins that I use for the treatment of these conditions.

"I think that whether or not they are alcoholic they have to be treated the same way. If they're alcoholic, it's vital that they stop drinking. The best way to achieve that is to try to get them to join Alcoholics Anonymous."

8
$\mathscr{I}$NSOMNIA

Although we spend roughly a third of our lives sleeping, the essential nature of sleep still isn't fully understood. Brain longevity expert Dr. Singh Khalsa reminds us that "recent studies have shown that you don't need to sleep as much as you think. In the last two hours, you have weird dreams and the rapid eye movement sleep is very intense. This raises cortisol levels and can actually cause you to awaken with stress and anxiety, which can lead to memory loss and other illnesses. In fact, people who have heart attacks have them most often in the morning. Ancient and modern thinkers recommend that you don't get up, take a shower or have your coffee first thing. Take a little time for yourself—this has been scientifically shown to be one of the most important things you can do to put on a suit of armor against stress and have a great day."

Many people wake up tense because they have been unable to sleep. Insomnia is a very common symptom of many of the disorders discussed elsewhere in this book, ranging from anxiety to schizophrenia and various other mood disorders. Typically, anxiety makes it more difficult to go to sleep, and depression can cause early waking. Insomnia can also result directly from physical symptoms such as pain or indigestion, or as a side effect of drug medication. People with chronic fatigue have serious sleep disturbance, are usually unable to fall asleep, wake up frequently and don't feel restored.

Some things that may help mild insomnia are calcium citrate and magnesium citrate, about fifteen hundred milligrams before you go to bed. About fifty milligrams of Vitamin B6 along with five hundred milligrams of inositol also helps promote sleep. For good herbs, investigate ashen flower, skullcap, valerian root and catnip.

Norman Ford, a health reporter and a researcher for 30 years, says that "tossing and turning and laying awake at night is not a reliable indication of insomnia. If you wake up each morning feeling fresh and recharged and you function efficiently during the day both physically and mentally, you probably do not have bonafide insomnia. The symptoms of true insomnia are feeling drowsy and uncomfortable during the day with a definite impairment in creativity, memory recall, cognitive ability, and mood, or falling asleep when you should be awake. Even though you believe you're getting adequate sleep, if all these happen together, you may have true insomnia."

There are actually six types of insomnia, Ford says:

"Subjective insomnia: you think you have insomnia, but you really don't.

"Initial insomnia: taking a long time—30 to 60 minutes—to fall asleep.

"Sleep maintenance insomnia: lying awake during the night between sleep cycles.

"Delayed sleep phase insomnia: you can't sleep before 2:00 to 3:00 a.m.

"Unfinished sleep insomnia you snap awake at 5:00 a.m. and can't fall asleep again.

"Disturbed sleep insomnia: when you are shocked awake by a terrifying nightmare, and this goes on night after night. It is quite rare.

"The most common one is subjective insomnia.

"The best way to improve your sleep is to cut out all day time napping and consolidate your sleep into a single night time unit. Get up at the same time every morning and don't sleep in on weekends. Go to bed only when you feel drowsy and tired, not when you think it's bed-time. Tire the body and mind by using both actively during the day. Watching TV is the most passive, inactive thing you can do, probably the greatest thief of sleep in existence. Instead, try to exercise abun-dantly every day and use the mind actively by studying, learning or playing mind taxing games like chess or anything else that makes you think, like creative writing or even surfing the 'Net. There is a huge difference between surfing the 'Net, looking for real information, and sitting in a stupor, hypnotized by a babbling television tube. So activi-ty is what sends you to sleep.

"Once you're in bed, relax in a comfortable position, take several slow, deep belly breaths, and then briefly review all the good, pleasant things that have happened that day. If they didn't happen today, they could have happened the previous day, so review them anyway. If you're not asleep within 10 minutes, get up, go to another room, and do something monotonous and repetitive. Write letters, pay bills, water indoor plants or practice deep relaxation. Return to bed only when you feel drowsy and ready to sleep. If you don't fall asleep again within 10 minutes, get up and go back to the same room and repeat the whole routine. Keep repeating it until you do fall asleep.

"The fact is, if you really need sleep, you will sleep, but many of us go to bed too early and we spend biologically inappropriate time in bed for the demands of our lifestyle. If our lifestyle activity demands that we only need six and a half hours of sleep and we spend eight hours in bed, we'll toss and turn for one and a half hours, it's just as simple as that. The answer, of course, is to lead a more active lifestyle so that you do need eight hours of sleep.

"If you don't have any daytime impairment of judgment or ability to drive or to calculate or to make decisions or to operate machinery, you probably don't have bonafide insomnia. Many people just worry about the fact that they can't sleep because we're conditioned to believe we need eight hours a night. The more we worry about not being able to sleep, the less we sleep and the more we worry. A good technique to overcome this is called paradoxical intent. It's based on the principle of the harder you try to fall asleep, the longer you remain awake. Para-doxical intent forces you to do the opposite—try as hard as you can to stay awake. The result is, you usually fall asleep. During a study at

Temple University, for example, a group of chronic worriers, people who normally took 60 to 90 minutes to fall asleep, were able to drop off in six to seven minutes. Every night millions of people lay awake worrying about how they will perform on the job next day. So one of the best ways to fall asleep is to try as hard as you can not to, and it frequently works.

"How much sleep does a person actually need? Another myth is that sleep needs decrease as we grow older, but that's not really true. One person in three age 65 and older complains of poor sleep, but the explanation is that as they grow older, most men and women use their minds and muscles increasingly less and less. When we function like an old, sedentary, unhealthy person, we get the sleep of an older, sedentary person, regardless of chronological age. A man of 70 who walks five brisk miles each day and spends several hours studying and learning will have approximately the same sleep needs as when he was age 25.

"Sleep needs decrease as we become less active physically and mentally. Worldwide, the average adult male spends seven and three quarter hours of sleep and the average woman sleeps for eight hours. Fewer than 20 percent of adults sleep for six hours or less, and about 15 percent sleep longer than nine hours. People are naturally short or long sleepers and not everyone will sleep the same time, but if you sleep less than five hours or more than 10 hours, it could indicate a medical condition.

"People over 40 complain that they wake up in the middle of the night and can't get back to sleep for 30 to 60 minutes. The reason is that every 90 minutes during the night, most adults wake briefly as one sleep cycle ends and the next begins. Each sleep cycle lasts 90 minutes. But after 40, inactive people may remain awake for 30 minutes at the end of a sleep cycle before they can drift back to sleep and into the next sleep cycle. This is actually a bonafide form of insomnia, called sleep maintenance insomnia, and it's caused by failing to exercise and tire the body by bedtime. It's also caused by failing to spend at least 30 minutes outdoors in the daytime. It's caused by eating a large, high fat, meat-centered meal late in the evening. It could be caused by consuming alcohol after 7:00 p.m. or going to bed feeling hungry or by daytime napping.

"If you do wake up after a sleep cycle in the middle of the night, the solution is to relax the muscles with deep relaxation and relax the mind with abdominal breathing—breathe deeply, use deep belly breaths; take several deep belly breaths slowly in and out. That will tame a racing mind. As the body slows, it slows the mind, and as the mind slows, it relaxes the body. In just a couple of minutes, these combined steps will turn on the relaxation response. The mind enters a calm reverie-like state and your brain wave frequency drops and you're on the brink of sleep.

"Another common form of genuine insomnia is when you snap awake at the crack of dawn and are never able to fall asleep again. That also can be eliminated by cutting out all daytime napping. Another good step is to go to bed later, perhaps an hour later. When you do wake up early, get up and begin the day, do nothing that is entertaining or pleasant, don't reward yourself, such as drinking coffee or fruit juice or watching TV. Having morning sex is one of the best ways to get back to sleep."

Dr. Samuel Dunkell is a psychiatrist, a sleep clinician working with an insomnia outpatient clinic and the Director of the American Sleep Disorders Association. His work concerning the position of the body in sleep is intriguing. He says that "the way we sleep at night reflects the positions that we take in our daily lives. Our general approach is reflected in terms of body language. Different types of people show different configurations. The person who sleeps on their back is a person who is ready to receive, who is used to being given everything; the world shares their products and wealth with them. A person who sleeps on the side sleeps between the face-down and the back position, so they are flexible. This position is characteristic of the majority of Americans. Sixty percent, I would say. sleep in the side position with the knees slightly bent, a semi-fetal position. Another group, quite large in number, sleep face down. These people like to know where they are at all times. They like to be in touch with their world and. to a certain extent, in control. Such people tend to be short sleepers, not to dream too much, to go to bed early and to arise early. They are somewhat compulsive, driven or active; their lives are geared for success in our society, which rewards that type of behavior. If we don't assume these positions we are restless, we can't fall asleep, we might even have insomnia.

"There is more. Most sleep research focuses on the individual sleeper, but most adults share beds with someone for most of their lives. This has not been studied too extensively because laboratory instruments used to study sleep are geared to an individual. I've seen that the way couples relate at night in terms of the configurations that they assume on the bed reflect not only their individual positions, but the relationship between them and their attitudes toward one another. Most people who have a new bed relationship, like newly marrieds who go to bed regularly with one another, sleep in the 'spoon' position. Both lie on their sides, facing the same direction, with one person behind the other. The person who generally takes the rear position has their arms over the partner. This is the person who sets the tone, the pace and is generally the nurturer in the couples relationship.

"My studies found that after three to five years of an ongoing relationship, gradually the couples disengage from one another in bed. They go into their individual personal sleep positions, knowing that their partner is there for them and ready to give them the security, love and contact that they need at night. During the night, from time to time, they assume that original 'spoon' configuration temporarily.

"Sometimes, people have trouble sleeping because one person encroaches on the other too much and one of them feels hemmed in. If that partner has a problem with intimacy, they may want to pull away. They will try to do things to try to discourage the partner from assuming too close contact and that's bad for intimacy. We'd rather have the couple share their life together at night as well as during the day. Whenever there are instances of discord and attempts to diminish intimacy, these should be recognized and discussed and dealt with.

"Senior citizens have particular problems. They fall asleep easily, but wake up too early. From fifty on, we need about six and a half hours of sleep or less per night. As we age, the so called body clock shifts in a direction which makes us want to go to bed earlier and get up earlier. That is a biologically inherent tendency. Socially, as we get older, our need to get up early is diminished because most of the senior group are retired. There is something of a contradiction there that has to be faced. I've found that most seniors get up about four or five hours after they have gone to bed, pass the time and then go back to bed again. In those extra couple of hours, they claim to get a very good rest. This is in error because it throws off our timing mechanisms and leads to insomnia. We should try to sleep in one full stretch at night. Staying in bed too long should be discouraged; one of the major errors is trying to make up for loss of sleep by staying in bed too long.

"The environment in which you sleep makes a difference, too. It should be a soothing decor. Loud colors, surfaces that reflect light, stimulating types of objects in the room—all distract from the ability to fall asleep.

"A number of different relaxation techniques can be useful. The main problem is to get the mind off of the worry. The worry acts like a magnet that pulls our thoughts and when that magnet starts going, it starts the worry machine going. That keeps us aroused and awake. So the main trick is to occupy our minds with something else that's less stimulating, even somewhat boring, but that keeps us busy and away from the danger zone. I have an interest in geography, so if I have trouble sleeping or I wake during the night and can't fall back to sleep, I try to remember the names of the various states of the union or the major rivers of the U.S. or the major rivers of Europe. I even go down the alphabet and try to name bodies of water. The same general principle can be used by others—if they are interested in sports, they can try to name teams and players and years and averages and things like that. They might try to remember the names of certain books they've read or movies they've seen or actors. Whatever is important and relevant to the individual can be drawn in. It's a very effective technique and before you know it, you're asleep.

"There are gender differences in sleep dysfunction. Pregnant women, whose abdomens have become extended during child birth, can't fall into their usual sleep positions or have their usual contact with their bed mates. There is also an increase in insomnia caused by the pregnancy toward the end of the pregnancy period. Postpartum, women often have difficulty falling asleep for a number of days or weeks.

"Men generally have most of the insomnia that occurs before the age of fifty-five but in the post menopause period, women catch up. This may be due to the loss of sex hormones or to physical problems that easily add to the inability to fall asleep.

"There is a period just prior to falling asleep when we sort of give up the world that surrounds us. Because this period of giving up the world means a kind of loss of activity and structure, it has a certain element about it that we call regressive anxiety. The presence of the bed partner whom we sleep with night after night reassures us. Being close, in touch, experiencing their breathing, their heart beat, their warmth—all this will overcome that anxiety producing phase and allow us to fall asleep much more easily.

"If we go to sleep with a sound going on, like a fan, the noise will grab our attention, wiping out all the other sounds we are accustomed to as part of our environment. That is called masking and when it happens, it creates anxiety. To overcome this, we try to structure the world in a way that we've found in the past has given us stability. We create a world from our past experiences that we know will help us to face the unknown. That is the masking phenomena. The world gets covered over with a mask and then we project a set of ideas or a structure formation in order to make sense of the world. It's the idea behind the so-called ink blot test. We see a kind of blob of ink and we try to make something out of it. The organizing principle each of us projects is what identifies us as individuals. The technique of unveiling the masking that I use with patients helps me find their essential approach and how they view the world.

"Sometimes the sleep problem is not psychological, but physical. The amount of times a person has to get up to urinate during the night breaks up their sleep and frequently leads to insomnia. As we get older, sphincters in women weaken and men have prostate enlargements, so it's important to avoid having too much fluid before you go to sleep. Avoid types of fluid during the day that cause a tendency to urinate, like caffeine, which is not only in coffee, but most soft drinks. If you do go to the bathroom and have difficulty falling back to sleep, use some of the relaxation techniques."

Dr. James Pearl has done a number of sleep and insomnia studies. He is a member of the Sleep Panel at the Presbyterian St. Luke Medical Center in Denver and in private practice as a psychologist. He finds that "about one out of three adults have occasional problems with insomnia and about half that group, one in six, have severe or constant sleep problems. After age forty or fifty, it becomes harder staying asleep through the night and people sleep more shallowly. Many different organ system disorders can affect sleep, respiratory problems in particular. There is a disorder known as sleep apnea, which is respiratory impairment. If you or your sleeping partner experiences problems with snoring, it's important to explore whether there might be some kind of breathing disorder. Sleep apnea is an episode in which your breathing is interrupted for about ten seconds. The person will stop breathing. Ten seconds later, you hear them suddenly gasp for air once. That causes them to awaken and typically, fall right back to sleep again. A sleep apnea episode can happen as many as several hundred times a night, without the person knowing it. If you are older and overweight, if you snore and are sleepy during the day, it is important to talk to a physician about the possibility of sleep apnea happening.

"Another physical problem is 'period limb movements,' where the person's legs, sometimes arms, but especially legs, twitch uncontrollably for a few seconds. These also become more common with age. Sometimes you don't even know when you are having these movement disorders. So if you awaken in the morning with your bedcovers in disarray or if your sleeping partner says that you are kicking him or her during the night, it is very important to talk to a physician

"Different substances can effect sleep, starting with sleeping pills. Both over the counter and prescription sleeping pills can improve sleep for a short period of time, but if you take sleeping medication for too long, you can build up tolerance. If you continue to take the same amount of medication, your body doesn't respond as strongly, so you need to use more and more. If you suddenly stop taking the medication, your sleep is going to become worse than it was in the first place. It's a good rule of thumb to not take sleep medications more than a few times a week or for more than about a month at a stretch.

"Other kinds of medications as well can sometimes influence sleep. Some have caffeine in them, so it might be worth a call to the pharmacist to see if yours does and whether it might be better to take it some time other than bedtime.

"Most people know that caffeine can influence sleep and for most people, it's okay if you don't take caffeine within about five hours of bedtime. But for some people, the drug is so strong that they have to stay off caffeine for about twelve hours before bedtime. The term 'nightcap' came about because so many people traditionally used alcohol to help them fall asleep. Alcohol is very effective to help yourself become more relaxed and drowsy and it often does help you to fall asleep. But as the alcohol is metabolized through your system during the night, if you had too much shortly before bedtime, it is likely to awaken you during the night because of withdrawal symptoms. Your body is wanting more. Drinking alcohol also makes sleep disrupted—you awaken more often and don't sleep as deeply. Generally, it is good to avoid alcohol for at least two hours before bedtime. You need to see how it effects you.

"Tobacco is a stimulant, people who smoke should not smoke in the evening. It stays in your system and keeps your physiology aroused.

"Cardiovascular disorders affect sleep. Angina, in which the heart muscle receives insufficient oxygen, can cause a person to awaken during the night with a choking pain. Coronary artery disease and hypertension or high blood pressure, can also influence your sleep. Medication prescribed for hypertension—usually diuretics—can cause you to awaken frequently during the night to urinate.

"Then there are the digestive disorders that interfere with sound sleep, starting with heartburn, a relatively common condition that tends to increase with age. It is also known as acid reflux because the sphincter that separates the esophagus from the stomach doesn't function properly and causes stomach acids to seep back up into the esophagus. Lying down flat will aggravate this condition, so it is good to elevate your bed. Place blocks as high as six inches beneath the head of the bed or arrange pillows from your waist to your head so you're not lying flat on your back. It is also good to eat dinner earlier in the evening, to allow the food to be digested before bedtime.

"Ulcer patients often experience insomnia caused by the effects of the stomach acid that is secreted during sleep. So if you have an ulcer and sleep difficulty, talk to your physician about what you can do to minimize that.

"There are many good therapies to help people sleep. if you are feeling like you are under a lot of stress and a lot of anxiety, it's important to take a look at that either with a self help book or with a therapist to see what you can do to minimize the problems. One powerful way to improve your sleep is to maintain a regular sleep-wake schedule. Getting up at the same time everyday is helpful, even on weekends. If you don't have problems with insomnia, it is fine to sleep in, but if you do have difficulty falling asleep or staying asleep, keep a regular sleep-wake schedule. Some sleep experts say you should go to bed at the same time every night and some say go to bed only when you're sleepy. Do whatever feels right for you. But it is really good to try to get up at the same time everyday.

"Sunday night insomnia is a common problem, especially for people under forty. Let's say you normally go to bed at eleven o'clock and get up at seven. On Saturday, if you sleep in an extra hour, your body rhythms are one hour behind. If you sleep an extra hour on Sunday, until nine, then your internal sleep-wake rhythm is two hours behind. Sunday night, if you try to go to bed at eleven o'clock, you are not sleepy because your body clock is two hours behind. If it is really important for you to sleep in on weekends, don't go to bed that Sunday night until you feel sleepy. You might sleep one or two hours less than usual but that won't hurt you.

"Light therapy has been proven to help. Studies show that people who spend a lot of time indoors away from windows, away from sunlight, have a disproportionate amount of insomnia. They have difficulty sleeping for the same reason that blind people do. Nine out of ten blind people have severe sleep problems because they are not getting sunlight into the retina of their eyes, into the brain to tell the brain that it is time to be awake during the day. The more light stimuli you can give your body during the day, the stronger your sleep-wake rhythm will be. I am talking about sunlight in particular. Indoor light is not going to make any difference. You need to expose yourself to bright, sunlight—just your eyes. There are artificial sun boxes that are commercially available. But if you have insomnia, get outside as much as you can, during your lunch hour, during your breaks. Don't wear sunglasses, unless you've got an eye condition that requires it.

"Another powerful way to improve your sleep is exercising in the late afternoon or early evening. When you do aerobic exercise for half an hour, you raise your body temperature. Five or six hours later, your body temperature drops. So working out after work or before dinner is an ideal way to get your body ready for bed. A lazy way to get that same benefit is soaking in a hot bath. It has to be really hot, at least 102 degrees. When you use passive body heating, the drop in body temperature occurs just about three hours later.

"A lot of people intuitively know that stressful experiences during the evening can disturb nighttime sleep and research has confirmed that. So it is important to think of the evening as a transition period between the day's troubles and the night's rest. Get ready to wind down. Try to leave your work at the office. If you have to bring it home, get it done early in the evening. Do stressful things like planning your schedule early in the evening or else wait until the morning.

"Visualization is one of the things you can do to slow down your mind. Counting sheep is just one example of mental imagery—forming pictures in your eyes along with sounds and sights. Some people do well by imagining that they are floating along on a cloud or on an air mattress in a warm sea, but just imagining that you are floating is one image that relaxes a lot of people. Or imagine yourself walking slowly down a staircase or riding down an elevator or an escalator. The farther you go down, let yourself sink more deeply into relaxation. Finally, you can count down to relaxation. Count very slowly beginning with 100 and visualize every number. When you come to each number, release tension in your body and relax more deeply. Visualize a number in a downward progression—each one on a staircase, for example, one step lower than the previous one.

"It's not only mental stress, but physical stress that can interfere with sleep. If your muscles are tense and tight or your breathing fast and shallow, try abdominal breathing. Take breaths that are increasingly deep and slow, so deep that it makes your abdomen push out. Hold it for a few seconds and let it out slowly, breathing away the tension.

"Finally, if you can't sleep despite everything you have tried, do something else. Switch on the light and read; watch a tape or clean out a drawer. A lot of people think that missing sleep is going to hurt their health, but losing sleep has very few effects. Many studies show that when people sleep less than normal, their performance the next day in most cases is just as good as when they had a good night's sleep. Highly creative tasks do sometimes become more difficult when you have lost sleep, but, for most of us, even if we go a whole night without sleep, we can get along fine the next day. Don't be afraid of insomnia. Don't lie in bed trying to sleep. Some people like to imagine sleep as a wave in the ocean and themselves as a surfer. Position yourself in this warm ocean and wait. The wave will overtake you and sweep you away."

Dr. Robert Atkins points out the efficacy of tryptophan, which isn't currently legally available in the U.S., in the treatment of insomnia: "Tryptophan is very valuable for sleep disorders because serotonin is the sleep chemical. If you take it right when you are ready to go to bed, when your serotonin level is on the upswing anyway, you are really fitting in physiologically with your body's chemical rhythms."

Most of the doctors I interviewed shared similar experiences in treating insomnia. A major cause of insomnia, especially if it's chronic, is reactive hypoglycemia. This is frequently exacerbated by eating late at night, especially if you eat foods with a high glucose level, such as pastries, candy, or even fruit juice. Such foods cause your blood sugar level to go up and then plummet, a fluctuation that can contribute to insomnia. Also, overindulging late at night in highly fatty foods can cause sleeplessness. That's because foods with a lot of fat take four to five times longer to empty from the stomach and be digested than simple or complex carbohydrates do.

Another big factor in insomnia is intake of stimulants, such as the caffeine in coffee, tea, chocolate, and even colas, which people consume at all hours without much thought as to the stimulant effects. Alcohol, although generally considered a depressant, can have stimulant effects in some cases.

In addition to food and drink, certain medications as well can be culprits in insomnia. Drugs that interfere with the natural sleep cycle include Prozac, the newer drugs related to it, and Xanax.

Exercising late in the evening is another possible bane for the insomnia-prone in that it can overstimulate adrenal levels and excite the musculoskeletal system, resulting in difficulty getting to sleep. Likewise, overstimulating the mind by thinking about unresolved conflicts can be a problem when the goal is sleep.

Herbs that are nontoxic and have no contraindications can be a real help to those challenged by insomnia. Unlike sleeping pills, herbs won't leave you in a fog in the morning, or feeling like you haven't really slept. Passionflower is an important relaxant herb popular in much of Europe. Other possibilities include valerian root, a natural calmative used by orthomolecular psychiatrists for people who tend to be anxious, and hops. Letha Hadady recommends that people who can't think clearly during the day and wake up at night sweating, with their hearts beating too fast, consider remedies that balance the adrenal glands in the heart. "The Chinese remedy called Ding Xin Wan is very good for people under stress—if you're working against a dead line or going through a divorce and are so overwrought you can't think clearly during the day but at night, especially, your heart is pounding and you can't sleep."

Other things to try: foods with naturally occurring tryptophan in high amounts; calcium citrate and magnesium citrate—1200 mg of each taken any time after dinner; 50 mg of the B complex; and 200 mg of inositol. Also, 200 mcg of chromium in the evening will help stabilize your blood sugar level.

For those with a partner, a gentle neck and head massage for 15 minutes may do the trick in conquering insomnia, and 15 minutes in a warm bath may be helpful as well (no partner required).

Along the lines of positive affirmation, writing in a diary shortly before bedtime can be extraordinarily beneficial. It can be a way of really seeing what you've done that's affirmed your mental, spiritual, and physical health, as well as any deeds you've done that have had positive effects on others. If a person spends some time at the end of each day reflecting on what they've done in the past 24 hours that's been positive, and on plans for the next day, he or she gains a sense of completeness about the day. In a sense, then, diary-writing legitimizes going to bed; it's as if you can now see that you really deserve the good night's sleep you're about to get.

9

*T*HINKING DISORDERS

According to Peggy Ramundo, co-author of the book *You Mean I'm Not Lazy, Stupid or Crazy?!*, "When people think of Attention Deficit Disorder, they generally think of hyperactive boys hanging from the light fixtures, running their parents and their teachers ragged. However, we now know that this disorder does not go away after childhood. Many adults have it."

The primary symptoms are impulsivity, inattention and hyperactivity. Ramundo's useful concept is "disregulated activity"—too much or not enough. Some of the more obvious manifestations are "chronic tardiness, argumentativeness, being unable to wait for a traffic light to change, jumping from activity to activity—having 14 projects started and none finished." It is often accompanied by substance abuse and "lots of disorganization."

"It is not unusual," she says, "to see someone hopping from one thing to another, one job to another. To those watching, this behavior looks like laziness or lack of motivation. They think of the person as hard to get along with, forgetful, irresponsible."

Attention Deficit Disorder per se only became part of our vocabulary in 1980, when the American Psychological Association identified it as a disorder. Although much of the focus is on children, adults suffer too. Ramundo's son was diagnosed with the disorder in 1987 and she herself in 1990.

Educational therapist Robert Bernstein says that parents "often have a child that they bring to me and I say, 'Well, this is the problem' and they say, 'Gee that sounds a lot like me.' Whenever I ask an adult, 'When did you realize there was a problem?' they always tell me the same thing—as long as they can remember, 'since I was four, since I was five.' That is very interesting because the official definition of Attention Deficit Hyperactivity Disorder is that it has to start before age seven. It's a problem that they've been living with their entire lives and haven't been able to compensate for it, which implies that it is an internal mechanism, not something that has to do with the parents or teachers.

"Recently, I saw a very successful adult who is very disorganized. His office was a total mess and he had to work sometimes all night just to kind of catch up on things that he needed to do. In the initial consultation, I gave him one of the simplest tasks you can do. It's almost embarrassing giving a forty-five year old a peg board, where he had to put the yellow pegs and the red pegs in the right places. There were five yellow pegs. He put four in perfect order. I would have bet any amount of money that he was going to put the fifth peg in, but he didn't. After he finished, I said, 'Why didn't you put this fifth peg in?' He said, 'Well, I knew it was going to happen eventually.' I asked, 'Is that the attitude you have on your job? You feel that you don't have to finish it because it's going to eventually be done?' He said 'Yes.' So that's his process—he can control that situation and put that last peg in and finish that job.

"I saw someone else who brought problems like: he cannot stand in line, he cannot be in a group. He never went out on a date. He never completed a class. His psychiatrist thought he had a learning disorder, but to me, it seemed that his problem was that he couldn't accept outside structure.

"Most people say they have learning problems. I confess I have no sense of direction. Fortunately, it didn't interfere with my academics. If it did, I would be labeled retarded. So the question for an adult is— is the problem really interfering with learning, doing a job or in a relationship? If it is, you have a problem."

For this, as for all disorders, nutrition is the key. People suffering from disordered thinking would do well to study all the general nutritional information about the brain throughout this book. Studies in the 1990s linked attention and activity disorders to zinc deficiencies, low essential fatty acids and very directly to artificial flavorings and other food additives like MSG and artificial sweeteners. There have been suggestions of effective treatment with tyrosine. Certainly eliminating caffeine from the diet is an essential first step.

Nutritionist Marcia Zimmerman points out that the timing of what we eat has a powerful effect on the brain. "There was work done in the 1980s at MIT and Harvard that showed how carbohydrates raise serotonin levels in the brain. Serotonin is a neurotransmitter that is calming and tends to put children to sleep. On the other hand, protein provides the necessary amino acids that are precursors of attention-grabbing neurotransmitters, namely norepinephrine and dopamine. No wonder children who have high carbohydrate breakfasts and lunches can't concentrate at school. And adults go off to work without an adequate breakfast, then eat donuts and coffee at 10 in the morning and wonder why everything is flashing past them and they're unable to concentrate or complete tasks. The timing of carbohydrates and proteins is very important."

Many people, including Peggy Ramundo, have been helped by vegetable chlorophyll green algae, a natural food that appears to stabilize the blood sugar level, provide amino acids in relatively balanced proportion and trace minerals in assimilable form, as well as concentrated sources of beta-carotene and vitamin B12.

Ramundo also finds adults helped by exercise—"very strenuous exercise, not just your three times a week, 20 minutes of aerobics, but an hour or two hours a day. Adults say it stimulates the action in the brain sufficiently that they do not need to take medicine. They are also finding therapeutic massage useful."

For many doctors on the cutting edge of brain longevity studies, attention problems can be early signals of declining cognitive power.

Dr. Richard Braverman has seen that "attention deficit marks a premature aging or dysfunction of the brain. There are many different kinds. You can have attention to detail. You can have failure of consistency on attention. You can have reaction time attention disorders. You can have impulsive attention deficit disorders. You can have blanking out or almost *petit mal*–like attention deficit disorders. Only when a doctor distinguishes which type of attention deficit disorder you have can he say which type of treatment is going to benefit you. This is what we see in depression, anxiety, all the psychiatric conditions, bipolar, schizophrenic. These conditions are all medical disorders of the brain with varying degrees of loss of brain function, metabolism, attention and memory.

"People with severe memory deficit have recovery if they are treated effectively. That can include everything including chelation. There are books on toxic metal syndrome describing the benefits of chelation on memory and research papers suggesting that if you do chelation you will pull out the aluminum and you will end up with improvement in memory. More work needs to be done in this area, of course."

10
TARDIVE DYSKINESIA

Tardive dyskinesia is a neurological condition which, as its name implies, is of late onset, that is, tardive. Dyskinesia refers to abnormal movement. Tardive dyskinesia describes the abnormal neurological movements that occur after a patient has spent a period of time on certain kinds of medicines. When the medicine is reduced or eliminated, the patient starts to demonstrate abnormal movements like involuntary blinking, smacking of lips, twitching around the face. They can occur at varying levels of severity and may involve the entire body.

Dr. Peter Breggin often testifies in court cases brought by people who have suffered these reactions to their medications. In 1998, a Louisiana judge ordered Bristol-Myers Squibb Company, the company that manufactures and distributes a drug called Prolixin, to pay $2 million to a 52 year old woman who had been prescribed the drug by her psychiatrist. (Prolixin is a "neuroleptic" drug, liked Haldol, Thorazine, Clozaril and others.) After five years, the woman had developed severe and disabling tardive dyskinesia. Muscle spasms and abnormal movements afflicted her face, neck, shoulders and extremities, as well as her speech and breathing.

"In 1973," according to Dr. Breggin, whose expert testimony in Louisiana was cited by the judge's ruling, "psychiatrist George Crane gained the attention of the medical community by disclosing that many, and perhaps most, long-term patients on neuroleptic drugs were developing a largely irreversible, untreatable neurological disorder, tardive dyskinesia. The disease, even its mild forms, is often disfiguring, with involuntary movements of the face, mouth or tongue. Frequently, the patients grimace in a manner that makes them look 'crazy,' undermining their credibility with other people. In more severe cases, patients become disabled by twitches, spasms, and other abnormal movements of any muscle groups, including those of the neck, shoulders, back, arms and legs, and hands and feet. The muscles of respiration and speech can also be impaired. In the worst cases, patients thrash about continually.

"The rates for tardive dyskinesia are astronomical. The latest estimate from the American Psychiatric Association in 1992 indicates a rate for all patients of five percent per year, so that 15 percent of patients develop tardive dyskinesia within only three years. In long-term studies, the prevalence of tardive dyskinesia often exceeds 50 percent of all treated patients and is probably much higher. There are probably a million or more tardive dyskinesia patients in the United States today, and tens of millions have been afflicted throughout the world. The disease affects people of all ages, including children, but among older patients rates escalate.

"Despite this tragic situation, psychiatrists too often fail to give proper warning to patients and their families. Often psychiatrists fail to notice that their patients are suffering from tardive dyskinesia, even when the symptoms are flagrant. In 1983, I published the first in-depth analysis of the vulnerability of children to a particularly virulent form of tardive dyskinesia that attacks the muscles of the trunk, making it difficult for them to stand or walk. Many or most tardive dyskinesia patients also show signs of dementia—an irreversible loss of overall higher brain and mental function.

"Indeed, it was inevitable that these losses would occur. The basal ganglia, which are afflicted in tardive dyskinesia, are richly interconnected with the higher centres of the brain, so that their dysfunction almost inevitably leads to disturbances in cognitive processes. A multitude of studies have confirmed that long-term use is associated with both deterioration and atrophy of the brain. Growing evidence indicates that these drugs produce tardive psychoses that are irreversible and more severe than the patients' prior problems."

According to Dr. Garry Vickar, "It used to be said that tardive dyskinesia was untreatable, but that certainly is not true now. Around 15 years ago there was a massive report that showed those physicians in orthomolecular psychiatry who were using vitamins did not have any patients with tardive dyskinesia. We tried to analyze what the factor was that prevented the emergence of TD. At one point, most of us thought that the addition of B6 might be the factor. Subsequent research has shown that it is probably vitamin E with its antioxidant capacity.

"The patients I've seen with tardive dyskinesia usually come to me after having been treated with drugs for a very long time. These are patients who have been on antipsychotic medications. If they're on an antipsychotic drug and they don't in fact have a psychotic or a schizophrenic illness, they're at higher risk. For example, somebody with a mood disorder given an antipsychotic drug is at higher risk for developing tardive dyskinesia.

"Typically those with tardive dyskinesia are patients who have been treated for schizophrenia over the course of many years. The ravages of the illness are combined with the cumulative effects of the medicine. The older antipsychotic drugs—Thorazine, chlorpromazine, Stelazine, Prolixin, Haldol—work in a certain part of the brain where the neurotransmitter function is tied in with movements. The implication is that treatment with these drugs over the long term can lead to movement disorders.

"Attempts to remedy this have resulted in the creation of newer antipsychotic medications such as Clozaril and Risperdal. These are allegedly less likely to cause tardive dyskinesia because they work on different centers of the brain. They relieve some of the schizophrenic symptoms without the potential for tardive dyskinesia. These drugs haven't been out long enough to know if they will cause other side effects. Clearly we haven't had enough time to know if the newer drugs ultimately will or will not cause similar problems.

"To treat tardive dyskinesia, you have to walk a fine line. You have to help patients reinstitute the very medicine that is implicated in causing it to relieve the dyskinesia. Sometimes I call neurologists in. They may have to use, in very interesting combinations, some of the antiseizure medicines that have antispasmodic effects.

"We used to think, many years ago, that the crucial missing ingredient in patients with tardive dyskinesia was vitamin B6. It turns out that it is probably vitamin E that is the protective element necessary with regard to TD.

"I treat TD patients with choline and lecithin and large doses of vitamins. The choline and lecithin are tied in with the presumptive mechanism of action of this abnormal movement. If there's an imbalance in the different neurochemical pathways, then it is thought that the choline and lecithin will help along what is called the phosphytotyl choline pathway. You add the lecithin so you don't have to give as much choline, because choline tends to lead to a very fishy smell in the body. It is presumed that this brings a balance back, or re-establishes the proper chemical balance in the brain to relieve the abnormal movements.

"If the chemical pathways in the brain were altered by the use of Haldol and other drugs, there may have been a disturbance of the intricate balance of neurochemicals necessary to coordinate smooth movements. The presumption is that choline and lecithin will help correct the imbalance that was created by the traditional antipsychotic drugs.

"In sum, I use a balance of B vitamins, lots of choline and lecithin, manganese where appropriate, and sometimes I have to call in a neurologist to see what treatments they might want to give, depending on the level of severity of the problem."

11

$\mathcal{B}$UILDING BETTER BRAINS

A good brain begins in the womb. While there are excellent reasons for pregnant women to take care of themselves by practicing good nutrition, an extra reason is the growing child. While not discounting the effects of environmental toxins, food additives, social conditions, lifestyles and allergies, recent concern over what has been called an epidemic of learning disabilities in young children has put some of the focus back on the mother's chemistry.

Marcia Zimmerman, a certified nutritionist in practice for 25 years, specializing in attention and hyperactivity disorders, says that part of the problem "could even be malnutrition before conception because neither young women nor young men are properly nourished when they conceive children."

"The brain," she explains, "develops very early. At between 18 and 21 days, the neural fold is developing in the young embryo. This later becomes the brain, spinal cord, heart and all the peripheral nerves. We know about the impact of folic acid this early, but we're beginning to get insights into the role fatty acids play. The brain is uniquely dependent on the correct fatty acids. These long chain, polyunsaturated, extremely flexible oils make up 60 percent of the brain issue. In particular, the developing embryo needs DHA, or docosahexaenoic acid, in very large quantities. The only source is to get them from the mother, but a lot of women are deficient in these fatty acids.

"During pregnancy, we want to emphasize a diet of whole grains and fish, especially fatty fish, which are rich in these Omega 3 fatty acids. You find them in salmon, cod, herring, anchovies, mackerel and tuna, although you should be careful of tuna because it is high in mercury. Most of the pregnant women that I counsel use DHA in supplement form, to insure that they get adequate levels. Flax seed oil is the precursor of DHA and you could use some on vegetables and salads or add the seeds to a smoothie in the morning. Canola oil and olive oil are good choices, rich in unsaturated fatty acids. Just stay away from generic vegetable oils, which are highly processed.

"Since food sensitivities affect the way the brain works, we eliminate milk, chocolate, eggs, wheat, corn, citrus, peanuts, sugar and artificial colors or flavors from the diet. We emphasize whole grains and fresh fruits and vegetables that are in season.

"While zinc and fatty acids are critical, baby formulas used in the past may have been deficient in these nutrients. They are plentiful, however, in breast milk, especially if the mother has been consuming a good diet."

Dr. Dharma Singh Khalsa, Board Certified by the American Academy of Anti-Aging Medicine, of which he is also the founder, has written numerous articles and two books on brain longevity. "When we talk about the brain, there is almost a schism in the way it's looked at these days. Many people in the medical establishment still look at the brain like it's a computer with certain files. I consider that very twentieth century. In the twenty-first century, the brain is going to be considered more like a symphony, an orchestration that is constantly changing and vibrating and moving and having deep rich colors.

"At a recent meeting of neuroscientists, the hottest news was about a protease inhibitor that might be able to effect the enzyme for Alzheimer's disease. They are still looking for the magic bullet. Information was presented on lifestyle, stress, the influence of things like that on the brain, but it didn't get the same kind of attention.

"The brain is a flesh and blood organ. It's just like other organs in the body. It's not a hard computer-like fixed organ. We cannot consider any longer that we are going to be able to impact Alzheimer's disease or any other brain disorder by trying to look at one specific enzyme, one specific gene or one specific gene or even one specific chemical. For example the multimillion dollars that have just been funded at the National Alzheimer's Centers to study the progression of early memory impairment in Alzheimer's disease are just looking at two chemicals. They are looking at the drug Aricept, which has been proven not to have a great effect except for a short period of time and vitamin E, which has been shown to have an effect, but they are not looking at the whole picture.

"The brain, as a flesh and blood organ, is dependent on blood flow. The brain is dependent on oxygen. Of course blood brings the oxygen. We need that. We have to have adequate nutrients like glucose. The brain thrives on glucose, so we have to have a good diet, not refined carbohydrates or sugars that do more harm than good. We have free radicals, these little products of metabolism that cause scarring of the brain. We have energy in the brain in the form of the power plant and the mitochondria. We have the synapse, a very important juncture where the electrical chemical energy is transferred from one cell to another to create the memory, to help us produce other memories, to draw up old memories, restore new memories and the emotions and all that.

"The brain is an organ, like the heart and I like to say that what works for the heart works for the head. When we think of the brain, we must think of lifestyle because there are things that we can do—exercise, nutrition, supplements, stress reduction, hormone replacement therapy. Don't forget the glands in the brain—the hypothalamus, pituitary, the pineal glands, so important for creating a healing environment in the body so we can regenerate ourselves, have more energy and vitality, even as we get older, rather than going in a spiral of degeneration and waiting for Big Brother to say, 'Hey, take this protease inhibitor.' It's just like the way they're looking for the one virus that causes AIDS, when a preventative approach is really what is needed.

"The endocrine system is primarily the hypothalamus, which is the brain's brain. The gland in your brain that controls just about everything, including aging, is not even the size of your pinky fingernail. It sends a whole bunch of hormones—called 'releasing hormones' or 'factors'—down to the pituitary gland, which is the master gland of the brain. This orchestrates secretions from all the glands in your body— the thyroid, the adrenal, the gonads (the testicles or ovaries). When you are young, it's responsible for growth and development and as we get older, it's responsible for reproductive functions and then, after a certain age, these hormones decline. The pituitary gland, in response to the hypothalamus, produces human growth hormone, one of the most important, if not the most important hormone to keep in good shape as we get older. But unfortunately, all these hormones peak at age 30, start to decline a little around 40 and at about 50, start to plateau down.

"All of these hormones affect our emotions, our moods, our sex drives. The most important thing that is coming out these days in terms of staying vitally alive is that everything is important: nutrition, supplements, the way we perceive our life, the way we respond to stress. Exercise is important, both physical exercise and mental exercise. If someone wanted to achieve and retain optimum mental potential, I'd work on their nutrition. Heart disease is a very high risk factor for developing memory loss in Alzheimer's, so we know that high fat in the diet will contribute to hardening of the arteries in the heart, the large arteries in the neck and the small arteries in the brain. Therefore it's critical to move away from these high fat diets. Our nutritionist works to construct a diet that has about 15 to 20 percent fat, so it's very tasty, but it's not the 30 to 40 percent fat that you see in the standard American diet or some of the high protein diets. Our supplements are like an all-purpose insurance policy of multiple vitamin mineral pill that has vitamin E, vitamin C, vitamin A, the B vitamins, and the minerals. Vitamin E is well studied to slow the progression of memory loss.

"We go with ginkgo too. The ginkgo tree is the oldest tree on earth. The leaf actually looks like the two lobes of a brain, the left and right hemisphere and so they call it a bilobal or ginkgo biloba. This herb enhances circulation to the micro capillaries, oxygenating the tissues in the brain. The medical establishment still says that not enough studies are done. Soon they will come out and say, 'Yes, ginkgo is okay to take.' Well we've been saying for a decade that ginkgo is a good brain-specific nutrient.

"We also use coenzyme Q10, which is still not well known. It is a very energetic cofactor that works in the brain's power plant, the mitochondria. The leading researcher in coenzyme Q10 told me he thought we should put it in the drinking water, it's that powerful. The studies are excellent showing that the old style phosphatidyl serine or PS, from bovine brains, was excellent, even with patients with dementia. The newer types of phosphatidyl serine which are synthesized from soy beans are proving excellent in reversing memory loss and rejuvenating the brain by about twelve years. Phosphatidyl serine has even been shown to improve seasonal affective disorder. Now there are some other nutrients that I like—like fish oil or DHA is an algae. You can get if from salmon. For children, it has been shown to improve ability to focus.

"Everything I've talked about is regenerating or protective, not stimulating. I stay away from compounds like DMAE and acetyl carotene because I think they are not good for everybody. They are way too stimulating. There is a new compound called hooperzene A that, in combination with vitamin E, can be very effective in blocking the enzyme that destroys the memory compound. It can be taken in capsule form, 50 micrograms to 100 micrograms twice a day. I don't think it should be taken by everybody because most normal people have enough of this memory compound.

"Anybody who does not have regular stress management program that is pro-active, something like a daily or almost a daily practice of meditation, does not have to worry because they won't enjoy good health. If you don't have some type of stress management tool to reduce the nasty chemicals, such as cortisol, that come from the chronic unbalanced stress we're all feeling as we go into the new millennium, you can count on having early degenerative disease. Cortisol attacks the memory center of the brain. It's like battery acid. Stress doses of cortisol come from chronic, unbalanced stress, not the acute stress of walking across the street and almost getting hit by a car. We are talking about daily stress over years, unresolved conflicts, anger, difficulty in the work place, difficulty at home—these all have an effect on your brain.

"Taking care of your brain requires exercise. I don't understand why the Alzheimer's groups don't emphasize this. There was a study looking at people who developed Alzheimer's Disease that showed that individuals with a regular exercise program, compared to those who did not, did not develop as much memory loss. If you exercise on a regular basis—you don't have to be Mr. Universe or run a marathon, you can do brisk walking, or jogging, or play tennis, or go on a treadmill, or go to the gym, work in your garden, do anything you want as long as you're getting your heart rate up and sweating three or four times a week. This has a very positive, healthy effect on the brain. It increases blood to the brain, it increases oxygen to the brain, it dilates blood vessels up there. It lets in everything that you need—because what good are nutrients if they don't get to the brain? There are many studies showing that growth factors injected into the brain can be very restorative, but you don't have to get them injected. You can produce your own growth factors just by going out and getting some exercise on a regular basis.

"Combine physical exercise with mental stimulation like reading a book, listening to a book on tape, or listening to an informative show and then discussing it with someone else. Combine mental and physical exercise sometimes—riding on a stationary bike and reading the newspaper or listening to a book on tape. You can actually make new connections in your brain this way. I saw a video the other day showing the neurons stretching out, looking for connections. Our brains are just hungry for connections, hungry to communicate, hungry to reach out and make new neuronal connections so that we can maintain our intelligence."

At his Institute in Tucson, Arizona, Dr. Kalsa teaches "Mind Management for the 21st Century" or "preventive medicine for the brain." "It is imperative to help people with age-associated memory loss," he explained, "because fifteen percent of people with what used to be thought of as a benign disorder progress to real dementia."

The Brain Longevity Program consists of four pillars:

1. Nutritional modification, including a fifteen to twenty percent fat diet. Adding breast of chicken, fish and non-animal protein products such as tofu is helpful. Certain fish are especially good for the brain. These fish include salmon, tuna, trout, mackerel, and sardines.

2. Stress management. Meditation decreases cortisol and enhances many aspects of mental function. Massage and guided mental imagery have also recently been shown to lower cortisol levels in the blood.

3. Exercise. Like ancient Gaul, there are three parts: mental exercise, physical exercise, and mind/body exercise.

Dr. Kalsa notes,"Aerobic reconditioning enhances mental function by twenty to thirty percent. The ancient art of brain regeneration, and of innovative mind/body exercises, derived from my twenty years practice of advanced yoga and meditation, are important in enhancing global brain energy."

4. The final phase comes from the white hot forefront of anti-aging medicine. "Among pharmaceutical drugs used to help regenerate the brain cells is L-Deprenyl Citrate. Deprenyl is a medicine that has been shown to increase longevity in animals and increase important biochemicals in the brain. In recent studies of patients with moderate Alzheimer's Disease, Deprenyl improved attention, memory, verbal fluency and behavior. Side effects associated with Deprenyl may include anxiety and insomnia if the dosage is too high. It may be contra-indicated in patients taking anti-depressants such as Prozac, and in those individuals suffering from heart disease. Deprenyl should only be prescribed and taken under the supervision of your doctor.

"Hormone Replacement Therapy with pregnenolone, DHEA and melatonin are also part of the therapeutic options in the prevention and reversal of memory loss. Pregnenolone has been clinically shown to be useful in patients with memory loss, especially those who have difficulty finding the correct words. DHEA is currently controversial because of concerns over long-term use. Dr. Kalsa continues: "When I prescribe DHEA as part of my program, I always have a blood level measured. If the patient is a male, I will also check their PSA blood test (prostate specific antigen) because of concern about the long term effects of DHEA on the prostate. Melatonin is useful for insomnia, jet lag and re-normalizing the body's biorhythms. It is my clinical observation that the generally recommended dose of 3-6 mg is too high. I prescribe 0.1 mg to 0.5 mg as a beginning dosage. Side effects with the higher dose include uncomfortably vivid dreams, morning headache and grogginess

"While it is very true that the Brain Longevity program can help us prevent and reverse memory loss as well as develop and maintain high levels of brain power, it can also allow us to tap into a very special part of our being. We can enjoy discovering who we really are and exploring the true nature of life. Along the way we will be sure to create a lifetime of peak mental performance."

Dr. Ray Sahelian, the editor of *Longevity Research Update*, is known for the evaluation of leading edge nutrients and hormones and he has been actively involved in research on the use of pregnenolone. "We heard first," he says, "about DHEA, the hormone made by the adrenal gland, which is the mother of testosterone and estrogen. Pregnenolone is the mother of DHEA. The body uses pregnenolone to convert into DHEA, which in turn converts into estrogen and testosterone or other antigens. Pregnenolone can also convert into progesterone. In fact, all the hormones made by the adrenal glands start out from pregnenolone and therefore, I call pregnenolone the grandmother of all the adrenal hormones.

"We have known about pregnenolone since the early 1930s. In the 1940s, some of the research included giving it to factory workers. They found that it improved work performance. People were more energetic, there was an anti-fatigue factor. Later on, they tested it in pilots in simulated flights. Concentration was better, performance was better. Eventually, researchers realized that pregnenolone had anti-inflammatory abilities and testing started on rheumatoid arthritis, lupus, osteoarthritis and other auto immune conditions. They found it had some benefits. However, about the same time, another hormone called cortisol was being evaluated. Cortisol is also made in the adrenal glands and has powerful anti-inflammatory abilities. Cortisol basically stole the limelight. Scientists doing research on pregnenolone put it aside. There are quite a few studies in the '40s, and in 1950 and 1951, then hardly anything up to 1996, 1997.

"If it weren't for the 1994 Dietary Supplement law that allowed a lot of these natural hormones and nutrients to be marketed, pregnenolone would have still been ignored. It's a shame because there is so much potential in this hormone. I was familiar with some of the studies done on mice and rats concluding that pregnenolone was one of the most potent memory enhancers. So when pregnenolone came on the market, I called up a lot of my colleagues and asked them, 'Have you ever tried this?' None of the health professionals I called had tried it. I called a lot of people in the vanguard of using new supplements and nobody seemed to know anything about it. I thought since it was available to the public, is a hormone, since I had written about melatonin and DHEA, people were going to use this hormone and I'd better learn more about it. Before I write anything, I take it myself because I need to know what it does in my own body. If I'm going to recommend it for somebody else, I need to take it.

"I bought a bottle of 10 milligram pills and started in the morning. I took it for about a week and honestly, I didn't feel much. The year before, I had taken DHEA, also I starting with 10 milligrams. I had felt a little bit of energy, a little bit of mood elevation, so I thought maybe pregnenolone didn't have the ability to cross the blood brain barrier in the brain. Maybe it just didn't do anything to the human body.

"About a week later, I increased the dosage to 20 milligrams, two pills in the morning. I thought I felt a little more energetic and alert. I could stay up a little bit later in the evening and still be active, but I still wasn't sure if that was a placebo effect. About a week after that, I went up to 30 milligrams, three pills in the morning. That day, I was really busy. I forgot that I had taken the 30 milligrams. I take a walk every evening, about four-miles, so I was walking in Venice, California on the oceanfront walk, about six or seven p.m., when I realized that a pleasant, harmonious, almost continuous sense of mild well being had come on. It wasn't euphoria, just a mild sense of well being. When I looked around, it suddenly seemed that everything was sharper, clearer. Colors were brighter. When I stopped and looked at a rose, a pink rose, it wasn't just a pink rose, there were shades of pink within it. Everything seemed like the best vision I'd ever had.

"I thought this was really strange. I kept walking, noticing patterns, windows, more flowers. It seemed that my perception had increased. Instead of just going up to my normal two mile mark and turning around, I kept walking and walking. I did six, seven or eight miles, came home, put on some music and the music even sounded better.

"The next day I didn't take any pregnenolone. I went to the library and got the research published in the '40s and '50s, all of it, read it all, word by word. I couldn't find anything about visual and auditory enhancement. One thing they did mention in the study of factory workers was that quite a number had noticed an enhanced sense of well being.

"The study of the pilots in simulated flight also mentioned an enhancement of well being, but nothing about visual and auditory enhancements. So I wasn't sure if it was just me experiencing this.

"Over the next few weeks and months, I recommended it to quite a few patients and friends. I talked to other health care practitioners who had heard about pregnenolone and were starting to use it. Quite a few had noticed clarity of vision on it.

"It became a passion for me other the next few months to learn as much as I could. I've tried pregnenolone in dosages from 5 milligrams to 60 milligrams. I've tried it in a variety of products over the counter. I've tried it in a variety of forms. It comes in sublingual, regular pills, micronized pills, cream, all kinds of forms. It comes in combination with DHEA and other nutrients like ginkgo and phosphatidyl serine and many others.

"The most significant area for using pregnenolone is as replacement therapy in our older years, our 40s, 50s and beyond. Our concept of hormone replacement is going to expand to include more than just estrogen, or testosterone. It can be used for an enhanced sense of mood, slight memory improvement, awareness, mental ability enhancement,. clarity of thinking, maybe a little more creativity. A lot of aspects of our mental condition will be helped because pregnenolone is made in the human brain, like DHEA. The enzymes are available that convert cholesterol into pregnenolone within the human brain, so these neurosteroids are within the brain, they have a function there. As we age, their levels decline and it would be appropriate in our older years to take tiny doses of these things.

"But until we learn more about this and DHEA and melatonin, the dosages need to be minimal. We do not know the long term consequences of giving high doses. Generally, my dosages are between 2 milligrams and 10 milligrams. I definitely do not recommend dosages as high as 50 milligrams of pregnenolone or DHEA. I've heard of cases of heart irregularities when people took 50 or 100 milligrams of DHEA or pregnenolone. An 80 year old woman felt palpitations in her heart the very day she took 25 mg of pregnenolone.

"I have urged all health food stores to not sell pregnenolone in dosages greater than 10 mg. Many buyers are buying the 25 and 50 mg pills and popping more than one a day. More is not necessarily better and is not a motto to live by when it comes to hormones. Besides my concern with the rare instance of heart irregularities, we have no idea how high dosages will influence tumor formation especially of the prostate gland, breast, ovary, and other tissues. You can go up to 15 or 20, but on a regular basis, stay on the very low dosages.

"In 1997, I attended a natural health show where I walked around the hundreds of booths set up by vitamin companies. It was amazing how many new supplements had been introduced—stevia, pyruvate, NADH, CLA (conjugated linoleic acid), silica, chitosan, androstene-dione, shark liver oil, 5-hydroxy-tryptophan, ultimate protein powders, stinging nettles, DHA (not DHEA, but docosahexaenoic acid), and others. Outlandish claims were made about a few of these supplements by some of their promoters. What were these claims based on? Nothing convincing. Sometimes a simple laboratory study done in an obscure part of the world on a small group of mice.

"Many of these nutrients, hormones, and supplements have not necessarily been proven safe before their introduction to the market. It may take months and years before any of their side effects are noticed. Often, these side effects occur when high dosages are consumed for prolonged periods."

For cell biologist Dr. Parris Kidd, the "single most important nutrient for good brain functioning is phosphatidylserine. It is part of a class of nutrients that is probably as fundamental to our health as the antioxidants are because, like the antioxidants, phosphatidylserine and its related substance phosphatidylcholine help protect our cells and tissues. They detoxify and support replacement of dead and damaged tissue, including brain cells.

"This class of nutrients used to be called lecithin, but now we have far more potent sources of PS. PS is a crucial building block for the nerve cells that make up the networks in the brain. It works particularly well because it is part of the membranes, those thin ribbons of material that are wound back and forth within the body of the cell. These enclose the cell and work inside it as surfaces on which the enzymes function to carry out metabolism, which is energy conversion. So PS is involved in the synthesis, the transport, the recycling and the functional action of all the chemical transmitters of the brain. All of these rely on the membranes working right, and nerve cell membranes rely heavily on PS to work right.

"As the brain ages, it fails to make phosphatidylserine or it substantially decreases in efficiency. As we get older, we seem to need more of it. There is not very much of it in our foods except in brain and people don't eat brain very often. Brain as a food is not so safe anymore. When people in their 50s, 60s and older receive supplemental phosphatidyl serine, all of their measurable brain functions improve. Energy consumption by the brain improves, electrical currents improve, the different brain zones are better integrated functionally, the chemical transmitters go back into the normal range. Dysfunction of memory, learning, concentration and even mood and coping with stress—all seem to benefit.

"There have been more than 60 human studies on PS, of which 18 have been conducted double blind. Numerous animal studies confirm these benefits and it seems that PS works at such a profound level of function in the brain through the cell membranes that it can support just about any aspect of brain renewal. Very definitely, the human brain can renew itself. New nerve cells can be made, and existing cells can re-extend their networks and rebuild to full levels of cognitive function.

"In clinical trials, PS was able to turn back the clock on memory loss by 12 years. That is, in matching up names and faces. People were testing at about 64 years of age and at the end of the trial, they were testing 52 years of age. So it actually turned back the clock on a measurable aspect of memory loss. It can also benefit persons who have motor problems and tremors as well as hallucinatory dysfunctions. It seems to be very good for mood as well.

"The recommended dosage can be from 100 milligrams to 300 milligrams per day, depending on the severity of problems. The clinical trials used 200 to 300 milligrams in two divided doses per day with meals. In some people, doses up to 600 milligrams may be necessary and these are tolerated without any significant problems. Benefits often begin at around three or four weeks, but they continue all the time the person stays on PS. In the trials, even after being taken off PS, people sometimes continued to improve. I think they should probably stay on it because it is a very safe nutrient. It has a very good benefit-risk type of profile and is not at all incompatible with other nutrients or even pharmaceuticals. I think PS is very, very good news for the brain."

Linda Toth has a Ph.D. in communications from UCLA and is a senior staff health writer for the *Journal of Longevity Research.* Increasing memory or brain power is one of her major concerns.

"Remember," she says, "that half of all the body's nerve cells are located in your head. Actually, a young baby has many more brain cells than an adult. Around age 10—we don't know why or how—the brain itself starts snipping away brain cells. We think it is so the cells don't continue growing and put pressure on the skull, which won't be enlarging too much more after the age of 10.

"The adult brain only weighs three pounds or less, about two percent of your total body weight, and yet 25 percent of all your body's energy is used to conduct memory activities. The brain reacts to any incoming signal in 1/30th of a second. It has about 100 billion nerve cells and each nerve cell shares information with up to 10,000 other tiny nerves in just the flick of an eye.

"People compare our brain to a computer. It really ought to be the other way around because even the laser computers they're developing now can't compare. The brain has evolved over the eons. Lower forms of life, like a reptile, just have a brain stem. But as the brain developed a mid brain and then the fore brain—that's where the cerebral reasoning function is—a very important center was developed deep inside the brain called the limbic system. If you were to take the brain out and spread it out, it would cover about three square feet. The brain in its evolution is like a piece of thin fabric that has been folded inside and molded into a ball to fit inside the skull. Deep inside that outer covering, what we call the gray matter, is the limbic system.

"Until about 10 years ago, we didn't know very much about the limbic system. For most of the 20th century, people thought it wasn't important. in the last 10 years with sophisticated electronic surveillance devices of the brain, we know that the limbic system controls our emotions, it controls short term and long term memory, and it is a very important part of the brain to protect.

"Memory usually fails today because of nutrient deficiency—high levels of salt, sugar, or processed foods are a big problem for the brain, because it needs enzymes. It's one gigantic laboratory of chemical reactions and various substances. We're not even exactly certain how many amino acids, we think it could be as many as 5,000 various amino acids in the brain, and these amino acid reactions are going on all the time. The brain is like a wheel, it never stops turning until you die.

"So nutrient deficiency is a big cause of memory loss. To save our memory, people can make sure they get live food and limit the foods that are highly processed in any way with heat. The second area is any kind of drug abuse, including prescription drugs. When you use recreational drugs like cocaine or speed, it's like putting a blow torch on your delicate brain cells. People who have a chronic long term use of these kinds of drugs tend to lose memory much faster than other people. Other causes are depression that comes from stress, alcohol abuse, brain disorders or injuries, or a tumor.

"But the most common reason for memory loss is some kind of cardio-vascular dysfunction, where the blood vessels that carry oxygen and blood and food substances to the brain are stopped, either by a narrowing of those arteries or a blood clot.

"The culprit might also be free radical damage. free radicals are extremely small ions that are on the loose, looking for a positive marriage or bonding with another electron in order to be stable. When they're unstable, they go looking for another ion and will actually steal an electron from a healthy cell. Free radical damage is caused by pesticides—in our foods, in the air, in the water, pesticides that we might touch. Also, by heavy metals in water, smog, air pollution. Household chemicals with chlorine, bleach or ammonia. I warn people never to mix ammonia and any kind of chlorine bleach product together, it is extremely neuro-toxic.

"The hypothalamus is critical. In the limbic system, it regulates weight and temperature. It also is the place where immune function starts, signaling the bone marrow to produce killer T cells and white blood cells to fight poisons in the body. If the hypothalamus gets damaged by mercury, aluminum or other chemicals in the environment, the brain doesn't have any way to protect the body. The immune system can be entirely compromised.

"Lest this sound like doomsday, let me predict that within 25 to 50 years, medical science will be treating most illnesses through the brain. We wont be needing surgery or prescription drugs so much. We will be able to stop disease before it begins. We're not there yet, but it's coming.

"Food allergies can cause memory loss, as can candida and yeast infections, the toxins from that yeast get into the brain. Certainly intestinal parasites, which also overgrow in the intestine for various reasons. You'll be told, well these are large molecules, there's no chance of them passing through the villai of the stomach or even the blood brain barrier, but research in Germany in the last 25 years has clearly demonstrated that large molecules can pass through these various membranes in the brain.

"Another big area of unsuspected memory loss are taste enhancers. These are chemicals that actually exist in the brain, glutamate, cystine, aspartic acid, but they put them in food because it excites the brain, the brain knows these amino acids, but when you get an imbalance in the brain, what happens is, it's like burning the filament out on a light bulb and so people need to watch taste enhancers. If you look on food packages, you'll find that these things are being hidden very cleverly. They very seldom tell you anymore, "monosodium glutamate," they say things like "natural flavoring, natural seasoning, herbs and spices, or spices." Be suspicious that that is a taste enhancer. In the mid '80s the food industry went to the FDA and got legislation passed under something called proprietary rights, which means they can hide their formula in food substances, they don't have to tell you that this is MSG."

Dr. Joseph Debe suggests that anyone who is concerned with mental/emotional symptoms and also protecting themselves against Alzheimer's disease and other neuro-degenerative diseases investigate a variety of special evaluative tests. One of these is an organic acid analysis. "Organic acids are metabolic intermediate compounds. They are compounds produced by the body in the course of metabolism and normally shouldn't appear in the urine in any concentration. When any particular one of these organic acids is elevated, it has a meaning. Some organic acids play a key role in producing energy, which is required to produce neurotransmitters. If we don't have adequate energy production, the neurotransmitter levels will fall. The organic acid analysis helps us get an idea as to whether serotonin levels are too low, whether dopamine or epinephrine levels are too low and then therapy can be more precise.

"The organic acid analysis also gives insight into the body's ability to detoxify. It shows the possible need for specific nutrients such as individual B vitamins, alpha liopic acid, coenzyme Q10. With this test, you can be sure that you need a particular nutrient rather than just using a shot gun approach. And the organic acid analysis also measures waste products from different organisms from bacteria, yeast and parasites.

"Anyone desiring a work up for mental/emotional disturbances should have a hair analysis, which measures toxic metals and also mineral levels as well. Another important test is the adrenal stress index, a salivary test that measures levels of long-acting stress hormones, cortisol and DHEA. If you take DHEA when your body produces enough of it, it can increase the risk of imbalance of other hormones including testosterone and estrogen. That can be related to certain cancers. So it's important that you have these hormones measured before you engage in any therapy to modulate their levels.

"The red blood cell fatty acid analysis involves taking a blood sample and measuring the concentration of the different fatty acids. Two of these are very important for mental/emotional functioning. One is called DHA and the other one is called arachadonic acid. Probably most Americans are deficient in DHA because we are not getting it from our foods. DHA is found in highest concentration in cold water fish. But most Americans don't eat enough of it. The body can also make DHA from flax seed oil, but there are a variety of conditions that impact the body's ability to do so and the red blood cell fatty acid analysis can tell us whether the body is actually making that conversion or not.

"Another test that is very important for evaluating mental/emotional disorders is the amino acid analysis. The amino acids are the building blocks, the precursors for the neurotransmitters. Tryptophane is the precursor for serotonin. Tyrosine is the precursor the body uses to make dopamine and norepinephrine. These different neurotransmitters are deficient in depression, in schizophrenia, in ADHD, very common neurological conditions. With the amino acid analysis we can determine if we need to supplement for those particular compounds. And the amino acid analysis also gives us insight into nutrient deficiencies."

Herbalist Letha Hadady points us toward a couple of good memory herbs. "The simplest one is gotu kola, which helps rebuild our nervous system and our brain. Take gotu kola capsules all day for better clarity during the day and better sleep at night. I have a good memory soup that re-nourishes the brain and has a number of moistening blood building herbs. The recipe is:

"A handful each of polygonatum, which nourishes blood vessels and bone marrow; lycium, a blood builder; cornus, a bitter dried form of cherry that strengthens adrenal glands; schizandra to keep moisture and strength in and prevents excess sweating from weakness; acornus, polygala, these work also to strengthen the adrenal glands; hawthorn, fuling, that also help in digestion.

"This soup builds blood, rebuilds bone marrow, which nourishes our brain, and keeps us from sweating too much by strengthening the adrenal glands. It's a way of building energy and holding it in so we don't lose it. That's a good approach with herbs, build energy and hold it in. With our breath and with our mind, breathe in healing energy and send out love, that will open all the doors for our self healing."

II
$\mathcal{D}$ISORDERS
IN CHILDREN

Often, those most susceptible to environmental illnesses and to misdiagnoses by conventionally trained physicians are also those who are least able to protect themselves from the dangers these problems pose. Our children live in environments we create for them, and they either benefit by or suffer from the changes we make in those environments. A range of behavioral, affective, and mental disorders affects children primarily. They are discussed in the following chapters.

In many cases, the culprit is found to be environmental toxins of one type or another. Dr. Harold Buttram has been pointing out since the early 1990s that "while most of our knowledge of the effect of environmental toxins comes from reports of occupational exposure in adults, there is no doubt that developing children are at even greater risk for developing environmental toxin-related illnesses. It is a known fact that pesticides are toxic to the nervous system. Most of our knowledge in this area comes from studies of occupational exposures in adults. What is not known—and all the texts say this—is how toxic are the continual low-dose exposures that are commonly incurred from the environment, and especially, how toxic they are to children. The evidence suggests that there is sufficient toxicity, from residual pesticides in foods, air, and water, and in homes and yards, to cause neurotoxic damage—particularly to children or to the fetus during pregnancy.

"All the scientific literature emphasizes that the fetus and young children are far more vulnerable to toxic chemicals than adults are," Dr. Buttram adds. "And yet the government standards for limitations of pesticides are set by adult standards, which do not take into account the heightened susceptibility of children.

"In order to assess the damage caused by pesticides and other toxic chemicals to the nervous and immune systems in children, every educated person should read a government publication entitled *Neurotoxicity: Identifying and Controlling Poisons of the Nervous System*. It points out that behavioral problems are one of the earliest signs of chemical toxicity, which is what we are seeing in children today. In fact, researchers in the field of chemical toxicity are extremely concerned about the impact of environmental chemicals on children."

12
*A*GGRESSION

A Personal Account of Aggression:
"Brittany"

I am Brittany's mother. Just after she was born, when she was about three weeks old, she started having recurring ear infections. She was always going on antibiotics—literally every two weeks—until she was about two years old. At that time a friend introduced us to an allergist in Massachusetts, who put her through allergy testing and treatment. We changed our daughter's diet after finding that there were certain foods to which she was severely allergic, such as chicken, sugar, and dairy.

After a year of allergy therapy, she is doing much better. She is a relatively calm child; she can play nicely by herself and has a very good temperament. She is one of these kids that, if you have to give her an injection, she'll just sit there and maybe giggle. But when she has sugar or chicken, she turns into a little animal. She becomes extremely cranky, gets almost violent. She will want to hit you; she will cling to me and to her father.

We didn't understand what was happening until we started to see a pattern. When we found out she was allergic to these things, we started to understand that eating these foods was what caused the tantrum-like behavior. Also, her infections completely stopped during the treatment. When she went off of the allergy treatments for a little while, because our insurance would not pay for them, her ear infections immediately returned along with the other symptoms.

Before we went to the allergist, I had talked to several doctors. We had gone to the best doctors and to different children's hospitals. Their answers were operations for her ears and medication to help calm her down if necessary. After a while the doctors started to treat me like a neurotic mother, implying that I must be doing something wrong for my child to be doing this. Or else they said she was going through a phase and would grow out of it. Both those kinds of attitudes got very frustrating.

This experience has taught me to trust myself. As a mother, you absolutely know your child, and if you feel that the physician you are talking to isn't correct, then you should question it, and go with your gut instinct because chances are you're probably right. As a parent, you know your child best. Since we've been working with Dr. Buttram, Brittany is doing much better, staying on the diet and avoiding foods to which she's sensitive. The main thing I would say is, trust your instincts and keep looking until you find what works.

As Dr. Doris Rapp explains, aggression, an important issue for some children, often has an environmental root cause. "Aggression can be due to dust, pollen, molds, foods, and chemicals. Any of these things can turn an absolute angel into a tyrant in seconds. A frequent clue to an allergic reaction is that affected children develop red earlobes, wiggly legs, red cheeks, a red nose, and sometimes a spacey look in the eyes. At times these children can be very nasty and aggressive, with a frightening demonic look in their eyes. They throw out their lower lip and their eyes are half-shut and they look as if they are going to kill you. I've seen this in three-year-old children who eat the wrong food, or if we just take one drop of an allergy extract containing a substance to which they are sensitive and prick their arm with it.

"We have videotapes documenting what we're talking about. However, insurance companies are very reluctant to pay for this kind of medical care, even though many times specialists in environmental medicine can see patients and relieve symptoms that haven't been helped by all the other medical specialists. They pay for medical care that does not help and don't pay for care that does help. We must ask why. Insurance companies say environmental medicine is experimental and anecdotal. If we take two hours taking a history and do extensive patient or parent teaching to show them how to figure out answers so they can finally detect what's causing the problem, on a long-term basis, it is time well spent. That individual stands a chance of remaining well and not needing drugs or hospitalization once the true cause has been identified and eliminated. Insurance companies should be delighted because, in the long run, this approach saves an enormous amount of their money, as well as preserving the well-being and preventing the heartache for so many patients and family members.

"Insurance companies are reluctant to pay the environmental specialist, but will very quickly pay the hospital. Each day in the hospital can cost $1000. The total cost for environmental treatment of a serious condition would be much less than a week in the hospital.

"I have seen a number of children who have been so difficult in school that they have been singled out by school officials. First, all the usual quieting drugs were tried, and when nothing helped, they were told that they would have to be institutionalized. We have videotapes showing that these same children can be turned around. They act great, until we give them a particular food to eat or skin test them with one drop of an allergy extract solution containing the item that bothers them. Within minutes, they are absolutely uncontrollable. Four people have to hold them down. They are spitting, hitting, kicking, and then we give them the right one drop, the correct dilution of that same substance that caused the problem, and they are right back to normal. This newer, more precise, allergy detection is called provocation/neutralization allergy testing. No, we can't explain why this happens. The body is smarter than the doctors.

"I have a number of patients who were going to be institutionalized and who did not need to be. I have seen many other children who were put in classes for the learning disabled because they've been classified as learning disabled or as having conceptual understanding problems or perceptual disorders of various sorts. Many times they fall between the cracks. The school doesn't know how to classify them, if, for example, they display 'autistic-like' behavior. Some (although certainly not all) of these children have responded beautifully to allergy care. Their grades go up significantly. One child's IQ changed from 57 to 125 in a period of 19 months. Some of the children have been returned to be in the classroom with their peers. Many of them can switch from home teaching to school if the parent can pay to have an air purifier put in the classroom," Dr. Rapp concludes.

An even more disturbing cause of aggression in children, teen-agers and adults, too, can be traced directly to the numbers and kinds of psychiatric drugs they have been taking. Dr. Peter Breggin, a leading critic of Ritalin and Prozac and medical consultant in several lawsuits brought against the pharmaceutical companies that manufacture those and other drugs, calls Attention Deficit Disorder "a disease of the professionals rather than of the children." The "professionals" remind him of the authorities in Aldous Huxley's *Brave New World*, except "actually, in *Brave New World* the children did not get drugs. We have reached a level of obscenity in the way we treat our kids that was not even imagined in that fantasy.

"All of these drugs can produce psychosis and violence. I went back and took a good look at the literature again. I found a controlled clinical trial at Yale in which a twelve-year-old boy dropped out of school. This little boy was on Prozac and he quit because he was having nightmares of going to school and killing his classmates and being killed. These were getting worse. He was losing track of what was reality. His symptoms went away when the Prozac was stopped. In the same study, a girl who was taking Prozac developed a violent psychosis and was attacking her stuffed animals. She did not recover when the Prozac was stopped.

"Both cases were published in a major medical journal as probable Prozac reactions. Yet the experts, my colleagues in psychiatry, get on the radio, TV, newspapers, and say there is no evidence at all for this reaction when there is a great deal of evidence. Prozac, in one recent study, produced mania in six percent of the children and they had to drop out of the study. Luvox, which is another antidepressant very similar to Prozac, caused a four percent rate of mania in a similar study.

"These rates are occurring in little four to six week trials, where the kids are carefully monitored. When you have somebody out in the community taking these drugs and not being monitored every week, their parents are not as involved as the ones whose children are in clinical trials, so your rates of kids getting out of control are going to be even higher in the general population. We are creating thousands and thousands of episodes of manic psychosis in our children.

"My colleagues are so unwilling to face the truth. They end saying that these kids have manic depression. So if your child gets manic on Prozac, instead of being told—Hey, I'm sorry, we gave your child a drug that induced mania—the parents are going to be lied to and told that the child's manic depressive disorder just happened to come out now. We won't even stop the Prozac. We may increase the Prozac, Zoloft, Celexa or the Paxil, these knock-off Prozac drugs. We'll increase it and we will give the child Lithium or Depicot or something else. In my clinical practice, I see kids on three and four drugs by the time they are twelve. The doctor declares the child to have one or the other disease or disorder when it is, in fact, drug induced."

Drug-induced aggression and violence nearly made it into the headlines as a result of what seemed like another epidemic—school shootings. "A large number of the kids that have been committing incredible acts of violence have been taking psychiatric drugs," Dr. Breggin says: "Kip Kinkle, the Oregon shooter, was taking Prozac and Ritalin some time before the shooting; T. J. Solomon, who did the shooting in Georgia, on May 20, 1999, was on Ritalin. Eric Harris, the leader in the tragedy in Colorado in April, 1999, was taking the psychiatric drug Luvox at the time of the murders. Luvox is approved for children and youth with obsessive compulsive disorder, but doctors often give it for depression, since it is in the same class as Prozac, Zoloft and Paxil. While psychiatric drug use is only one of the contributing factors to the episodes of school violence, it is one of the most easily prevented factors. There is strong scientific evidence to support the view that these drugs should not be given to children and teenagers."

Dennis Clarke, chair of the Executive Advisory Board of the Citizen's Commission on Human Rights, expands our understand of drug-induced violence to include some well known mass murderers. "In Austin, Texas in 1966, Charles Whitman went up into the Texas Tower, the first school shooting in the United States. Forty-eight hours later, the FBI held a press conference and said no drugs were found in Whitman's body. This is the same report that we got on the incident at Columbine High School with Eric Harris. No drugs were found in the body. Now we learn that, in fact, Whitman had been on prescription amphetamines. He was displaying a classic amphetamine psychosis. According to the FBI, he had been eating amphetamines like popcorn while he was up on the tower shooting people. Had we learned that at the time, it would have changed the whole course of what we're doing with amphetamines and amphetamine-type drugs like Ritalin in this country.

"When we go back and inspect the Richard Speck murders in Chicago 1966, we find out that Richard Speck was on a combination of LSD, which was a prescription psychiatric drug in 1966, and amphetamines, which were a prescription psychiatric drug in 1966 and still are, and that he was also drinking alcohol. Without these powerful mind altering drugs, we would not have the violence that we have in our society today.

"No one has a problem attributing increases in violence within the inner cities to the use of crack cocaine. That's 'those people over there' for the majority of the Americans. But the fact is that the rise of senseless violence among white children and young adults is directly connected to drugs, only they are legal drugs."

13

ATTENTION DEFICIT DISORDER AND HYPERACTIVITY

A Personal Account of Attention Deficit Disorder: "Tim"

I am the mother of Timothy, who is five years old. Since his birth, I've been trying to find out what was wrong with him. It's really been a personal battle. Many people looked at me cross-eyed and said that he is a normal little boy, he is just growing; or he is immature; or it is my fault because I don't discipline him properly; I am not stern enough, they said, and I should introduce physical punishment.

Since Tim was my first child, I had nothing to compare his behavior to and since I was coming out of the corporate world, I didn't really know with whom I could share my doubts and insecurities. I felt very vulnerable exposing myself to other mothers and saying, "I can't do this. What's wrong with my child?"

By the time Tim was three, there were times when I just couldn't stand being a mother. All I did was say "No, no, no" all the time. He started doing dangerous things to his younger brother, such as pushing him down the basement stairs in a walker. And I thought, "This is not Timothy. He knows that that is not right." There was a look in his eye, and I thought, "What has possessed him to do this?" I knew something wasn't right, but I was told he was acting out because of his new brother, that this was typical, and not to worry, to discipline him as necessary.

When he was four, his schoolteacher said, "I'm having a difficult time with this child. He is extremely bright, but he can't color in the pictures and he doesn't know how to socialize with other children." So I decided that it was time to go to a child behavior specialist. He said that when Tim could sit still, he demonstrated a high IQ, but he was extremely immature and needed to be observed.

By the time he turned five, his pre-kindergarten teacher suspected an attention-deficit disorder, with hyperactive tendencies and suggested medical care. We brought him to the hospital and the behavior specialist said that Ritalin would be necessary, along with counseling.

Based on our family history of chemical dependency, I felt that Ritalin was not a good option. So I started looking for other possibilities. Two weeks after the diagnosis, we had a birthday party, and I served my boy ice cream, chocolate cake, and a glass of milk. He went totally off the wall. To try to control him, I had the children play school and I asked Tim to recite his ABCs. He stopped at "D." Now, he had known the whole alphabet for a year and he just panicked. He looked so scared, absolutely horrified. He said, "Mommy, I don't know what to do. What comes after D, what comes after D?" I knew it was the food, and that from there, I needed to find an answer.

I happened to see Doris Rapp on a television show, and I picked up her book. I gave my son the multiple-elimination diet that she suggested and the results were unbelievable! The doctors were surprised. The chief of the pediatric staff was extremely intrigued, but because of the way he was trained, he wasn't able to offer me any medical support. But he did support my going to Dr. Buttram until he could learn more himself.

Now that I have figured out that my son's problem is food allergies as well as allergies to environmental substances such as pollens, it really bothers me that medical doctors don't have this fundamental knowl-edge of nutrition. Reviewing the first five years of Tim-othy's life, I notice a pattern. He has always been at his worst during July and August. Now I realize he is severely allergic to ragweed, to the grasses, and to dairy and corn. When he came in contact with these substances all at once, it just gave him a full-barrel effect. In the summertime we would eat fresh corn on the cob, and after, as a wonderful treat for the whole family, we'd jump in the car and go Dairy Queen, with all the ragweed blowing around. As soon as the frost hit, he was much better.

After six months under Dr. Buttram's care, Timothy is a totally changed child. The kindergarten program he will be entering next year has tested him and, in their opinion, he is a normal child and shows no evidence of an attention deficit. Plus there is no hyperactivity and has been none for at least four months.

Attention deficit disorder is a term that describes a wide range of learning problems. Since 1980, hyperactivity has been included in the diagnostic category instead of being treated separately, as it had been before. The list of symptoms includes: short attention span, inability to concentrate, inability to sit still, difficulty following instructions, destructive behavior, tendencies to talk too much or interrupt, inability to wait one's turn, being accident-prone.

It is a very controversial diagnosis. A child is considered to have ADD if they meet eight out of 14 behavioral standards, as observed by their teachers. Since no teachers see a child in the same way, the subjectivity is a big problem. While practitioners agree that we are in the midst of an epidemic of troubled learning and behavior among children, few assign the same kinds of cause to the problem and few are in accord about effective treatment. Opposition to the most common orthodox treatment—the prescription drug Ritalin—has been increasingly widespread and vocal.

Dr. Harold Buttram, who helped Timothy and continues to help other children with many of these symptoms, says that the problem is reaching epidemic proportions. "I always make a point of asking patients of mine who are schoolteachers and have been teaching for 20 or 30 years whether there has been a change in the behavior of children during that time. The replies are consistently emphatic—that there has been a drastic change in children. There are more hyperactivity and attention deficit problems, more learning disorders, and more behavioral problems."

On the other hand, many experts, especially since the late 1990s, are challenging the idea that this is a real mental disorder and objecting to the way children are being stigmatized by it. Some call ADHD (Attention-Deficit Hyperactivity Disorder) a myth or a "wastebasket diagnosis" for everything else the doctors can't find another name for. Many find social and political factors at the root of the epidemic— overcrowded schools, the desire to replace family and teaching with a pharmaceutical control of youngsters, and the profit motive of the drug companies always in search of new markets.

Some of the children's so-called symptoms, they say, are often normal childhood behavior. Or the product of boredom in un-challenging school situations. "The fundamental problem," as Dr. Peter Braughtman puts it, "is that the diagnosis is entirely subjective. Let's say the first period teacher is given a behavior check list, the third period teacher is given a behavior check list, so are a counselor and a playground attendant. You come up with four different views of the child.

"There is no physical marker making this a disease, so it is wholly inappropriate to talk of it having a cause or a treatment or a chemical defect or an allergic basis. As a neurologist for 35 years, it was my duty to each patient to determine whether they have a disease or not. I haven't proven that a patient has a disease until I demonstrate that they have some abnormality. That might require a brain scan to show a mass or a tumor, a chest X-ray to show a tumor, a biopsy to further define the character of the tumor, or a laboratory test to show a chemical abnormality of the blood, urine or other body fluid. When one has a patient with symptoms that persist but no abnormality can be found, one has not proven that there is disease.

ADHD, invented in committee in 1980 at the American Psychiatric Association, has never been proven to be a disease. The whole concept of how to define "attention" is problematic. There is no specific work to refer to to show us what it means. Dr. Tractman points out that the main researcher in the area of attention in the 1970s, Dr. Thomas Mulholland, described a conference of the major experts in this area around the world, none of whom could come up with a satisfactory definition of attention. The methods used to diagnose attention and hyperactive disorders, then, by its very nature, are completely subjective. There is a laundry list of about 100 adjectives to describe a child with attention deficit or hyperactive disorder. Do you need three, do you need five? Is there a hierarchy, which ones are important? You just have a myth.

"Still, there is no question that we see children who have trouble learning in school. This is a reality and this we know is true. In my experience, these children have a very high intelligence. Their intelligence, however, is in the area of creativity, a right brain activity. In school, reading, particularly, is a left brain activity. So what we have is children who are learning with their right brain, trying to do something in an intellectual, cognitive way, and not able to do it."

Dr. Joseph Trachtman tells us that a historical link between brain defects and learning disabilities has colored our view of the problem. "In the scientific literature, starting in the early 1860s, we find a French anatomist named Brocha reporting two people with lesions damaging the left side of the brain. These people had lost their speech—this came to be known as acquired aphasia, aphasia meaning loss of speech. Shortly after that, there were a number of reports about children who had trouble learning and they were labeled with 'congenital aphasia.' From those early reports of congenital aphasia, we get to the label that we have now of ADHD. It has the implied connotation of brain damage, carried over from Brocha's research. In the 1970s, the same condition in children was called 'minimal brain damage,' or MBD. The physicians' handbook for screening MBD was published and supported by Ciba-Geigy, the manufacturers of Ritalin."

When there is a real learning problem, the "number one cause is poor nutrition," says nutritionist Howard Pleper, author of *The ADD Diet Book*. Again, the problem is our lifestyle. Because "we believe in instant gratification. It's easy to go out and get foods with chemicals and additives, especially preservatives, so that if we decide not to eat it today, we can eat it three years from now. Also, the soil in which our food is grown is depleted of the essential nutrients. Even the soil in which 'organic' fruits and vegetables are grown. There are some organic farmers who do not re-mineralize their soil.

"Among the environmental contaminants at play when children have learning or behavior problems are insecticide and pesticide residues in our food and water and metal contamination, especially aluminum or lead toxicity. A holistic pediatrician in Florida says the lead toxicity he finds in children comes not from paint in older homes, but from piping and solder through which lead leaks into the water itself. Indoor air pollution, food allergies and repeated use of antibiotics, which promotes the overgrowth of yeast and leads to candida, are among the causes of this."

Dr. Joseph Debe adds that a recent study of children diagnosed with ADHD found "65 percent had parasites, one-third had yeast over growth and 75 percent had a condition called Leaky Gut Syndrome. Leaky Gut Syndrome is when the intestinal lining is weakened. Normally, the intestinal lining serves two purposes: it allows for absorption of nutrients and at the same, time it keeps toxins from the intestinal tract from making their way into the blood stream. In the 75 percent of these children who had impaired intestinal barrier function, toxins were making their way into the blood stream at greater than normal concentrations. Some of these toxins impair energy production when they become involved in biochemical reactions. One of these chemicals in particular —from yeast—has been associated with childhood autism."

As Dr. Michael Schachter notes, these conditions are frequently improved by cleaning up children's diets and removing fluoride: "Some of these children are sensitive to fluoride, which may cause headaches, hyperactivity, and problems with attention. Fluoride is often present in their drinking water and toothpaste! Some children are prescribed fluoride tablets or given fluoride treatments at their dentists' offices or at school. Some of these children are benefited by removing all sources of fluoride. Additionally, vitamin and mineral supplements, such as magnesium, may be quite helpful.

"Homeopathy can also be extremely useful. I saw one little boy who suffered from recurrent ear infections and was hyperactive. When we gave him the proper homeopathic remedy, removed sugar from his diet, and gave him a little cod liver oil, the pediatricians and specialists who had been following him for his ear infections and asthma were amazed at how beautifully he did; he turned out not to require tubes in his ears, which they had recommended. Also, his attention deficit and concentration span improved."

Dr. Judithye Reichenberg-Ullman has treated hundreds of ADHD children homeopathically. She is worried, first of all, about over-diagnosing. "We hear so many stories from parents about children who have been in a classroom for just two or three weeks and they' re called into a teacher's conference and the teacher suggests have you thought of putting your child on Ritalin?

"Some of these are just active, normal children, and many of them are gifted. Imagine if you had an IQ of 150 or a photographic memory, you'd probably be bored to tears in some of these classes, wanting to find other things to get your attention and to keep you stimulated. It is shocking how many precocious and intelligent children are being diagnosed with ADD. Some of them are put in special education classes. One of the things that happens with homeopathic treatment is that the children get out of those classes, are back in normal classrooms, and they get their imaginative natures and their creativity back. It's very rewarding.

"But we definitely do see children who are bouncing off the walls, completely unable to concentrate, legitimate examples of children with ADD. The characteristics are: drifty, driven and daring. Drifty, as in, 'calling planet earth, do you read me?' Drifty means difficulty concentrating. Many children cannot understand what they read or what's being asked of them in class. They are very, very slow to comprehend and very absent minded, spacey. Their parents have to give them the same instructions four or five times, which leads to a lot of frustration. Driven is 'wired for sound,' impulsive, not thinking before a child does something. Many children grow up to be adults with these same or similar characteristics—unable to sit still, fidgety, squirmy, wandering around the room. Daring actually being reckless. These people can put themselves and other adults or kids in danger of being hurt.

"There is no question that homeopathy can help many of these children. If parent and child stick with treatments for at least six months, we estimate about a 70 percent effectiveness rate in the hands of a experienced homeopathic practitioner.

"Many studies correlate ADD with abnormalities of specific neurotransmitters. A study at the University of California at Irvine in the late 1990s found that children with severe ADD had a decreased sensitivity to dopamine. The homeopathic point of view would be that the neuro transmitters may indeed be found to have a correlation, but that this is a result of the imbalance in the person. Whether you talk about a neurotransmitter imbalance, or something physical like candida, whether you talk about fibromyalgia or a strep throat, from a homeopathic point of view, these are not the causes, these are the results. Homeopathy seeks to go to the root of that energetic imbalance in a person, to address the cause. When the cause is addressed, all of these other things will fall into place.

"Sugar consumption is part of the problem. Many parents say that the day after Halloween, for example, their children are bouncing off the walls, that they notice a definite difference. However, it's not enough in the case of most ADD children to decrease the amount of sugar in the diet. We have very conscious parents in our practice and many of these parents have made these dietary changes. The same is true of allergens—from a homeopathic point of view, this is the result of an imbalance in a person, not the cause of the problem. Most of the kids that we see have seen allergists or addressed the allergies and they're still having problems.

"In homeopathy, each person is treated as a unique human being. There are over 2000 homeopathic medicines. A word of caution: it has taken me about 15 years to really understand homeopathy to the level that I do and we do not recommend self treatment for ADD. It's one thing to self treat colds and flus, you can learn to do that, but not with ADD.

"Here's an example. A 16-year-old named Sherry was referred by her family practice physician. She had a five year history of ADD. She had been on Ritalin since the 6th grade. Without Ritalin, she couldn't focus, she was distracted by noise, by movement, she couldn't concentrate taking tests, she stared off into space and stopped in mid sentence. No matter how much she tried to be quiet she couldn't. She was frequently embarrassing her friends. She would be driving and miss seeing another car because she didn't notice it. She was always fidgeting and fiddling and clicking her nails and tapping. Ritalin had given her hives. It also made her feel like she didn't know herself, that's what she said. Her tendency to procrastination wasn't affected at all by the Ritalin. She also loved pickles, ate them straight from the jar, and she loved to suck on ice. The medicine she needed was called *baratrum album*, it's a plant, and for her that's what was really helpful.

"Another child was brought in because she had lots of problems in school. She was even getting an F in PE. She was getting a D in math. Her mother brought her in because she was being self destructive, mutilating herself, scratching her face, pulling out her hair. She felt that people hated her. She would lash out at her mother verbally, could kick and punch and even threatened to hurt herself with a knife. She had a very different situation and she needed a remedy called *liacin*, which is actually made from a very dilute preparation of rabies. So these children need all different kinds of homeopathic medicines.

"There is a medicine called *stramonium*, which is thorn apple, that we often give to children who, in addition to having difficulty concentrating, have a lot of fears and can be quite violent. So it depends entirely on not just the symptoms of that individual, but the states, in other words, really understanding a person in depth."

Dr. Lendon Smith summarizes some of the history of treating hyperactivity in children, and then describes his own clinical experience: "The man who discovered the paradoxical effects of stimulant drugs on hyperactive children was Charles Bradley from Portland, Oregon. In 1937 and 1938, he found that most children with 'hyperactive syndrome' came from difficult pregnancies, especially those which ended in troublesome deliveries. The hyperactive children were the second of twins or born with the cord around their neck. They were premature, or born with a collapsed lung or too much bilirubin. A number of things might have interfered with the oxygen supply to the brain. The problems had not been enough to hurt the child's intellect but just enough to hurt the part of the brain that has to do with self-control. This was Bradley's original concept.

"Then, in 1938, a mistake was made. Charles Bradley was in charge of a home for problem children when he asked a nurse to give an overly active girl some bromide. The nurse accidentally used the next bottle, Benzedrine, and the girl promptly went to sleep. The doctor commented to the nurse that the bromide sure worked well and the nurse responded by saying, 'What did you say?' The doctor asked, 'What did you give her?' It turned out that this was the first time anybody had ever used a stimulant drug on somebody who already seemed to be overstimulated. That started the seemingly paradoxical treatment approach of giving stimulants to hyperactive children.

"Researchers have since found that the part of the brain primarily affected in hyperactive children is the limbic system. Hyperactive children don't seem to have enough norepinephrine, a brain neurotransmitter, in their limbic system in the little cells that have to do with inhibitory control. That's why Ritalin, Dexedrine, Benzedrine, caffeine to a certain extent, and some other stimulant drugs have a calming effect on these children. They prevent the reuptake of norepinephrine at the synaptic cleft. This is something all neurologists understand.

"I was working with a lot of hyperactive children in my practice in Oregon," Dr. Smith continues. "One of the children I was treating was affected by this syndrome. We found that speed, methamphetamine, was helpful to her. Teachers would send children they suspected of having the syndrome to me.

"I began to notice that these children had certain traits in common.

They had short attention spans and they were unable to disregard unimportant stimuli. Everything came into their nervous system from their eyes, their ears, their skin, and their muscles with equal intensity. They were unable to selectively respond to certain stimuli and to ignore others. They couldn't just pay attention to the teacher, the board, or what was in their workbook.

"We found that many of these children would calm down after being placed on five or ten mg of Ritalin or Dexedrine. If they responded we diagnosed them as having the hyperactive syndrome. If that didn't work then we believed something else to be wrong.

"We had trouble ruling out psychological disorders or problems at home. You can imagine these children disrupting not only the classroom but the home environment as well, resulting in their parents either beating them or finding some other rigid disciplinary measure in their attempts to get these children to settle down and pay attention. Over a period of ten years I saw seven or eight thousand of these children and I noticed a pattern that interested me. I found a ratio of 5:1, boys:girls. This rules out Dr. Bradley's theory that hyperactivity was a result of a hurt to the nervous system. If he was right the ratio would have been 50/50.

"I also found these children to be fair most of the time. They were blue-eyed blondes and green-eyed redheads. We did see some African Americans but in general they were fair-headed and light-skinned. I concluded that some genetic factors were involved here. I also discovered that these hyperactive children generally were very ticklish, goosey, sensitive. When I shined a light in their ears to check their eardrums, the light would bother them as if they could hear a light and see sounds. It was incredible how sensitive they were. The stethoscope was always cold on their chest even though I warmed it up. My gentle hand on their abdomen to palpate the liver and spleen was an irritant and made them giggle and jump off the examining table. They noticed everything.

"As time went on, I started to incorporate nutritional testing and discovered that every single hyperactive child I saw had low levels of calcium and magnesium. I became interested in controlling behavior with diet after I noticed how my daughter responded to foods. If she ate sugary stuff she'd have trouble, but if she ate complex carbohydrates or protein, her level of activity was fairly even. I found that hyperactive children did well when eating five small good meals a day.

"I was hoping to discover a sugar causation and not a hurt to the nervous system. I found that about 15 percent of these children did have some hurt to the nervous system, but that most of them came from family backgrounds of alcoholism, diabetes, and obesity, all sugar problems. I thought, 'Aha, I've got an answer here for hyperactivity. We should just stop the sugar.' It worked in a few cases, but not all.

"Then I saw that most of these children had had ear infections as infants. We know that ear infections in general indicate food sensitivity, usually to dairy products. I discovered that their present diets were usually laced with milk, cheese, ice cream, and lots of other dairy foods. Stopping all dairy helped some of these hyperactive children but it still wasn't the whole answer. It showed that some of these children had trouble absorbing calcium from dairy products because they were allergic to them. Almost all these children had circles under their eyes and had had their tonsils taken out. They had retracted eardrums and would constantly clear their throats. That indicated a sensitivity to dairy products. Their intestinal tracts prevented the uptake of calcium from the milk they were drinking. Their blood and hair levels of calcium and magnesium were very low. Also, they weren't getting the calcium and magnesium they needed. We all know that calcium and magnesium have a calming effect on people.

"After many years of investigation, I had learned that hyperactive children are often ticklish, goosey, and sensitive. They come from a family that has diabetes, obesity, or alcoholism. Generally, they're boys. Their teachers say they're in trouble. An especially important point is that they are usually okay one to one with their mother or father at home alone, but in a class of 30 other kids they cannot function. These children do better in small groups or one-on-one situations. That is ideal for them.

"Drug therapy helps them disregard unimportant stimuli. I found I could produce the same effect in most hyperactive children by giving them the right dose of calcium, usually 100 mg a day, and the right dose of magnesium, usually 500 mg a day. After receiving these minerals, usually 60 to 80 percent could manage without drug medication. It all seemed to fit. There was good evidence to indicate that hyperactive syndrome is related to food allergies, sensitivity to sugar, and not having enough calcium and magnesium.

"The next thing I noticed was that parents and teachers would report that many of these children were off and on, like Jekyll and Hyde. The parents would latch on to that little phrase as being almost diagnostic. That to me meant that it was not a psychiatric condition but a blood sugar fluctuation. It could come from eating sugar or from eating foods to which they were sensitive. We know that if people are sensitive to dairy products, for instance, the blood sugar will rise and get up to maybe 180 mg after eating a dairy food and then drop precipitously down to 60 mg. Then they crave these same dairy products again. They go up and down, up and down.

"If a teacher reports that a child is fine on Monday morning, doing his work and sitting still and then for no good reason on Monday afternoon he is all over the place, falling asleep or being disruptive, we can have a good idea that his behavior is related to something he ate for lunch. We have to carefully monitor the meals he eats and make sure the child doesn't get any particular food he is sensitive to. Along with milk the usual offenders are corn, wheat, soy, and eggs.

"The diet we recommend incorporates good foods as much as possible. Too much fruit may be detrimental due to the sugar. We recommend whole grain foods. We eliminate white bread, white rice, and empty-calorie foods. We don't have candy bars around. We don't have white soda crackers. We don't offer desserts to these children. We suggest good foods, complex carbohydrates, and vegetables, cooked as little as possible. Nibble, nibble, nibble is the rule we emphasize for hyperactive children. The whole family has to change their way of eating. Many of the parents find that they feel better on this diet as well.

"Once people change the diet of the hyperactive children, they find they can get off drugs, the Ritalin, Dexedrine, or whatever else they are on, or reduce the dosage, or take it only on tough exam days. My results showed that 80 percent of these hyperactive children were made 60 to 100 percent better. Most of the children and their parents would notice a change for the better but still feel that something was missing.

"Then I found, as I got more into a nutritional approach, that I needed to incorporate more vitamins. I was missing vitamin B6, pyridoxine. I found that 50–100 mg of pyridoxine was very helpful, especially if the child had trouble with dream recall. This is also good for children who can't seem to concentrate.

"So there were two clues I looked for. I would ask teachers or parents of these children, 'Is he goosey, ticklish, sensitive?' If they were, I would know it had something to do with calcium and magnesium. If they said, 'He has a Jekyll-and-Hyde personality. He's on and off, good and bad,' then I knew the problem was related to diet. As I became more nutritionally aware, I found out that many of these children had trouble with their intestinal tracts. I gave them vitamin shots. They sting. If it really stung and really made them hyper, that was because they weren't absorbing enough calcium. That was another clue. If you have enough calcium in your muscles then the stingy shots aren't so painful.

"Many parents said the vitamin shots were very important and that they really made a difference to the child, but I had no way to figure out how much B12 and B6 to give. It was helpful to me to find out that that could make some difference.

"In the past ten years I have been working with a chemist from Spokane named John Kitkoski who has discovered that most people in North America are somewhat alkaline. This may be the key as to why this condition had become more common in the past couple of decades. The earth is aging and has become more alkaline. The increased incidence of this condition, even though obstetrical management has gotten better, is because our foods have gotten worse and more processed.

"This alkalinity, from which many of us are suffering, is often the key to this problem. If people are somewhat alkaline, the minerals, like calcium and magnesium, are less soluble. It's more difficult for the minerals to work with the enzymes to do all the things that they're supposed to do for the body if the minerals—especially the calcium and the magnesium—are not soluble enough to be usable.

"This is the way we figure out whether someone is alkaline: When we evaluate the blood test, we add the levels of sodium and potassium in the blood, the alkaline elements, and we get a certain sum from that. Then we add the CO_2 and the chloride; these are acidic elements. That sum we subtract from the sum of the sodium and potassium. We should get a value between 6 and 12. Most people are above 12. This accounts for aches and pains, a narrow face, crowded teeth, certain allergies, a spastic colon, trouble absorbing foods. They could be eating the best food in the world, but if they're somewhat alkaline the nutrients in the food may not be available to them.

"This is why many people have found that becoming vegetarian has made a difference for them. Vegetarianism tends to make people more acidic because vinegar is produced. Most vegetarians don't have trouble with high blood pressure.

"We can sometimes spot these people. Say a child of nine or ten is somewhat hyperactive. He has circles under his eyes and he's got a nose full of junk. He's got a nasal sound. We look at his jaw and it's narrow. His front teeth are crowded. We know that this child probably was not breast-fed and that he probably is alkaline and probably drinking cow's milk, to which he is sensitive. Therefore, he's not getting the calcium/magnesium he needs. He's probably craving calcium and magnesium because he knows somehow that he needs it. He doesn't know, however, that he won't be able to absorb it.

"It's been pointed out that most prisoners drink five times the amount of milk that ordinary people do. It may be the same phenomenon. They're looking for the calcium that they cannot absorb although their bodies are telling them they need this.

"So often at bottom it's a whole bunch of things causing the hyperactivity; it's never just one thing," Dr. Smith adds. "We were trained in medical school to make a diagnosis and to treat with a drug. The drug Ritalin is a standard for this. If it works that's a clue to me. If a stimulant has a calming effect then something is wrong with this person's ability to manufacture the right amount of norepinephrine for his limbic system. Therefore I can work on the diet and at the same time slow down the use of the Ritalin, which has side effects, such as leading to shortened stature. As this child grows up he is going to have to face the fact that he has got to change his diet."

Dr. Allan Spreen's approach to treating hyperactivity in both children and adults is very much in line with what we've been hearing from Dr. Smith. As Dr. Spreen states, "I have seen particularly hyperactive children who have an attention span of about two seconds. Often they are called autistic because they can't linger on any subject matter long enough to even begin to learn anything, much less give their parents a moment's peace. Often they are irritated by chemicals in their food that their system wasn't designed to handle: artificial color, artificial flavor, highly refined sugar, and flours and sugars that have had the nutrients required for their assimilation completely removed.

"My approach to hyperactivity is to try to get the individual biochemically in the best nutritional shape, and we usually get really nice results. Some people can have a very slightly sluggish thyroid that might not show up on blood tests. But with very low doses of thyroid, they feel so much better, even though their blood levels still remain normal on blood testing. Their whole emotional make-up improves. Their concentration gets better, and their energy level improves."

Dr. William Crook is on the side of those who believe the disorder belongs to the modern world. "One of the advantages of having treated two generations of children since I left Johns Hopkins in 1949 is that I can say quite clearly that we did not see these children in the 1950s and early 1960s. Children now eat more fast foods, they drink more sodas, they spend more time looking at television than they spend in school, 28 hours per week. Television promotes junk food, television promotes violence. Children are indoors, not exercising, playing kick the can or riding bicycles. They're not getting full spectrum light that they get from sunlight; they're sitting in shaded rooms.

"Children need one-on-one attention. They need to be held, looked at and listened to. In our rushed world today, many parents struggle to do this, but they can't give their children the bed time stories, the hugging, the rocking to sleep, a lot of the things that I grew up with.

"Another big factor is the rise of antibiotic drugs. We were taught in the 1950s, parents and professionals, that antibiotics were wonder drugs. Parents would come in: 'My child has a fever, has an earache, give me an antibiotic,' and most doctors gave them antibiotics, which knocked out some enemy germs, but also knocked out friendly germs, disturbing the normal balance of bacteria in the intestinal tract. This leads to the overgrowths of a number of unfriendly organisms, including not only the common yeast, but other bad bacteria.

"This also creates what is called a leaky gut, so these children absorb food allergens that they would not ordinarily absorb. Food allergens are clearly related to ADHD. There are reports going back in the peer reviewed literature 70 years and double blind studies in the 1990s proving that children with ADHD are clearly sensitive to dietary ingredients. These included not only food but also the food coloring and additives. Also, pesticides in the food. John Wargo from Yale University in a 1996 book describes what is happening to American children because some of the foods that look so beautiful on our supermarket shelves may have been imported from Mexico or other countries where we've shipped DDT and other pesticides.

"I do think discipline is appropriate for misbehavior in hyperactive children. The term discipline, from the Greek, comes from disciple and it really means teaching. You've got to teach the child and there are clear scientific studies to show that rewarding good behavior, even with a smile or a pat, is much better than punishing a behavior that you disapprove of. Some children are difficult and hard to raise and you have to learn that the two to three year old is always getting into things and you don't punish him for doing the things that two to three year olds do. You have to think about what the child is saying, what the behavior means, and then you will be less apt to feel like you have to punish.

"The main danger of prescribing drugs is that you do not get at the cause.

"Suppose someone has a headache. You can relieve it with aspirin or Tylenol, but suppose this person has a slow-growing brain tumor that is not recognized after you mask the pain? The second danger is that the child who takes long term Ritalin is apt to become a juvenile delinquent, to be put in jail. There was a 1987 study in the *Journal of Child and Adolescent Psychiatry* with two groups of Caucasian middle and upper class boys. One group received only Ritalin, the second group, multi-modality therapy, including psychological and educational counseling. Over a number of years, 22 percent of those that received only Ritalin ended up in a mental hospital or a jail. None of the others were institutionalized. There was, I should note, no difference in the two groups in terms of vandalism, marijuana use, alcohol use or petty crime.

"There are many, many nutrients, minerals and vitamins that are useful in treatment. Recent scientific studies support use of omega 3 fatty acids, found in flax seed oil. We know about zinc. Studies of the effect of magnesium go back to at least 1922, when McCollum at Johns

Hopkins put some rats on a low magnesium diet and those who did not get enough magnesium were irritable, had convulsions and some of them died. Much has been publicized for all of us about our needs for calcium, but magnesium is a very important nutrient for children. So are the B vitamins. One study of autistic children, a double blind study, showed that vitamin B6 helped them. In another study, in 1979, one group of children were given vitamin B6 and another group of children were given Ritalin. The children on vitamin B6 did just as well as the children on Ritalin, so again, we have to treat the cause.

"The child's brain or the child's body is like an automobile and if an automobile is putting out blue smoke and getting six miles to the gallon and jumping and jerking, would you not look at the kind of fuel you're putting into the gas tank? We should look at the same thing for our children."

Dr. Mary Ann Block finds that 90 percent of the time, low blood sugar and food allergies or hypersensitivities are the underlying causes of behavior and learning problems. "You find behavior problems commonly in a child who eats too much sugar, doesn't eat enough protein and doesn't eat frequently enough. When they get hungry, they get irritable and agitated and when they eat, they calm down. The number one most likely food allergy—for behavior, eczema or asthma—is cow's milk. From there, it can be many other things—wheat, corn, certainly sugar—usually the food the child likes best and eats the most that is causing the symptoms."

Nutritional supplements are the backbone of her practice. "I recommend magnesium to all my patients because it has a calming effect, it relaxes the body, and if allergies are part of the problem, it can help with that as well. Seventy to eighty percent of the American population is deficient in magnesium, but for the ADHD child, it's imperative. Essential fatty acids are extremely important as is vitamin E—those work together. The mineral chromium is an important nutrient, often referred to as the blood glucose tolerance mineral. It helps the blood sugar stabilize. Almost every single hyperactive child I've seen has had a B vitamin deficiency too.

"I also recommend osteopathic manipulation. This is directly working with the nervous system of the body, very, very gently—it almost doesn't look like they're doing anything—so it's a nice treatment for children. The sympathetic nervous system causes the release of chemicals in our body that make us more hyper and sometimes osteopathic manipulation can help slow that down and get the nervous system more in balance."

Many practitioners, myself included, reserve our severest criticism for the drug Ritalin. Manufacture of Ritalin rose from 3 tons in 1990 to 8.5 tons in 1994, 90 percent of it prescribed in the U.S. By 1996, the International Narcotics Control Board (an agency of the United Nations) reported that 10 to 12 percent of American boys between the ages of 6 and 14 were taking the drug. It was estimated that by the year 2000, Ritalin would be prescribed for more than 8 million children in the United States and that in the future, 22 million children may be placed on it or other activity-modifying drugs. Some doctors prescribe iit for three year olds, although it is not meant for children under six.

Ritalin does provide temporary answers—65 to 70 percent of the children show positive reactions to it—but the question is, what are the side effects?

Howard Pleper says, "This is scary. As I lecture around the country, parents come up to me and say 'my child has been on Ritalin and here are some of the side effects.' One of the biggest is anorexia—children absolutely lose their appetites, they stop eating. Anorexia is an extremely dangerous disease that weakens the immune system. It starts to look like chronic fatigue syndrome. Because Ritalin is a class two drug, like cocaine, withdrawal is extremely difficult when somebody has been on it long term, whether it is a child or an adult. The drug stunts growth. We have found children who have stopped growing, and I've seen some adults on Ritalin for several years who have stopped growing and are close to dwarfism.

"Ritalin causes serious depression. Children become little robots, they sit in class, and teachers love it because they don't cause problems, but the children become so depressed that they go back to the doctor and get put on another psycho tropic drug for depression. A lot of children on Ritalin are not able to sleep at night, either."

Dr. Peter Breggin is even more angry. "We used to beat our kids and we used to think that was okay," he says. "Now that it is no longer generally considered okay to whip the daylights out of a child, more bizarre and potentially more destructively, we think it's fine to give a child toxic substances while the brain is growing.

"We have data on the dangerousness of these drugs. We know they can cause psychosis in children. Animal studies show that when you give amphetamines to animals in the same dose that you give to kids, after only a few times, you get brain cell loss and permanent changes in the brain. That is how these drugs become addictive.

"We have new studies in the late 1990s showing that if you take Ritalin as a child, you are more likely to abuse cocaine as a young adult. These stimulant drugs are considered so addictive that they are in a more addictive class that Valium and Xanax, which everybody knows are addictive sedative tranquilizers. It's astonishing to think that we are willing to do this to our kids.

"When you see what Ritalin does to an animal, it really demolishes the myth that the drug is correcting a biochemical imbalance in the child because there is the same effect on a monkey or a dog or a cat or a rat. These drugs suppress all spontaneity, all autonomy, all searching and exploring behavior. They suppress socializing behavior, they suppress the desire to escape and they enforce—probably because of their effect on the basal ganglia of the brain—compulsive, narrowly focused behavior. An animal like a monkey that was previously desperate to get out of its cage and play with its neighbor will instead sit quietly behind the bars picking at its own skin compulsively instead of grooming another monkey. That's what we do to our kids. We are making good caged children.

"I don't have language strong enough to describe how outrageous it is that literally multi millions of our children are already being suppressed with psychiatric drugs instead of having their needs met. Their needs for everything from nutrition to inspiring education, consistent discipline in the home and unconditional love. They are having their needs unmet while we drug them into submission instead."

Dr. Peter Tractman sees yet another grievous repercussion. "Among the children I have seen, 90 percent or more of those who have been diagnosed ADHD and are on Ritalin, have a vision problem. They have trouble processing information through the vision system and into the brain. Once we give them some remediation and teach them how to process information properly, within about 10 weeks, they are usually reading on grade or very close to grade and the problem is gone.

"The reading problem can actually be caused by the drug. Ritalin's side effects include stunted growth, loss of appetite, baldness, Tourrette's syndrome, nervousness, rapid and irregular heartbeat, and insomnia. It also affects the eye's focusing. So Ritalin inhibits a child's ability to focus on print that is up close, for reading. So a drug with no proven efficacy to improve either cognitive ability or academic ability is given to a child, who suffers these terrible side effects, including his inability to see clearly so he can read."

14
AUTISM

A Personal Account of Autism: "Jamie"

My son Jamie is now three-and-a-half years old. At about 15 months, he began to lose a lot of the qualities seen in normal children. He stopped talking, he stopped interacting, and he stopped making eye contact. All of this pointed toward autism. Before that, he had been very, very healthy and had developed well ahead of his milestones, except for a very long period of ear infections, which were treated by an equally long course of antibiotics. Over time, we became more and more concerned about him.

At about 18 months, he was diagnosed with severe language delay, meaning that he was not doing anything that the average 18-month-old child does to communicate. Also, he had developed a number of rather bizarre behavioral traits, including spinning and staring at the walls and only playing by himself. We saw a child psychiatrist in Maryland where we live. He thought we had a very serious problem, but he wasn't sure it was autism. He wanted us to look into the possibility of allergies and yeast infection. So we found various people to address those issues and Jamie began to improve.

As the improvement continued, he began to speak again, after about six months. But the improvement was somewhat limited. He still didn't interact with other children, even though a lot of the bizarre behavior had receded and he had perked up quite a bit. Looking for further help with the allergies and the developmental problems, because it still seemed as though there was a missing piece, we went to Princeton to see Dr. Baker. Dr. Baker has very thoroughly investigated Jamie's biochemistry and provided treatment and a lot of suggestions and support. Jamie experienced another big jump forward to the point that now his allergies are of relatively little concern, his development is almost on track (about six to eight months behind), and his behavior and his speech are vastly improved. In the fall, he will go to a normal nursery school, although the children will be six to eight months younger than he is. Aside from this, he will be back on track.

We realize that we are able to turn his symptoms on and off by simply modifying his diet, so we try to be careful with what we feed him. Sugar is the biggest offender. He can take it in very small amounts periodically. But if he gets too much of it, it is like shooting a rubber band across the room. He just flies around the house, becomes totally unreasonable, somewhat destructive, and very aggressive. He also becomes overly emotional. He realizes that we are going to try to discipline him for acting out, even though he is aware that his behavior is not really within his control.

> So I think he feels unjustly persecuted when he is
> punished.

Autism is a collection of symptoms usually characterized by a child's inability to use words for language, an absence of eye contact, and an inability to relate well to people—or even to objects. As Dr. Leander Ellis explains, "Little kids with autism don't play with toys; they are in a foggy cocoon of their own.

"An infant's brain is like a do-it-yourself kit that has to be built over a period of about 25 years," Dr. Ellis continues. "If you stop him at any point along the way, particularly in the first three years, you are going to have what we call an autistic child. If you stop him substantially beyond that, you get some attenuation but a child that is on a level that is much higher. If you stop the ones below the age of about three years, they tend to actually regress and lose some of the functions that they have already learned.

"I saw a four-and-a-half year old boy recently. His medical history showed that he had ear infections and multiple exposures to antibiotics, and that regression started around 20 months. Within two weeks after we put him on a milk-free and wheat-free diet, with no sugar and no obvious sources of mold or yeast, he began to talk and play with toys, to make eye contact, and to relate to other people. I put him on a mild anti-fungal agent and he regressed markedly. His mother cut down the dosage to about a quarter of how much I had given him, which was already a small dose, and in about ten days he brightened up. When he came back five weeks after the first evaluation, he walked in with a little spaghetti machine that he was pushing play dough into and cranking out play dough spaghetti, and he said, 'I'm making spaghetti.' He acted like a typical child, asking numerous questions of his parents about everything in the place. He had become a toy fanatic. They joined a toy-lending service, to meet his insatiable desire for toys.

"The child, who is now about six, is reading, drawing, and can sound out some words. He is still mildly hyperactive because he's reacting to the mold in the air, especially in the spring, but he is markedly improved. We also use nutritional support and his mother has him in an intensive tutoring program."

Dr. Sidney Baker offers additional insight into the nature of autism and the limits of our understanding of it. "All doctors are taught that if you get the right diagnosis, then you'll know the treatment for that person. My patient Jamie illustrates an essential problem with this belief. He was originally diagnosed as being autistic and there was relatively little discussion questioning the accuracy of that diagnosis. He really exhibited the classic symptoms of autism. But to say that because we know the diagnosis, we know the treatment for all the people in that illness group, is not a very useful approach. In Jamie, the pattern of biochemical abnormalities was not especially characteristic of autism. Jamie had a subset of problems that may go with that group, including disturbances of digestion (probably a disturbance of the germs that live in his digestive tract, which may be the mediators of the sugar response) and a bunch of other biochemical markers. My approach to treating him was simply to find everything that was out of balance and, keeping an open mind, to say, 'Let's measure as many things as are reasonable to do, step by step, and fix the imbalances where they occur.'

"I don't think that we entirely understand autism, even using this approach. I think that autism is the single most elusive diagnosis to make, at least in terms of finding the key to it. But when you approach children with what you could call this naive approach of fixing imbalances where you find them, it really works quite well. Part of the corrective action involves helping the child to stay away from things that he or she is bothered by—either foods to which he or she is allergic or sugars—and helping him or her get enough of the nutrients that seem to satisfy a particular biochemical need. Early intervention really helps a lot in the future of such children."

Dr. Michael Schachter describes some of the research currently being conducted in autism around the world. "There is some really good research, especially in France, that shows that magnesium and B6 will help considerably—though not cure—autism, much more than some of the drugs that are commonly used, and with fewer side effects. Some ten or 12 double-blind, placebo-controlled studies have shown that magnesium and B6 are helpful for autism in children. I'm working with one young man now who's autistic, and we seem to have run up against some interactions with some of the drugs that he was on (including Inderal and Haldol). But the controlled studies indicate that autism can be helped with magnesium and B6. DMG, dimethylglycine, also seems to be helpful, not only with autism but also with reducing aggressive behavior."

Dr. Jay Lombard admits that "autism is a very tough disease, as any clinician who treats it or any parent who has a child with autism knows. It's a very common disorder because when you incorporate all of the different manifestations of autism, the incidence is much higher that what we previously thought and seems to be increasing. One of the things involved is neurotransmitter abnormalities, in particular serotonin, which is derived from the amino acid tryptophane. Autistic children have too much circulating serotonin, but it is not performing its duties properly, so you get symptoms such as anxiety and sleep disorder. One of the strategies of treating autism is to enhance the beneficial effects of serotonin. This can be done either nutritionally or pharmaceutically. Some of the nutritional compounds that increase brain serotonin levels include L-tryptophane, obviously, because it's a precursor to making serotonin; the herb St. John's Wort acts as a serotonin enhancer in the brain; and a relatively new compound that has gained wide popularity—the modification of the amino acid SAM-e or S adenosyl methionine, which has also been shown to increase brain serotonin levels.

"The other part of treating autism has to do with the immune system, which is over-activated in a lot of children with autism who have chronic ear infection and chronic bowel problems. One of the things that we look at in our practice is excessive yeast involvement. We use probiotics like acidophilus, which helps increase the natural intestinal bacteria in the gut and reduce the amount of yeast.

"There is some evidence that autistic children have problems with the mitochondria in the brain, that they are not making enough brain ATP levels. Two compounds that are particularly effective are cretonne—which should only be given under a doctor's supervision—and a compound called CDP cauline, a form of cauline that helps build up brain cell membrane."

For Dr. Alan Cohen, autism is "basically, a severe behavioral problem, where a child has difficulty interacting and connecting with their environment and with people in general. There really are not too many things done conventionally to help, but there are behavioral programs, behavioral modifications and certain medications.

"A lot of these children have problems with their immune system. They have an increased sensitivity to infection, hyperactivity to vaccinations and as a result, they need to be on repeated courses of antibiotics. This leads to a whole cascade of effects which need to be addressed.

"Number one, there could be problems with the gastrointestinal tract as a result of the repeated courses of antibiotics and poor diet. There could be abnormal digestion, pathological alterations in the bowel flora and, as a result of an upset in the normal bowel flora, increased permeability to antigens, peptides, and microbial toxins, which are produced by the abnormal bacteria in the intestinal tract. The gastrointestinal tract is directly related to the brain because the circulatory system connects both areas. If these toxins, antagonists, and peptides that normally should be secreted are re-absorbed into the blood stream, they can go to areas in the brain and cause disturbance in normal brain function.

"One area I would like to look into is the presence of certain biochemical abnormalities which can be tested. Autistic children may have low levels of certain sulfur amino acids or, very importantly, their livers may not be functioning well either. We always build up our own internal toxins from the food that we eat and also external toxins that we take in from the environment. The main organ that handles all these toxins is the liver.

"The system needs amino acids, vitamins and minerals and other such nutrients to function properly. If this is not functioning properly, these toxins both internal and external will again build up; instead of being excreted into the stool as they should, they will be re-absorbed into the bloodstream. Again, the circulatory system connects our entire body and these potentially harmful molecules and chemicals can end up in the brain, where they cause local inflammation and interfere with normal brain function. You see the effects of this in autistic children, as well as hyperactivity and attention deficit disorder.

"These children also tend to have certain mineral deficiencies, especially zinc and selenium, and this can be tested. A certain group of them tend to have problems with heavy metal toxicity, which at times can be noted on hair analysis and these include antimony, aluminum and arsenic. They also may have a history of subclinical hypothyroidism. The thyroid is extremely important for brain function.

I have a number of children who had hypothyroidism detected based on their body temperature and when they were treated with natural thyroid hormone replacement, their will to concentrate, their behavior, their focusing and overall ability to function improved as well.

"There are certain treatment modalities that people can do. I would have to say this should be supervised by a medical professional. There is a very important consensus report called 'Defeat Autism Now' that people can get information from. Some basic, simple, inexpensive approaches can be tried that may bring a response from the child within 30 to 60 days.

"One is diet. The diet should be very fresh, varied, totally free of additives and preservatives. Avoid gluten, which is in wheat, oats, barley and rye, as well as milk protein. These sometimes cause food allergies, which can also affect the brain. Inflammatory components from allergies can end up in the brain, causing inflammatory reactions. I also suggest eliminating yeast and mold.

"I would advise a trial of avoiding certain common food allergens, including milk, corn, soy, eggs, tomatoes, beef, peanuts, and there are several more, but that should be individualized. Sometimes these children have difficulty breaking down protein and they reabsorb these peptides which are amino acids that tend to mimic or exacerbate neuro transmitter difficulties within the brain. Simply utilizing the enzymes that you get from papaya or pineapple can help to a certain extent.

"At least 18 studies show 30 to 40 percent of children with autism respond to B6 replacement. That dose depends on the child's size and age but could be from 100 to 600 milligrams a day. Also magnesium is extremely important, approximately 200 milligrams a day. Calcium, approximately 200 to 300 milligrams a day. Zinc, between 20 and 40 milligrams a day. Selenium, between 100 and 200 micrograms a day. A multi-vitamin is important, as well as essential fatty acids, including flax seed oil or fish oil. There is also a vitamin-like compound called dimethylglycin which helps oxygenation to the brain.

"In addition, children with a history of being on repeated courses of antibiotics have an alteration in their normal bacteria flora. They have an overgrowth of yeast, which can produce toxins that get into the blood sugar and interfere with normal brain function. Sometimes, a trial of antifungal medication or either Nystatin or Diflucan can be helpful. Other natural approaches that can help keep down the growth of yeast include garlic and citric seed extract and caprolic acid.

"I have seen a large percentage of children treated with traditional means, not benefiting, then switching to a more complementary or holistic approach and making major improvements. This is a little bit more difficult to follow because it requires a lot of input on the part of the patients and the children to follow these dietary recommendations and the supplemental regimes. This takes a family effort and children very much have role models in what their brothers and sisters and their parents are doing. Everyone really needs to follow this approach. All I can say is that it is a very healthy approach for anybody to have a diet free of additives and preservatives, organic as much as possible, pesticide-free. A lot of these children have problems with the detoxification process in the liver and toxins build up. You want to minimize the amount of toxins that they are exposed to, by using organic food, with no pesticides and increased nutrients. A number of vitamins and minerals I talked about are increased in organic foods. All these things could be helpful for a lot of people in the family."

Dr. Alan Cohen is among many people now looking at the possibility that vaccines are at the root of autism. He sees a connection between autism and hyperactivity in kids and attention deficit disorder as well. "It is interesting to note that the epidemic of autism, ADD and ADHD really did not take place until the onset of childhood vaccinations. There may be a connection between certain vaccinations and the onset of these symptoms."

15

ℬEHAVIORAL DISORDERS

A Personal Account of a Behavioral Disorder: "Maria"

My daughter, Maria, has been helped in a dramatic way by alternative medical approaches. A couple of months ago, Maria became wildly uncontrollable. She's only nine years old, but she was going out at five and six o'clock in the morning to shop with homeless people. She would go into violent rages and would sleep only about four or five hours a night. Finally, I couldn't keep her home anymore and so I put her into a psychiatric hospital where they determined that she was suffering from manic depression. They started her on lithium but she wasn't herself; she wasn't conversational the way she usually is, and she was still depressed. She had elevated liver enzymes which, at the hospital, they failed to follow up on. She also had elevated levels of thyroid hormone, which they also failed to follow up on. After three weeks in the hospital, she had calmed down somewhat, and I was able to take her home. She still wasn't well.

I had been consulting with Dr. Slagle while Maria was in the hospital because I have the utmost respect for her and knew that if anyone could figure out what was wrong with my daughter, she could. As soon as Maria came out of the hospital, she had several blood tests done, which showed she had antibodies against her thyroid and that her thyroid levels were fluctuating up and down. Also, she had probably had some sort of liver virus that had precipitated this auto-immune reaction in her thyroid. Dr. Slagle prescribed amino acids, B vitamins, and several other vitamins, as well as a homeopathic cortisone and baby aspirin to help shrink the swelling of her thyroid.

On the second day of her taking the aspirin and the homeopathic cortisone, her behavior became completely normal. It was a miracle. For close to a month and a half, my daughter had been completely out of control, unable to have a conversation, alternating between being hysterical and being completely quiet. I had been so terrified. It was as if I had lost her. And on the second day of the medication, she began to be able to hold conversations; she was completely normal—like herself again. I know that had I not gone to Dr. Slagle, she would have continued on lithium and been somewhat controllable, but not herself.

Dr. Slagle also found that she was highly allergic. My daughter had very allergic reactions to various foods that she was eating on a regular basis. It was clear that her problem had been her immune system and not a psychiatric disorder, which never would have been taken care of had she just stuck with traditional medical doctors, even though she was being seen by some of the best in the country. So thanks to

Dr. Slagle and the alternative medical field in general, I have my daughter back.

Dr. Harold Buttram describes how behavioral disorders in children, such as hyperactivity, are caused by chemicals, and the history of successfully identifying and treating the problem:

"If you spend an hour in a room with a full-blown hyperactive child, you will never forget it. These kids are literally off the wall. They are constantly moving, as they are incapable of spending concentrated attention on any given task, even playing. They're irritable and very often aggressive and hostile. Doris Rapp has shown pictures of some of these children biting their mothers, trying to destroy toys, and this sort of thing. These are extremely disturbed children.

"Parents often use the term Jekyll-and-Hyde to describe their children. When they're doing well they may be sweet and lovable little children. Then, if they eat something to which they're allergic, very often a junk food, you get the Jekyll-and-Hyde transformation. They become ugly and belligerent.

"What actually happens here is the cerebral cortex, the higher center of the brain, literally shuts down and control gets thrown back to the more primitive centers. There is a center at the base of the brain, for instance, that has been shown to be a center for anger. What stimulates this center? Chemicals."

Dr. Buttram points out the link between an increase in environmental toxins over the years and a corresponding increase in behavioral disorders in children. "It is important to point out that there has been a drastic increase in behavioral disorders in children since World War II. Dr. William Crook, a retired pediatrician from Jackson, Tennessee, commented in a talk that when he went into practice as a pediatrician in the early 1950s he never saw a hyperactive child. I think people of my generation—I went to school in the '30s—in thinking back don't remember seeing a child with the hyperactive syndrome.

"It is really an ominous situation. I talked with a psychologist consultant for our school district not long ago and mentioned this subject. She stated that she has noticed among children increasing evidence of autistic tendencies. This is something that she has never really seen before. Thinking it might possibly be a local problem, she called other school districts and found they were observing the same thing.

"What has happened in the past 50 years that has brought about this increase in behavior disorders? According to published reports, before World War II, less than one billion pounds a year of organic chemicals were produced in the United States. By 1963, that number had increased to 163 billion pounds per year. Today it is somewhere around 250 billion pounds per year.

"According to an official publication, approximately 70,000 chemical compounds are now in commercial use. Of these, only about ten percent have had any testing at all for neurotoxicity. Among this ten percent, only a handful have had thorough testing.

"An interesting study was performed on residents of North Carolina, North Dakota, and New Jersey. The investigation assayed the chemicals in indoor air, drinking water, and exhaled breath of 400 subjects. Ten volatile chemicals were found to be present in the exhaled breaths of most patients. These chemicals are therefore extremely prevalent.

"Organic volatile chemicals are lipid or fat soluble. Therefore, they have an affinity for the fatty or lipid tissues of the body. The brain is a primary target because it consists largely of lipid or fatty tissues. It is also a target because of its rich blood supply.

"The primary symptoms of volatile organic compounds are therefore cerebral. They include headaches, dizziness, difficulty with concentration, memory lapses, feelings of fogginess or spaciness, drowsiness, and fatigue.

"It's important to point out that in your standard text of neurotoxicology one of the earliest signs of chemical toxicity is that of behavioral changes. Therefore, I think there are very good reasons for tying in environmental chemicals with the epidemic we're having of behavioral problems such as attention deficit disorder and hyperactivity. The massive increase of environmental chemicals to which these children are exposed is connected to their symptoms.

"A combination of subtle brain damage from environmental chemicals, nutritional deficiencies, a crippling of the detoxification systems of the body, food allergies, and an overgrowth of candida in the system will produce a very sick child. The manifestation of this will be a crippled immune system. This means the child will have more allergies. He or she will be sick a lot of the time and on antibiotics. The brain function cannot possibly be normal; it would be a miracle if it were. The hyperactivity, attention deficit, and behavioral problems, in my opinion, are all actually a continued spectrum of the same thing."

Dr. Buttram identifies several specific groups of environmental chemicals. "Group One consists of toxic heavy metals, of which lead, of course, is the best known. This category would also include mercury, cadmium, aluminum, and others. Our concern here is more with the other category, the volatile organic compounds, which are made up of carbon molecules. The commercial uses of volatile compounds break down into three major classes: formaldehyde, organic solvents, and pesticides.

"Formaldehyde is present in many, many commercial products. It is present in new homes in the building materials, paneling, floors, and ceilings made of plywood or particle board. It's also present in the carpets, fixtures, and furnishings. The bad thing about formaldehyde in a building is that it is very slow to dissipate. Its half-life may be six, seven, or even ten years. It takes this long before it is dissipated to the point at which the building is safe to live in. Formaldehyde is also used in fabrics and is found in many of the clothes we wear.

"Organic solvents are present in hundreds, if not thousands, of products. They are found in perfumes made from synthetic musks, for instance, and in caulking, paint, varnishes, and cleaning solutions, which are often very toxic.

"Pesticides, our last category, may be the most dangerous of all. They are used, of course, to exterminate in homes or out of doors. If you live in a farm or orchard area you may be subject to pesticide drifts. There are also often significant residues in foods, especially in foods imported from countries where there is no regulation in the use of pesticides."

The treatment of the wide range of illnesses arising from environmental chemicals, according to Dr. Buttram, must include education, enhanced nutrition, and nutritional supplements. "The pioneers in this field used to be called clinical ecologists, but they've now changed their name to the American Academy of Environmental Medicine. These are the people who have really broken ground in this area. They're leagues and leagues ahead of the more conventional medical doctors, and they've set the standard for several of the approaches to treatment we recommend.

"First, we educate parents on how to avoid chemicals. For virtually all of them this is a first, because nobody has ever talked to them about these things before. Identifying and eliminating poisons in the home is not usually that difficult. We take a history of the home environment in regard to the building of the home and other possible sources of chemical exposure to the child. We teach parents how to reduce exposure to the more toxic chemicals, such as formaldehyde and volatile sprays.

"The problems that arise often occur due to exposure in school. If you have a cooperative school administration, the problems can usually be solved. But from what I have seen, school staff and administration don't usually recognize the potential hazards to children of chemical exposure and their ignorance of the risks sometimes presents additional obstacles.

"Second, we do nutritional counseling in which we emphasize just plain simple food without chemicals. I detest the term 'health foods' because it's so misleading. I think 'plain foods' is a better term. I ask parents, who are now in their 30s and 40s, to think back about how their grandparents ate two generations ago. In many instances their wasn't ideal, but it was vastly superior to the way people eat today. They ate mostly plain, unadulterated food.

"So the prime emphasis on diet is the avoidance of chemicals. I attended a meeting in Dallas one time where Dr. William Rea was the speaker. He is certainly one of the most highly respected men today in the field of environmental medicine. Dr. Rea said that it's secondary whether a person is a vegetarian or a meat eater. What is far more important today is the avoidance of chemicals—both chemical additives and residual chemicals.

"In our area there are new markets called Fresh Fields that specialize in organic foods. If you're fortunate enough to live near markets such as these you can shop there, especially for organic fresh fruits and vegetables. Doctor's Data has some very good studies showing that organically grown food compared to market food has significantly higher levels of nutrient minerals and lower levels of toxic metals. Eating organic food, then, may be the most important thing of all. Beyond that, you need to focus on balanced nutrition.

"For children I think it is imperative to get organic fruits and fruit juices even if you can't do anything more than this. From the figures

I've seen, fruit and fruit juice tend to be more highly contaminated with pesticide residues than other classes of foods. Children eat more fruit and drink by far more fruit juice than adults. From this source alone, they could very easily ingest toxic levels of pesticide residues.

"There was a book published a few years ago called *Pesticides in the Diets of Infants and Children*, sponsored by the National Research Council, which is one of the highest scientific advisory boards. This book, although scientifically written, really raised Cain about our present screening processes for pesticides and didn't mince words about it either. It claimed that the uncontrolled exposure of our children to these pesticide residues is highly prevalent.

"Third, for practically all children, we recommend a high-quality hypoallergenic multiple vitamin. We use one by Klaire Labs, which makes vitamins separate from minerals. We don't recommend giving large doses. We offer other nutritional supplements in special situations. When candida is present from antibiotic overuse, lactobacillus acidophilus and bifidus are given. When lead and other toxic heavy metals are found, we add a very simple detoxification component to the program, which includes vitamin C and garlic. Garlic is added because it is high in the sulfhydryl amino acids.

"We recommend using a high-quality flaxseed oil. This provides the essential fatty acids for the development of the brain, nervous system, and cell membranes. We emphasize nutrient minerals such as calcium and zinc since we know that these minerals can replace the toxic metals in the body. We particularly recommend beans and lentils, which are also high in sulfhydryl amino acids, because of their detoxification potential. The sulfur in these amino acids actually binds with the lead or other toxic heavy metals and helps to carry them out of the body.

"Food allergy testing is another important component," Dr. Buttram concludes. "Most of these children are allergic to certain foods and some of their major symptom complexes can be related to their food allergies. We can approach this either through elimination diets or else through skin testing, which we commonly do. We find neutralizing doses and treat with sublingual drops. This can work very well. When it does work you have some very grateful parents."

16
CHRONIC DEPRESSION

Just as Dr. Leander Ellis insisted that more children today suffer from behavioral disorders than in the past, Dr. Lendon Smith asserts that more children today suffer from chronic depression. And like Dr. Ellis, Dr. Smith also cites the toxic overload created by environmental chemicals as the cause. Dr. Smith is particularly adamant about the importance of magnesium, and the magnesium deficiencies that have occurred in many children as a result of environmental poisoning.

"Today there are more children who are chronically depressed than there were in the past," begins Dr. Smith. "Our chemistry seems to indicate that chemical deficiencies are involved, e.g., magnesium deficiencies. Mr. Kitkoski, the chemist from Spokane, Washington, whose research I've shared, has spent a lot of time studying the function of electrolytes in the human body. He figured out that we all need the right amount of electrolytes to act as a buffering capacity for the blood. The electrolytes—sodium, potassium, bicarbonate, chloride, a little bit of sulfur, a little bit of magnesium, and some calcium—are all the things that become electrically active when they are dissolved. Electrolytes have to do with controlling the pH, the acid/base balance, which controls what the minerals are doing, which brings us back to magnesium levels.

"I think that all the artificial chemicals that are in our environment and food are exerting a toxic overload on children. It's not just lead, but all the things that we are inhaling and eating, that are in our water, and all the things that are in our food that shouldn't be there, as well as the things that are removed from our food that we need. All these things are having an effect on our children.

"For example, I've visited classes of 25 or 30 children sitting there, restless, shuffling their feet, and I ask, 'How many of you have headaches once or twice a week?' and every hand goes up. I look around and see this sea of pale faces with circles under their eyes, as if they had all just been hit in the stomach. I ask them what they had for breakfast, and while they all said that they had eaten breakfast, it turns out to have been a donut or some other cake or pastry because their parents had no time to fix them a decent meal. Or, if the parents did fix them a decent meal, they wouldn't eat it anyway because they chose to get some candy on the way to school instead.

"I used to speak at the Reading Teachers Association meeting in California every year. Three thousand reading teachers would get together and have a meeting to decide what textbooks and what reading method they would use. They always had their meeting in the first week in November because they all knew they couldn't teach any of the kids until all the Halloween candy had been eaten. The kids were just...gone! So teachers certainly know about children's poor eating habits.

"Stephen Schoenthaler, a sociology professor at the University of California, did an experiment from 1979 to 1984 with almost a million New York City school kids. The kids were given breakfast and lunch, without sugar, color, or flavor additives. Over a period of five years, the achievement scores of the children went up significantly—without a change in the teaching methods. Only the diet had been changed. The kids who were getting the best grades at the end of those five years were the kids who were eating the school foods, so the researchers knew they could have a positive impact with diet. Obviously diet isn't the whole answer to educational problems, but it's a start," Dr. Smith concludes.

17

*F*OOD
ALLERGIES

A Personal Account of Food Allergies: "Alison"

As Alison's mother, I can honestly say that Alison was born crying. She cried for the first two years of her life. I took her to a clinic at the time and found out she was allergic to corn, wheat, and bananas, which caused her to cry every day, all day long. I took her off those foods, and she became a normal, happy two-year-old. She did well for quite a while until she got a problem with a vitamin deficiency, which caused her to be uncontrollable. I couldn't do anything with her. If I wanted her to get dressed she would scream, rant, and rave. It would take me three hours just to get her dressed. After reading an article on vitamins, I put her on vitamin supplements. That's when we realized that she hadn't smiled in six months. Then she was fine again, until two years ago, when she started to scream at me all the time, day in and day out, no matter what I wanted her to do, over absolutely nothing. She would scream at me that her shoes were wrong, her hair was wrong. It would take me all day long just to get her into the shower. At this point she was ten years old. She should have been bathing on her own. I would go pick her up at school and when she was 70 feet away from me, she would scream, "Mom, you are early!" And she would go on and on about why I was early. The next day she'd look at me and she'd scream, "Mom, you are late!" And she would scream the whole way home, until she went up to her room and I would go off somewhere else to get away from her. She got worse and worse all summer, and in the fall, almost two years ago, I took her to Dr. Buttram.

Dr. Buttram diagnosed my daughter as having food allergies: to corn, potatoes, chicken, egg yolks, rice, and chocolate. They put her on these sublingual drops and now I have my normal, happy daughter back again. It was a dramatic change. She had become extremely difficult to live with. She would just scream at me about the most ridiculous things. Nothing was ever right. If she got out of bed—Why didn't I wake her up?—Why didn't I let her sleep?—And she would shriek at the top of her lungs. Some days were worse than others. Now I know that on the days she had a combination of foods or a lot of the foods she was allergic to that she was at her worst. The way that I figured out it was food again was because every once in awhile we would have a great day or two and every once in awhile her diet just happened to not include these things. Then she would be fine. But the next day she'd be right back again with the behavior—totally out of control for long periods of time.

When my mother found out about Alison's behavior, she told me that I myself had been an absolutely horrendous child. Now that Alison had been diagnosed, she understood that I had had food allergies too. Now I understand that children's behavior problems are not always due to what the parent is doing with the child, as far as discipline is concerned. I've had a lot of children; I've been a foster parent for years. When Alison first started this behavior I tried everything in the book and nothing worked. And the thing that told me that something was controlling her, instead of her doing this, was the fact that we would have good days. And it didn't matter what we were doing on a bad day. If I would sit and play with her all day long, and it was a bad day, we would have a bad day. And discipline meant absolutely nothing, because something was controlling Alison. It was a chemical imbalance in her brain that was controlling her because she had absolutely no control over what she did. It was like the food was controlling her. I related it to the behavior of a manic-depressive or a paranoid schizophrenic who has no control over what they are doing.

Now, when I go to the shopping mall, I see kids who I know have food allergies by the way they are crying. My husband used to say I was crazy, but when Alison was two years old and she would cry, I could tell if it was a food-allergy cry or a two-year-old cry by the sound of her voice. It was a different kind of crying. I have friends who complain about their kids constantly and one child in particular I know has food allergies. And the mother will not take him in to be tested. She'd rather complain about it. The biggest obstacle I see to helping children with behavior problems caused by allergies is making parents understand that there is an alternative. You don't have to live like this. You have to ask yourself, "Do I really want my child to live like this?"

I feel bad that Alison was so miserable for so long.

> There are so many kids out there that are this miserable. There are kids in learning disability classes and the parents just don't look any further than their nose. Some parents do make an effort and take their kids to standard allergists who test them, but those doctors may not be able to locate the problem. A friend of mine took her child to a regular allergist who tested him for all the standard things and said he was fine. But he never tested him for half the things to which Alison is allergic and the doctor never questioned the mother about the child's diet.

When people think of child allergies they think of hay fever, asthma, eczema, and hives. But there are many other areas of the body that can be affected by allergies. As Dr. Doris Rapp informs us, "Allergies can cause headaches or stomachaches; they can affect the bladder, causing your child to wet the bed or to have to run to get to the toilet in time. Allergies can cause leg aches, muscle aches, joint aches, sleep problems, behavior problems, and learning problems. Some children will become tense, nervous, and irritable. Others will become withdrawn and unreachable, hiding in corners and pulling away when you go to touch them. Still others will become very hyperactive and aggressive. Often they will bite, hit, scream, and do all kinds of nasty things.

"Most allergists—including myself for my first 18 years in practice —would not recognize this host of physical and emotional symptoms as having been caused by allergies. But I now recognize that dust, molds, pollens, foods, and chemicals can affect almost any area of the body and can cause all of the problems mentioned above in some individuals.

"Now it would be going too far to suspect that every time a child has a headache it is an allergic reaction, or that every time an adult has a bellyache it is due to food sensitivity. But currently, with conventional medical practitioners, this diagnosis is never even considered and is therefore missed too many times. People will have headaches for years and never once consider whether there might some underlying reason for the headache.

"Environmental medicine wants patients to start to take more control of their health. We want you to pay attention to how you feel. If you don't feel well, or you suddenly can't think correctly; if you're confused, or unusually irritable, or emotionally volatile; if you cry or become upset or angry for no reason; you have to start to ask, 'Why am I having this reaction now? What did I eat, touch, or smell?' Our whole society is geared to go to the medicine cabinet for a painkiller or an antihistamine when we should be geared to get a pencil and paper to record what could be causing this problem at this time.

"After we have educated the parents, they often come in to see us knowing exactly what is causing their child's problems. They can tell if it's something inside or outside the house, if it's a food or a chemical. They can pinpoint the cause.

"Basically, why would a child have allergies or environmental illness? One of the main reasons is that their immune system is not up to par. If the immune system is inadequate, we can develop allergies and environmental illness. One way to strengthen the immune system so that your child is less prone to environmental illness or allergy is by using various nutrients. A helpful resource is the book, *Super Immunity in Kids,* which says, basically: If you take the correct nutrients in the correct amounts, you can strengthen the immune system so that you are less apt to become ill from natural things such as pollen, dust, and mold exposures. You will also be less apt to become ill from exposure to infections.

"Now how can a parent tell if their child's learning problems are related to environmental factors? Think back. Does your child say, 'When I go to school in the morning I feel great!'? Or does the child say, 'I feel great when I leave the house and by the time I get to school I don't feel right.'? Or does he say, 'I feel nervous'? Or tired, or irritable, or, 'I have a headache.'? If that happens, you have to think, it might be the fumes on the school bus, or what he ate for breakfast, or what he uses to brush his teeth, or the soap that he uses. You've got to think of everything that he came in contact with before he got on the bus, and then what happened when he was on the bus.

"One way for parents to figure out what's causing the problem is to drive the child to school. If you find he can eat, bathe, wash, and do everything else in the usual manner in the morning and you drive him to school and he's fine, then it's probably the bus that is causing problems. And you can check back and forth a couple of times and try to confirm or negate your suspicions. Now, children who are sensitive to things in the school will frequently notice that their headache starts within an hour. And the headaches frequently become more intense during the day. By Friday afternoon, the headache will be much worse than it was on Monday morning or on Sunday night. At first the headaches may disappear one to four hours after your child leaves school, but later on, if there are too many exposures during the week, you may notice that they don't get better at night and that it might take the whole weekend for the headache to go away.

"Another clue that certain exposures are making your child feel worse is when your child can smell everything before anybody else. She smells natural gas, or smells that perfume across the room, or she can smell food cooking before anybody else. She can smell disinfectants. If these odors bother your child and she can perceive them faster than anybody else, it means that she is probably becoming sensitized to the abundance of chemicals that we have now managed to put in our food, air, water, clothing, homes, schools, and workplaces.

"What else do you notice if a child is sensitive to something in school? The child may get an A one day, and an F the next day in the same subject. It isn't that your child lost brain cells within 24 hours, but it does indicate to me that you should investigate that school to try to find out what could be causing the problem. Is the school dusty or moldy? Are the ventilation ducts open and clean? Was the basement of the school ever flooded? Does it smell worse on damp days? There is nothing worse in present-day schools than some of the synthetic carpets. They are made of chemicals that cause problems. In addition, they use adhesives that are full of other chemicals that cause even more problems. Many of these chemicals are neurotoxic, which means they damage the nervous system, or carcinogenic, which means they can cause cancer.

"Here is a list of symptoms you may recognize from your child's behavior: The ability to hear, talk, or speak clearly is impaired. Your child suddenly speaks too fast—is hyperactive—or doesn't make sense when he talks. An environmental sensitivity can alter children's ability to write, read, or see clearly. Some children develop blurred vision or double vision by the end of the day because of chemical exposures at school. Some develop red earlobes or cheeks, wriggly legs or dark circles under their eyes. All of these signs and symptoms can be caused by an environmental illness.

"If you suspect that your child may have been exposed to neurotoxic substances—those that actually damage the nervous system—ask your doctor to send you to specialists who can tell you whether the nerve conduction time in your child's body is normal or not. They can do a variety of blood tests to find out if the chemicals that are in the carpets and the adhesives are in the blood.

"The doctor may even make an allergy extract of the air in a room that smells of chemicals. Sometimes the child is exposed to just one drop of the allergy extract of the air of a room—a particular room in the home or school—we can actually reproduce a headache, a stomachache, or problems thinking. The doctor makes the allergy extract the same way one would bubble air through a fish tank: Using a pump to bubble the room air through a salt solution in a tiny test tube. The air bubbles for about eight hours and at the end of this period a solution remains that contains some of the chemicals that were in the air. Then an allergy extract is prepared from this solution which can be injected in the skin, or placed under the tongue. If it causes numbness in the arms, tingling in the fingers, a headache, stomachache, problems with remembering, or a change in activity or behavior within ten minutes, we have probably collected the problem chemical from the air within the solution.

"Using the new and more precise method of allergy testing called provocation/neutralization, the doctor can then make dilutions of that chemical solution and probably eliminate those same symptoms with one drop of the right dilution of that solution. In other words, if the child develops a headache in a certain room, you can put a drop of the air allergy extract under the tongue and provoke the headache in three to eight minutes. Then you can give the child a five-fold weaker dilution of that same solution and often you can eliminate or neutralize the headache in less than ten minutes.

"After you have done a skin test with the allergy extracts, and shown that there is a cause-and-effect relationship between the child's behavior or physical symptoms and a chemical in the school, the next thing is to determine what the school can do to eliminate the problem. One of the things they can do is not put carpets in schools. If they do have carpets and they're causing problems, they can take the carpets up and put in hard vinyl tile. In such cases, it is important to insist that they use adhesives that are safe when installing the tile.

"Another big problem in schools is poor ventilation, especially in the winter. Due to the energy crunch we had in the '70s, many schools closed down their ventilation systems to save money and to cut down on the cost of heating. Dust, molds, and chemicals have accumulated at very high levels in these schools. The windows don't always open, and the result is that there has been a gradual build-up, so that more and more children and teachers seem to be adversely affected when they go to school.

"One of the things that you can insist on is that school officials check the ventilation system. There are fast and easy ways to measure the amount of carbon dioxide in a classroom, which can tell you whether the ventilation is good or not. The level should be 800 ppm or less. Relatively simple tests can also be done to measure for certain chemicals, such as chlorine and formaldehyde. Sometimes, because of poor cleaning of the ventilation systems in schools, the problem is dust and molds, not chemicals. Other times, they put chemicals in the duct-work while cleaning, which really causes trouble because the chemicals then circulate throughout the school, causing illness. Sometimes the intake for the ventilation system is too close to the area where all the school buses line up. The bus drivers let the engines idle for long periods, resulting in all the gasoline fumes and hydrocarbons entering the ductwork intake and circulating throughout the school.

"In one case I encountered, a school had a printing press, and the exhaust pipe from the printing press was at exactly the same level as the ventilation intake on the roof, with the result that all the chemicals from the printing press were going right back in and circulating throughout the school. Some printing press chemicals are toxic to the nervous system and cancer-causing.

"A patient I saw last week has three sons who came home smelling of mop oil, which is used to clean the school. The mother said that the children's clothes smelled so badly that she had to use very hot water to eliminate the smell. One of the boys developed a headache and a burning sensation in his throat. So I asked her to bring some of the mop oil and I just put it underneath his nose and let him take one whiff of the odor. Within seconds, he was complaining of a headache around his forehead on both sides of his temples and he said it was throbbing and that his throat was burning. I gave him oxygen for about ten minutes and the headache, throbbing, and burning in his throat gradually subsided. We videotaped this reaction.

"There was another child who had trouble only on the two afternoons a week when he went to school. He would be weak and tired, hardly able to stand; he couldn't hold a pencil, clung to his mother, but only on those two days. I sent the mother to the school and asked her to try to figure out what's different in the schoolroom that might be causing your son problems. It turned out that they used a very common disinfectant aerosol in the room, six times a day on the tabletops, to reduce infections. Then they used the same solution on the cot that he napped on. All she had to do was ask the school to stop using that disinfectant and install an air purifier, and the child improved remarkably.

"Then the mother noticed that he had similar problems when he went into the gym, and it turned out that they were using a certain kind of floor wax in the gym. We suggested that they use something that had fewer petrochemicals in it and the result was that he can now be in the gym for 20 minutes. That child had tics and twitches, which is another thing that you see in some children with these allergies. The symptoms disappeared after environmental allergy care.

"I have seen children from all over the country who have problems at school. Some of these children who come to see me don't come in complaining of allergies. But the affected teachers and the children almost uniformly have a history of hay fever, asthma, or eczema. And they have relatives that have these same conditions. Their immune systems are not up to par, or they wouldn't have allergies to start with. But they are the canaries—the first ones to become ill when a school is chemically contaminated, or is too dusty or too moldy. Many children who have these allergies also find that their problems grow worse after their school has been remodeled, repainted, newly carpeted, or refurnished with furniture made of materials that release formaldehyde or other chemicals into the air.

"Children who wheezed a little before, now wheeze a lot. Youngsters who were stuffy once in a while are now congested all the time. Not only do they get nose problems, but they start having infections in the sinuses and their ears. Many of them feel tired and weak when the schools are chemically contaminated. One parent said that their child was too tired to turn the pages of his book. Another said that her child was crying because he couldn't play football anymore because he was just too weak. These are some of the things that are happening in some schools throughout the country, mainly because of dust, molds, and chemicals.

"Schools also serve food, and much of the food is contaminated with pesticides. Ideally, your child should eat only organically grown food because it is less contaminated with pesticides, food coloring, or other chemical additives that may be causing your child's adverse reactions. However, in some places, it remains difficult—and expensive—to buy foods uncontaminated by chemicals. Organic foods may be readily available in New York City, but they certainly aren't in many other cities. I encourage people to grow their own vegetables so that they will have their own source in the winter and one which they know does not contain any chemicals.

"There is one very important and simple thing you can do to tell which area in a school or in your home, or which food, might be causing your children a problem. Ask your children how they feel before they eat a meal, or before they enter a particular room. Also ask them to write their name and to draw. You should do the same thing. And then, if you have asthma, blow into something called a Peak Pocket Flow Meter, which is a plastic tube with a gauge on it. If you blow 400 before you eat and half an hour later you blow 200, one or more of the foods that you ate is causing asthma or spasm of your lungs. Check out each food separately five days later and find the culprit.

"Another thing to do is to take your child's pulse before eating. If the pulse is 80 and suddenly after eating it is 120, a food has set off a silent alarm in the child's body, which has caused her pulse to increase. So check the writing, the drawing, the pulse rate, the breathing, and how your child feels and looks before a meal and then a half hour or so later. If any of these variables indicates a change for the worse after a meal, one of the foods your child ate may be the cause of the problem. If the change occurs after being in a particular room or area, something in there may be at cause.

"Wait for five days before the attempt to find the problem food. It is critical that you wait for five days to get all that particular food out of the body. So for five days, if you have noticed your child had a reaction after eating corn, don't feed your child corn (and tell her not to eat any at school either). Then at eight a.m. on a Saturday, give her the first of the foods she may have been reacting to, and at ten a.m. give her the second possibility one, at noon the next one, and at one p.m. the next. In this way, you check each food all by itself. Again, check the breathing, the pulse, the writing and drawing, and how your child feels and looks before and a half hour or so after each food.

"You can apply the same principles of food isolation to every room in your house and at school or every room at work. Check your breathing (or your child's breathing) before you enter a room, do all the things that I suggested above, and then do them again several hours later. If you find that a particular room is a problem, then you have got to ask, 'Why? What do I smell in this room, what am I touching in this room, what is in this room that could be bothering me? Is it the heating system, the covering on the furniture, the carpet, the floor wax, the furniture polish? Are there items that have been dry-cleaned in this room? Is there an odor?' You'll be surprised at how much you can figure out on your own.

"Also check out the car. Notice how you and your children feel before you get in the car, then check again half an hour later. Compare indoors with outdoors and you'll be able to tell whether it's the outdoor pollution, the lawn spray next door, the mold, pollen, or pollution in the air that is causing problems outside versus inside. You can easily figure out many, many answers by checking your child's pulse, his breathing, and how he writes, draws, feels and looks. Check these same parameters on yourself as well. If you have high blood pressure, you can even use a blood pressure cuff and check your pressure before and after each of these exposures and you'll turn up answers. By keeping detailed records, you can often figure out the reasons why your children are ill, and many times you can then get rid of the cause and make them feel much better.

"Don't forget to check lavatories. Many children go into the lavatories at school feeling fine, and when they come out they can't think at all because of the chemicals in the disinfectants and deodorants that are used in the lavatories. Don't forget the garage, which has many chemicals in it. Don't forget the attic, which is dusty, and don't forget the basement, which is dusty and moldy.

"Keep in mind: The indoor and outdoor factor that causes more problems than any other is molds. If you live in a moldy house and you are always wheezing, on cortisone, always sick and in and out of the hospital, it could be the moldy house that you are living in that is causing the problem. Sometimes if you live in too much mold, it doesn't matter what kind of treatment you're on. You have to move or get away from the thing that is causing the problems.

"In the workplace, don't forget all the areas that have chemicals which could be affecting your brain. Remember: Excessive chemical exposures can and will damage the body. If they can't be excreted, they can be stored in the fat, and sometimes these fatty tissues get an overload and develop cancer. When you breathe something, these chemicals can go straight through your nose, right up into your brain. There is no barrier there to protect your brain. And the brain is, to a large degree, fat.

"There are some new ways of doing brain imaging that can actually show changes in the brains of some of the people that are exposed to neurotoxic substances. For example, if a child sniffs glue or hair spray or aerosols, you can actually show a characteristic pattern of change in the brain imaging-pattern on the particular individual, which will look different from somebody who has epilepsy or someone who has schizophrenia or depression. They actually produce different brain pictures. I'm sure in a few years, many people who say they are always depressed, or tired, or nervous will be able to have a brain-image pattern taken that will show that specific areas of the brain have been affected by certain exposures or foods.

"Ask your children to write down or tell you their five favorite foods and beverages. The five foods and beverages that they write are probably the foods that are most likely to cause them difficulty. If they wrote down chocolate, cocoa, and cola—which are all different forms of chocolate—it means that chocolate could be the cause of their problems. If they wrote down bread, cake, cookies, pasta, and macaroni, chances are the problem is wheat. If they wrote down ice cream, yogurt, milk, cheese, and pizza, they are probably sensitive to dairy products. In fact, the food that causes more chronic and acute illness in all of society, to my mind, is, unquestionably, milk and dairy products," Dr. Rapp concludes.

III

ORGANIC CONDITIONS COMMONLY MISDIAGNOSED AS MENTAL DISEASE

18

BLOOD SUGAR INSTABILITY (Hypoglycemia)

A Personal Account of Hypoglycemia: "William"

I had been seeing a psychiatrist for depression and was on medication—and still am. I noticed that while the medicine took care of certain symptoms, it seemed to have no effect on an enormous number of them. I used to be a body-builder back in the early 1980s, so I had some experience with nutrition. I went to see Dr. Spreen because I noticed that my hypoglycemia was acting up; I noticed a direct correlation between what I ate and how I felt. When I went to see him, I was complaining of really severe panic disorders, irritability, and difficulty in concentrating. I went from having an excellent memory to no memory at all. Also I had such fatigue it felt like I was walking in Jell-O all the time.

I'd sleep 12 hours a day and get up with no energy at all after sleeping. I'd be tired the whole day.

The first thing Dr. Spreen did was to give me injections of B12. Immediately I noticed a difference. As soon as I'd walk into the gym to work out, my energy was there. In the morning I felt really good. But I was still plagued sometimes by panic attacks. So he put me on a high dose of tyrosine, which is one of the free-form amino acids. I took up to seven grams a day and noticed a real strong response. Tyrosine is also related to the thyroid because one of the products the thyroid needs for normal functioning is tyrosine. He also put me on a low dosage of thyroid, a quarter grain a day. I took that and noticed immediate results. With that and the tyrosine, I felt like a new person.

This experience showed me that even though a doctor may be treating you for depression, he might be missing the things that might have lead to the depression or that might go hand in hand with it. Many books that I've read—in particular, Carlton Frederick's *New Low Blood Sugar and You*—say that when there is any mental disorder present, hypoglycemia is going to be right there along with it. But the medical community doesn't accept that hypoglycemia is as predominant as some nutritionists say it is because the doctors are thinking about the organic forms, which are much rarer. But with the diet that we are eating today, which is high in carbohydrates and low in basically everything good for you, hypoglycemia is manifesting itself in great numbers.

As a child, I ate a diet that was full of simple carbohydrates—all sorts of sweets and sugars—and had a lot of the symptoms that are associated with hypoglycemia: I was hyperactive and had asthma. You see, hypoglycemia can trigger asthma attacks. Since I started working out and watching my diet, the asthma went away.

For the panic attacks, Dr. Spreen suggested vitamin C. I took vitamin C powder, which is ascorbic acid, in the morning. I probably took 15 to 20 grams a day. It was almost like taking a sedative. It calmed me right down. My thought patterns straightened out; I was calm; and I wasn't as irritable and fidgety as I had been. I balanced out the rest of my nutrients with a mineral supplement and a good vitamin supplement high in the B spectrum. I take an additional B complex with pantothenic acid on the side because Dr. Spreen thinks that most people don't have enough B vitamins in the diet. I'm inclined to agree with him, since I've followed his advice and noticed an enormous positive response.

According to Dr. Hyla Cass, people with hypoglycemia are often diagnosed as though they have simple depression and anxiety, and then treated for a psychological condition. "They are put on anti-anxiety agents such as Valium or Xanax. If they are extremely depressed as well as anxious, they are put on antidepressants such as Prozac. I've had people come to me on medication that wanted to go off of it. It turned out that they were hypoglycemic.

"You can replace antidepressants with amino acids, minerals, and cofactors, vitamins for amino acid metabolism," Dr. Cass adds. "When depressed patients come to see me who are also hypoglycemic, I put them on a hypoglycemic diet, which is approximately six small meals a day. Also, I have them take chromium for balancing their blood sugar levels. I also give them magnesium, glutamine, and tyrosine. Tyrosine is an excellent natural antidepressant. It's a precursor to the neurotransmitter norepinephrine, which is one of the brain chemicals that helps us feel good.

"Hypoglycemia can result from a combination of stress and poor eating habits, particularly in people genetically predisposed to this condition. The disorder can present itself in a variety of ways: depression, irritability, anxiety, panic attacks, fatigue, 'brain fog,' headaches including migraines, insomnia, muscular weakness, and tremors, all of which may be relieved by food. There can be cravings for sweets, coffee, alcohol, or drugs.

"In fact," Dr. Cass continues, "many addictions are related to hypoglycemia. Coffee and sugar consumed by recovering alcohol or drug addicts only prolong their problem, though in a less dangerous, more socially acceptable form. (It is interesting to note the large amount of these substances consumed at Alcoholics Anonymous meetings, for example, and on psychiatric wards.)

"Such individuals can often overcome coffee, drug, and alcohol addiction through correcting their hypoglycemia, with minimal withdrawal symptoms or later cravings. For recovering alcoholics, for example, I recommend the hypoglycemic regimen described below plus the amino acid glutamine, 500 mg, three to six times daily, which is particularly useful to counteract cravings.

"The following hypoglycemia program is designed to both strengthen the adrenals and maintain adequate blood sugar levels:

➤"Elimination of refined carbohydrates (sugar, white flour), coffee, and alcohol.

➤"Small, frequent meals of complex carbohydrates, high fiber foods, and protein.

➤Daily supplementation with a multivitamin/mineral complex that includes (otherwise add) 200–600 mcg chromium, 200–400 mg magnesium, 10–20 mg manganese, 500–1,000 mg potassium, 50–75 mg B vitamins, 500 mg pantothenic acid (vitamin B5), 3,000 mg vitamin C. These supplements can be divided into doses taken two to three times daily."

Dr. Leander Ellis suggests that hypoglycemia can be brought on by a variety of causal factors, some circumstantial, others stress-related, still others environmental. "Hypoglycemia," Dr. Ellis explains, "is a phenomenon that can be triggered by allergy, infection, exhaustion, or large amounts of sugar that encourage the growth of yeast in the intestinal tract, which then, in turn, gives rise to some allergic effects and a variety of other subtle effects. I see hypoglycemia as a symptom of a larger problem, rather than as a disease. Most of the time there are other important causes to account for the roller-coastering of the blood-sugar levels. The most common one is probably candida, yeast. The next most likely cause is food allergy. Often, a person is not only gorging on sugar, but is allergic to sugar, is not only gorging on chocolate, but is allergic to chocolate. So you get a curious combination of candida, yeast mold, fungus allergy, and allergy to foods. You usually have to control these several elements, as well as to get adequate nutritional support, in order to quiet these symptoms down.

"Candida is a major factor in hypoglycemia, depression, and chronic fatigue that the medical profession has continued to ignore, despite the research results that are available to the medical community. The major reason for this is that medicine is taught by prestige suggestion, meaning a doctor needs someone he or she trusts to tell him what is important. Unfortunately, the people that we doctors have the most contact with after we leave medical school are drug company representatives. Therefore, until a learned professor at an Ivy League medical school tells us that candida is a problem, it doesn't exist."

Dr. Warren Levin explains the basic physiology of hypoglycemia, as well as some of its special characteristics. "Hypoglycemia is a basic problem that is frequently stress-induced. When people take a large dose of sugar into the body (and one cola drink contains more sugar than the entire bloodstream), the level of sugar in the body goes way up. Now, the body's entire commitment is to maintain balance or equilibrium (the technical word is homeostasis). The body produces a basic hormone called insulin that is supposed to take the sugar from the blood and deliver it into the cells, and when the sugar goes up very rapidly the body reacts excessively, resulting in too much sugar being driven out of the blood, and that produces low blood sugar, or hypoglycemia. The body then has to correct the balance again, and it can be an emergency. If the blood sugar goes too high, it is not an emergency; the body can tolerate it. But the brain requires a certain level of blood sugar to function, so when the blood sugar starts plummeting—and it can sometimes drop at a frightening rate—the body calls forth its emergency hormone, adrenaline.

"Adrenaline was designed to protect us against the saber-toothed tigers back in the primitive world. It mobilizes all sorts of bodily functions. One of the things it does is to dump sugar from the liver into the blood very rapidly. However, adrenaline also causes what we call the fight-or-flight reaction, associated with the state of fear. We get a rapid heartbeat, dry mouth, sweating, fear, and a sense of impending doom."

Dr. Levin then concludes with a cautionary tale that contains precisely the kind of great wisdom and knowledge that the medical community needs to hear: "Now, suppose someone has an ice cream sundae and a few hours later he or she sits down to read the funny papers and all of a sudden he or she gets this terrible reaction. The individual goes to the doctor and explains that while just sitting there, reading the paper, all of a sudden the skin got sweaty and the heart started pounding. The doctor says that the problem is all in the head and that the patient must have a Prozac deficiency. 'With this Prozac prescription,' the doctor adds, 'you'll be fine.' We have to stop thinking that way. Headaches are not a Darvon deficiency, depression is not a deficiency of Elavil, and until doctors realize that the body's biochemistry is an exquisite balancing act, and start treating it with great respect, we are in a lot of trouble. Hypoglycemia is not a disease; it is a symptom requiring a search for an underlying cause."

19

$\mathcal{C}$ANDIDIASIS

Personal Accounts of Candidiasis:
"Ellen"

I have suffered from chronic candidiasis since I was about 13. We think it might have been linked to my taking massive doses of sulfa drugs for kidney problems when I was younger. I can't remember a time since I was 13—and I'm 31 now—when I didn't have a yeast infection. There may have been two- and three-week periods when I wasn't suffering from symptoms, but I always, to some extent, had a very severe yeast infection. I went to conventional doctors and they gave me the typical vaginal and topical cremes, and basically patted my hand and told me to come back and see them in two weeks. These medications seemed to help during the time that I used them, but invariably the infection returned, and was often twice as bad after

I stopped the treatment. So after a while, I simply avoided going to see any physician and just lived with the problem, except on the occasions when my symptoms got so severe that I just had to go see someone.

Eventually, I went for a Pap smear and a nurse practitioner suggested that I read a book called The Yeast Syndrome. It wasn't until I read the book and got Dr. Stoll's name out of it that I even connected my physical ailments with my mental health. I had always been moody and prone to periods of depression and there was a history of depression in my family. I never needed to be hospitalized, but I felt that some of these bouts, especially during my adolescent and college years, were extremely severe. I suffered mood swings and would have described myself as having a very volatile personality. But after going to Dr. Stoll, who started me on oral Nystatin, changed my diet, and used various supplements to correct my nutritional and physiological deficiencies, within about 60 days I felt like a totally different person. In fact, my husband commented that it was like being married to a different person. In hindsight, I can see that as my candidiasis symptoms were eradicated, my mental symptoms disappeared. So I use mental symptoms now as a red flag. If I start seeing personality changes within myself, I take a look at what I've been eating lately and how I've been feeling, and make some changes there. Then I seem to get back on track.

I have learned that conventional treatments that just treat the symptoms are not going to help you. You have to look for the root cause of your ailments. There is help out there to be found. You simply have to find someone like Dr. Stoll who knows how to treat your illness, and comply with their recommendations. You will get better.

Ever since I began modeling in New York about 15 years ago, I've had tremendous difficulty with depression and also with hypoglycemia, which was then a very fashionable disease. I was constantly on a diet and constantly in doctors' offices for yeast infections and digestive and stomach problems. I visited a lot of doctors who would tell me it was all in my head and send me to psychiatrists. I spent the better part of 20 years going from doctor to doctor for various things, having my husband tell me that I was a hypochondriac and feeling like one, and also working things out in therapy trying everything that I could.

Learning to take responsibility for my own health was a big switch in my life. Part of my health that was causing me a big problem was dental, so I went and had a lot of dental surgery done and came back to Dr. Stoll sicker than I have ever been, with severe headaches. I felt as if someone was banging a steel hammer inside my head. And I was angry all the time. Dr. Stoll had me do a stool test, and it came out that I had an abundance of candida. At the time, Dr. Stoll explained that dental work will exacerbate candida. In its way, this problem was a gift to me because in the past, I had only half-believed that I had candida. I didn't make a commitment to getting better. This time, within two months after taking Nystatin and vitamins, and doing aerobics, and going to a therapist to make sure that I got everything worked out, I was a different person.

I felt so totally different that it gave me the perspective to look back over the previous 20 years and say, "Oh, if only I had known all of this then, I wouldn't have done all of that." I had spent my life running down the wrong roads. And it was such a relief because the change allowed me to really begin to live.

Now I have my little ritual. I take my vitamins and do my aerobics, and make sure that I keep my house environmentally clean of gases and pollutants that exacerbate the condition. The change in how I felt was like going from 2 percent to 98 percent well. It was so dramatic.

"Nancy"

My youngest child was born with a lot of health problems—nothing life-threatening, he was just sick all the time. He lived on antibiotics from the day he was born until he was about five years old. He cried all the time and never slept. Most people don't think of an infant as being depressed, but when a baby cries all the time, you could say he's depressed, or in an anxious state, or in a state of pain. It was certainly very stressful for the both of us. As it turned out, most of his problems were allergy-related. He had ear infections, bronchitis, very severe eczema, and his digestive tract had become very permeable.

Within a month after I had taken my son to Dr. Stoll, and we had begun regenerating his intestinal lining through treating his candidiasis and watching his diet, I began seeing some improvement. Six months later, he was a totally different child. We were a totally different family.

My child had inherited his allergy problems from my mother-in-law. She had severe asthma and emphysema and she was extremely depressed because she thought that she was dying. She was so sick that she would crawl out of bed in the morning to a chair, and just wheeze and cough all day long in that same chair. She could do no housework, she no longer had a driver's license, and she didn't go anywhere. She spent more time in the hospital than she did at home.

So I took my mother-in-law to Dr. Stoll and within a month or two, she started showing tremendous improvement. Within about four to five months, she was a totally different person. The care she received literally turned her life around. She took the driver's test and got her driver's license again. She bought herself a car and became very active among senior citizens. The depression was gone. She had been on 13 different drugs, and he probably got her off three-fourths of them.

"Bob"

I had been sick for 25 years and was just slowly getting worse. At my worst, I passed out and wrecked my car. It was really hard to work and I was getting very depressed. I went to the local doctors, the local hospital, and even tried five days at the Mayo Clinic. They sent me back with sleeping pills and tranquilizers, and told me that it was all in my head.

Things had gotten so bad. My wife wouldn't leave me and I was dragging her down. I was borrowing money from my family just to keep going. I had no reason to think that I was ever going to get better and I was continually getting worse. So I decided to commit suicide. And I remembered when I was a kid that our dad always told us, "Kids, if you ever want to commit suicide, that is okay, but there is only one acceptable method. And that is starvation." So I said to myself, "Fine, all I have to do is stop eating for about three months and I will be dead. That sounds real good to me." So I did. I stopped eating, and of course after about two days of not eating my symptoms went away. At the time I didn't realize that it was the food that I was eating that was contributing to my being so sick and depressed.

Finally I went to Dr. Stoll, who was the tenth doctor I'd seen. He read over my history in about five minutes and said, "Well, I can almost guarantee you that I know what is wrong with you." He sent off a stool sample, which is an $80 lab test. When it came back, it confirmed his diagnosis. I had candida and giardia, little parasites eating holes in me. I went through this whole process of changing my diet and treating the candida and giardia and in about three months, I got better. I thought I was cured so I started eating the same old junk, and got sick again. I did that about twice. So it took me about a year to get totally cured.

No words can describe the joy of living in a healthy body after being sick for a long time. I can now eat almost anything except sugar—meaning sucrose—honey, and potatoes. I can eat fructose, corn syrup, and any other forms of sugar. When I was at the Mayo Clinic, we went through five days of tests and at the end of it I had a list of possibilities. One of those possibilities was food allergies. And I said, "I'm here, you have this nice big laboratory, why don't you test me for food allergies?" The internist, who acted like the director of the show, got mad. He said, "You don't have food allergies, and I'm not going to test you for them." So those are the kind of people I was dealing with at the Mayo Clinic. I have toyed with the idea of going back to the Mayo Clinic or writing them a letter, but I haven't because I'm convinced that they would just put my letter aside and say, "Oh, another hypochondriac."

"Dr. Stoll has been persecuted by the Kentucky Medical Board for years for that very reason. Some of his patients went back to their old doctors after they were cured and told them what had been wrong. Some of these other doctors got so embarrassed and mad that they filed charges against Walt Stoll with the Kentucky board. There has never been a patient complaint against him; the only complains were from other doctors. So going back to your old doctor and explaining can sometimes have very negative repercussions.

Dr. Ken Korins explains that candida is a yeast, which is a normal part of the constitution. "Usually, it lives harmlessly in the GI tract or the skin.

However, overgrowth can affect the GI tract, the genital-urinary tract, the endocrine system, and the nervous system. Some of the symptoms that yeast or candida can cause are fatigue, decreased energy, problems with libido, problems with thrush, which is a white coating on the tongue or esophagus caused by overgrowth of the yeast, bloating and gas, intestinal cramps, rectal itching, altered bowel function, vaginal yeast, urinary tract infection, menstrual complaints, depression, irritability, problems with concentration, as well as allergies, chemical sensitivities and decreased immune function in general.

"People with candida often crave sugars, alcohol and various carbohydrates. The patient is most often but not always a woman between the ages of l5 and 50. There might be a past medical history of vaginal yeast, antibiotics, birth control and steroids. Antibiotics are particularly important in causing problems with yeast. It used to be that antifungals were commonly given with antibiotics because of this reason. Many other drugs such as oral contraceptives, anything that interferes with hydrochloric acid and a lot of simple sugars in the diet can cause problems with yeast.

"People who have problems with candida often have PMS, food allergies and other environmental sensitivities as well as conditions like psoriasis and irritable bowel syndrome. The diagnosis is often made by a history of the symptoms, but it can be confirmed with a stool culture, which will show high levels of candida, and also by an antibody test.

"Although candida is usually a normal part of the constitution, stress interferes with the secretions, with the immunity, with the nutrition or drugs or impaired liver function. When this happens, the yeast products are absorbed by the body. On the one hand, toxins are produced, which creates a metabolic stress on the body, interfering with liver function and the elasticity of enzymes. Also, antigens are produced by the yeast which in activity with the toxins, cause activation and depression of the immune system. Antigens cause auto antibodies to develop, which can wreak havoc with the body, causing rheumatoid arthritis symptoms, among other things.

"So we have a condition that causes problems in the immune system, hormonal imbalances, and in general, multi-system involvement, including problems with food and other chemical sensitivities. This leads to a situation where people are more prone to infections. Therefore, they get put on more antibiotics, which gives the candida more opportunity to proliferate. It develops a vicious cycle.

"We have to reduce the predisposing factors that cause the growth in the first place. Some suggestions would be a diet with a low component of simple sugars, especially refined sugars. It is also important to limit foods containing honey, maple syrup, and milk because of the lactose. Even these simple sugars, the candida can thrive on. Foods containing yeast or mold such as alcohol, cheese, dried fruits and peanuts and known allergens should be avoided since they also weaken the immune system and leave less reserve to deal with these conditions.

"The digestive system is extremely important to deal with. Supplementing with hydrochloric acid, pancreatic enzymes, and other herbs, such as bitter herbs, which can help secrete bile, may prevent candida overgrowth. Pancreatic enzymes can be particularly important because incomplete digestion of proteins may cause food allergies. Also, the pancreatic enzymes help keep the intestines free of yeast, bacteria, protozoa, worms, and help break down the immune complex.

"The immune system is extremely important to address. Treatment for AIDS, cancer, or diabetes or treatments such as chemotherapy, steroids, or radiation greatly affect the immune system. Nutrition has to be addressed. Technically, a nutrient can cause problems with candida because there is no known nutrient that doesn't have a some effect on the immune system. However, studies have shown that nutrients that are especially low in patients with candida are vitamin A, B6, zinc, lignum, magnesium, essential fatty acids, folic acid, and iron. Of course, a high potency multi-vitamin should be added to the supplements.

"Any drugs that are compromising the immune system must be addressed, otherwise treatments are not going to work because you are going to be continually perpetuating candida overgrowth. Drugs like Tagament and Ranitidine, that are used for gastric ulcers and gastritis, decrease hydrochloric acid secretion, which is essential to control candida and also for absorption of nutrients.

"The liver is a very important organ in the control of candida. If the liver is overwhelmed with toxins, it cannot detoxify the body properly. These toxins are released into the system, creating problems like psoriasis and premenstrual syndrome. The liver is also important because of something known as the die-off effect. As the candida is being killed by the body, more toxins are released, causing an exacerbation of symptoms, even if the person is on the way to healing. So the liver must be in optimal function during the healing process."

There are many natural herbal remedies which can be very effective in treating candidiasis. Coprilic acid is a fatty acid with a lot of antifungal properties. One gram with meals can be very effective. Lactobacilli are well known bacteria; they are good bacteria that can decrease candida growth. Garlic is extremely active against many fungi and in fact some studies have shown that garlic is more active against candida than Nystatin. Barberry, in tincture form, stimulates blood supply to the spleen and activates macrophagen. It can be very helpful in maintaining the normal floor of the gut. It's active against many pathological bacteria including candida, including e-coli and salmonella. Common spices can even be beneficial—ginger, cinnamon, thyme and rosemary, all these things can help.

Dr. Aubrey Worrell also approaches the candida problem holistically: "The body is the source of the candida allergen. When there is more candida than there should be in the gastrointestinal tract, the body absorbs more of the candida antigen. You accelerate the problem by eating sugar and adding foods with mold and by breathing mold in.

"Over a period of years, I noticed that patients with candida manifest multiple symptoms. As an allergist, I would of course see patients with asthma, hay fever, and skin rashes. But I began noticing that many of these patients with allergies had other problems such as respiratory and gastrointestinal symptoms. Another complaint I see quite frequently is people just not feeling good. They're tense or headachy. They're tired and weak. They have a tendency towards depression and fatigue. They're forgetful and unable to concentrate.

"In actuality, these problems are often manifestations of a subtle disruption of immune function in which there's an overgrowth of yeast and an increasing allergy to the mold.

"I place patients with multiple symptoms on a mold-free and yeast-free diet that eliminates foods such as milk and dairy products, particularly cheese. Milk and dairy products are contaminated with mold, and mold is used in the process of cheese-making. I also eliminate yeast breads and yeast foods, as well as vinegars, since these contain a lot of mold allergens.

"If a person is eating a lot of sugar, if he or she has taken a lot of antibiotics, if he or she is not eating a good diet—then the candida is more apt to grow. And that person is likely to have more candida antigen released into their system.

"You have to use a combination of approaches in treating patients with candida. Number one, you have to have a good, nutritious diet. It can't be loaded with alcohol and sugar. It has to be composed of broad-spectrum healthy foods. Number two, you put them on the mold-free diet. Number three, you have to place them on Nystatin therapy for approximately two to six weeks."

Dr. Richard Tan confirms many of Dr. Worrell's insights. Dr. Tan also emphasizes a systemic and holistic approach: "I have been diagnosing a large number of patients with candida, and sugar affects them greatly. Quite a few patients that I am seeing have memory lapses, are forgetful and depressed, and they have seen other doctors who diagnose the depression and give them antidepressants. When I go over all the system reviews, I find that it is more of a systemic problem; along with the candida, they also have some sinus problems, achy bones and joints, stomach upsets, and gas. They often say that they have cravings for sugar or foods that contain sugar, as well as bread.

"I have a survey form that I go through. In my scoring system, after awhile, if the score is high, then I strongly suspect that they have candida. So then I explain my hypothesis and start to treat them. I put them on a diet program plus some anti-fungal medication. When they come back after two weeks, they usually say that they haven't felt so well in a number of years.

"This quick recovery is a revelation to me. I keep on seeing this type of patient. And every time I treat one, I am still amazed at how different they become after awhile, at how much they improve.

"It is estimated that about one-third of the population has candida. I would say that among my patients about 15 or 20 percent have candida in varying degrees.

"Patients with candida should avoid all processed foods, and especially those with sugar, such as soft drinks. Get back to the basics.

Grow your own garden if you can. If not, maybe go to a health food store, where you can buy organic, unprocessed foods. While most Americans eat too much fat, people with candida need to be more concerned with sugar than with fat. If you eliminate nutritionally poor foods, you will often be surprised at how your taste for things changes as your diet changes."

Dr. Ray Wunderlich emphasizes the link between depression and such physical imbalances as candidiasis and thyroid disease. "A very high percentage of the people I see who are depressed also have imbalances, such as an overgrowth of candida. Thyroid disease is another example. If you considered all the women whom I treat in my practice, from 70 to 75 percent of them would have thyroid disease, and an even higher percentage would have some form of candida, which is yeast overgrowth.

"A good example is a TV reporter I saw this morning. After coming into my office to film a segment on my approach to medicine, she got personally interested in what I do. She is 40 years old. We did a mineral analysis on her and found that she is deficient in five nutrient minerals. She is a perfectly normal, functioning individual of 40 years of age. But when you examine her carefully, it turns out that she has recurrent vaginal yeast infections, some bloating, some gas and indigestion, and she has taken antibiotics: a classic profile of a candida patient, which is all too common. In a place like Florida, where the weather is so humid and molds and yeasts grow so readily, problems associated with recurrent yeast infections are almost an epidemic."

Dr. Walt Stoll brings his understanding of the body's immune system to bear on his clinical approach. He describes his clinical experience using examples from candidiasis patients, with references to rheumatoid arthritis patients and others. As he explains: "The immune system sees the world in black and white. Something entering your body that it comes in contact with is either you or it is not you. If it is you, the immune system is not supposed to attack; if it is not you, then it is supposed to attack. One of the things that your digestive tract does is to break down things from the environment into particles small enough for you to absorb without alerting your immune system that they came from somewhere else besides you. But if, for example, your gut is not doing the job perfectly, it leaks a particle of protein (a peptide) that is large enough to alert the immune system, in your joints, muscles, or ligaments, for instance. Then your immune system can't tell the difference between the protein particle from outside and the one in your tissues, so it attacks both. Let's imagine that every time you have corn, for example, you don't break it down perfectly and one of those peptides leaks out of your intestine. Your body attacks the corn peptide, but it's also attacking the peptide—that is identical to the corn peptide—in your muscle, ligament, and joint. You'll feel that immune response as arthritis, tendonitis, or other conditions.

"If you stop the process," Dr. Stoll continues, "the immune system settles down in three and a half days, and you begin showing improvement. The first example I heard of was about ten years ago. If you took someone with rheumatoid arthritis or took a group of these patients and put them on a fast, 75 percent of them would improve within a week. You can't keep someone on a water fast forever, of course; but here was a dramatic illustration of the fact that there was another cause of rheumatoid arthritis that we could address. We didn't necessarily have to limit our course of treatment to gold shots, cortisone, and a crippling future for the patients.

"There are a number of things that make the gut more permeable to peptides. Stress is one of them. We know not to go swimming right after we eat, because there is not enough blood supply in the body to adequately supply both the intestinal tract and the muscles. When your blood supply is concentrated in your intestinal tract digesting your meal, going for a vigorous swim risks not getting enough blood in the muscles, resulting in cramps and, possibly, drowning. When you are chronically stressed—and most stresses are not psychological but environmental —your body deals with it with a fight-or-flight response, which makes your muscles get a little more chronically tight and active. Your body concentrates more blood supply into the fight-or-flight area and then takes away the blood supply from the intestinal tract. The intestinal lining replaces itself on average about every 14 hours, so it requires a heavy blood supply. If you are chronically stressed for long enough, eventually the intestinal lining functions less normally, which of course produces other imbalances. The normal bacteria that are supposed to grow sometimes get out of balance and allow candida to move in and flourish. This damages the lining further and so things leak even more.

"I've been practicing medicine with an awareness of these types of problems for 15 years and in my experience this food absorption syndrome is the main cause of brain fatigue, or 'brain fag,' as it is called. By the time I see most of my patients, they have had everything else tried unsuccessfully on them and a large percentage of them have this syndrome as their basic cause. If the patient is willing to follow directions, within a few weeks they already see enough improvement so that they know they are doing the right thing. Within a few months, they've usually improved enough so that they can handle it from there on their own.

"My procedure is to first collect all the medical records that the person has accumulated up to that time, so I don't have to repeat any tests that have already been done. If some things have obviously been missed, then I try to fill in the gaps. There are labs around the country that do a pretty good job of looking for parasites, candidiasis, low magnesium, and other disorders that are either not done or done poorly by conventional labs. I look at the entire chronological history of the patient for a couple of weeks before their appointment and try to think of any factor that might have influenced their health and that might be indicated as a pattern of change over time. Then we have the regular data bases that we use in conventional medicine to look for other kinds of patterns. I'll also ask the patient to keep a record of his or her usual diet and anything special that they ingest for a week or so. Then I put all those pieces together with a general physical exam and see if the pattern suggests some of these other causes.

"Finally, when I get a picture and it's pretty obvious what is happening, I educate the patient sufficiently so that he or she can make an informed decision about going forward with the therapy. I tell patients to make their decision very carefully, so that once having decided to go ahead they then are able to maintain that commitment. That way, we are sure that if the patient doesn't get well it is because we were wrong, and not because the patient was careless about sticking to his or her diet and regimen. Generally, I can predict within a few days how long it is going to take for the person to start feeling better. I have patients keep a record of their symptoms so that they can track their own progress and improvement. As you get better, frequently you forget how badly you were feeling before. Unless someone lives with a patient, it's hard to assess exactly where you are once a patient begins to improve.

"The treatment depends upon the cause, of course. If the person has candidiasis, then the treatment is relatively simple and straightforward. A strict diet is necessary for a while. I will probably have to give them some digestive enzymes to correct the poor protein metabolism, until they can do some relaxation techniques to get the blood supply back to the intestinal tract, which usually takes from three to six months. In the presence of candidiasis, I usually use some Nystatin, a prescription anti-fungal agent, to try to directly attack the candida problem. If the person hadn't been absorbing things too well for a while I might use some concentrated nutrients with antioxidants to try to replenish the body with what it needs to repair itself and to improve the immune function."

"Jack" (described by "Gail," his wife)

For ten years my husband suffered with what was diagnosed as acute, chronic gastritis and depression. For a long time, we didn't link the two. So he was treated for gastritis and suffered several endoscopies, and for his depression took lithium, Prozac, you name it. Neither condition got much better. We eventually decided that he should stop taking all those heavy-duty drugs because they seemed to be doing more damage than good. Finally, we heard about Dr. Stoll and he diagnosed my husband as having candidiasis. With the use of the anti-yeast medication Nystatin, and diet and vitamin therapy, he got better on both counts—the gastritis and the depression—very rapidly. We saw a change within about two months.

We had spent ten years, going from doctor to doctor and hospital to hospital, trying to figure out what was wrong. He had been hospitalized with panic attacks; he had really been put through the mill. After all of that, his treatment and cure turned out to be quite simple.

Dr. Michael Schacter points to the overflow of a candida problem into other diseases. "The overgrowth of the microorganism candida albicans is often an important factor in people who are depressed. Many patients who have candida problems are also depressed. Oral antibiotics, oral contraceptives, and steroids predispose a person to chemical imbalances and an overgrowth of candida, or yeast, which is frequently manifested as abdominal gas and bloating, chronic vaginitis in women, and depression. Frequently I will treat it with an anti-candida diet, eliminating sugar and yeast products and using a variety of anti-candida nutrients. Sometimes I'll use anti-candida medications. This regimen will frequently clear up the depression, as well as many of the other symptoms."

20

CHRONIC FATIGUE

Fatigue: Gary

I did an experiment. I wanted to see how far I could push my body before it would collapse. I kept very detailed records. My diet was absolutely the same, the amount of protein, fat, and carbohydrate, the amount of vitamins and minerals and enzymes, the amount of juices, nothing changed. Then I raced every single week. I did about 50 races a year. For 81 races, I had a personal record each week, faster than any that I had done up to that point and I had not changed anything. One day, there was a race in Central Park, a short little 3 mile race. I couldn't run that race as fast as a slow training session. I charted that. I said to myself maybe it was lack of sleep, maybe it was the flight, maybe it was all these things. The next week another race, same thing. I could not do it. I did not have the energy.

I had a full blood chemistry done. I tested for every virus, bacteria, parasite, hepatitis, everything. My blood was clean as clean can be. I had to ask why I had no energy when I stressed myself in competition. I realized that there is something that medicine does not talk about, science does not look at. I had looked in the Western model first, being a scientist, wanting to see if I had a virus or blood sugar imbalances. No, everything was normal. What I found I was deficient in at that point was the essential chi energy.

The chi energy is life force energy. It had been diminished by nearly 2 and 1/2 years of training and pushing nonstop. It doesn't show up in our blood or in our cells, but something is missing. It took almost 6 months before that was able to re-balance itself and rejuvenate. Then I was able to start all over again and, this time, compensate for it. The rule of health is compensation. We all cannot move out of a city that is polluted, move away from a job that's got high noise and dust particles or even away from working around sick people, as I do. By re-balancing and rejuvenating and compensating that's how we are able to be healthy. If you live in a very polluted environment, you put in antipollution devices. You balance yourself, give yourself time and peace and quiet. Training for a marathon is very immune depressive. Understanding the compensation factor, now I take some vitamin C drips. The amount I will have in my system is different than anyone else's because it's unique to my own system. Each person has their own unique needs. It deals with the energies and I'm not talking about viral or bacterial or blood sugar or glandular depletion.

Even when you rest and the muscles are recovered and the blood chemistry is normal, liver enzyme, everything is normal, it's possible that that vital energy still isn't completely balanced yet. That takes time, you cannot rush that. I have tried every form of compensation—nutritional, biochemical, biomedical, every possible thing—and that's how I help people today, based upon a real lack of energy in their system.

People who are working on things they really enjoy spend an inordinate amount of energy working—not just physical but emotional energy, spiritual energy—and that is not in and of itself depleting. I remember some friends who were building themselves a home and they would have friends up for work weekends. We would all chip in and help them. Everybody else would be exhausted after 6 hours and they would be happy working 12 hours later. There are ways that we can tap into inner resources within our body and within our mind that allow us to compensate for fatigue. It's the compensating energy of the chi, the sub-meridian that engages us in life. When you suddenly think about doing something you have not done that you are excited by, you have all the energy in the world. If we can keep ourselves positively focused and have goals each day to achieve something that is obtainable and within our reach, it gives us more energy. That helps us with other things that could be depleting us.

You can deplete your energy and become exhausted just by consumption or by the thought of consumption. In other times and other cultures you will never find someone with a closet packed with clothes. We deplete ourselves because we are not focusing on things that are energizing emotionally.

When someone tells me they have fatigue, I don't stop with just bacteria and viral panels or the blood sugar examination. I look at other things—what they've done in their life, what they're feeling, what they're believing, because that will affect an energy system that we can't measure, but is there. By re-balancing that system, you can frequently help a person have their over-all life energy improve and then you work on the individual glands and organs and blood chemistry.

I measure fatigue backwards, in increments. You felt tired, but you didn't have flu and you were not sore in your muscles or joints. You had intermittent fatigue: more energy in the morning, less in the evening or afternoon. You go to exercise or you want to stay up a little later and go dancing, but you just don't have any energy. You wake up and just don't seem to be rested no matter how much sleep you get. You really have to look at levels of fatigue. From that very mild form of fatigue to the very major, the information in this chapter will help all because someone who has full blown chronic fatigue syndrome may have multiple factors at work in their system, whereas someone else may only have 2 or 3.

It is difficult, but possible, to distinguish between feeling over-tired, constantly worn out and having chronic fatigue syndrome. All of these states affect our mental and emotional life. Sometimes, fatigue is caused by other diseases of either mind or body.

Most fatigue-centered conditions begin slowly. A person gradually feels less energized than in prior months or years. They just can't do the things they did before.

Dr. Jacob Teitelbaum actually lost a year in medical school due to his contracting chronic fatigue syndrome. For over a decade he's worked with chronic fatigue and fibromyalgia patients. He identifies chronic fatigue syndrome as a group of symptoms associated with severe, almost unrelenting fatigue. "Disordered sleep is classic—trouble falling or staying asleep. Severe achiness is usual in a lot of different parts of the body. For some people the most disabling and scary part of the disease is the brain fog—confusion, poor memory, trouble finding words, even names. Increased thirst is very common because of the hormonal problems, bowel disorders, recurrent infections. So if you have several of these together, I think you have the disease. The new fibromyalgia and chronic fatigue criteria show that there are about six million in the country with this disease." Other practitioners include, on the list of symptoms: recurring sore throat, lymph nodes swelling, headache, intestinal discomfort, depression and decreased concentration.

The first thing people do is usually the worst thing. "When people feel horribly tired and can barely function, they try to take coffee or caffeine to boost their energy. It feels better for a little while, but caffeine is a loan shark for energy. You'll feel better for a couple hours, and then crash four or five hours later. When people crash, they drink more coffee and then more, up to eight to twelve cups a day. They're wiped out. It's really important for people to come off the coffee so their energy levels can start to come back up.

"Also, caffeine aggravates hypoglycemia, which is very common in this disease because of the underactive adrenal gland. This can put people on an emotional roller coaster. The average American gets 150 pounds of sugar added to their food each year, which is 18 percent of their calories. This plus white flour, having lost most of its vitamins and minerals, results in a diet that truly is destroyed before people ever get started, and then this sets them up for chronic fatigue syndrome.

"The B complex vitamins are very important, so get one that has at least 25 mgs of B complex, selenium, zinc, chromium, copper. If your iron is low, treat that. The lousy diet decreases the immune function with this disease, so bugs that most people wouldn't get, like candida overgrowth, parasites, abnormal bacteria growing in the bowel, are common. These things get to the B12 before you can absorb it. Because digestion is poor, people are not absorbing the B12 they need. The body over-utilizes the B12 to try to heal the damage, and both of these things drive the B12 level down to very low levels. This causes fatigue and a lot of other problems. The B12 deficiency can also aggravate allergies, such as sulfite sensitivities. So getting B12 shots, even if your doctor says the levels are technically normal, would be a very important part of the treatment. B12 shots—1000 to 2000 micrograms once a day to once a week—a total of 12 shots can make a big difference, regardless of your level.

"Current evidence suggests that a major portion of these symptoms are manifestations of a poorly functioning hypothalamus. This is a very exciting area of new research. If you had to look for the missing link that ties this whole disease together, the hypothalamus is a good one. It is a very small area, called the master gland, in the brain that controls four major functions: different glands; temperature regulation, (if you have this disease, your temperature is almost never up to 98.6, it's usually 97); sleep; and blood pressure, pulse and blood flow. You usually find low blood pressure with this disease, which is why your spouse jumps to the other end of the bed when you put your cold feet on them. These all stem from the hypothalamus.

"The glands are critical. You see low DHEA because of the underactive hypothalamus in about 70 to 80 percent of people with the disease. The thyroid will often be low—even if the blood tests are normal, because blood tests look different if the thyroid is low from the hypothalamus not working than most doctors would expect them to be. So you have to go by the symptoms: fatigue, cold intolerance, dry skin, confusion, achiness, and a low body temperature. These call for a tri-

atal thyroid hormone. Low adrenal function causes, a loss of stamina and low estrogen in women (people often get this disease a year or two after a hysterectomy or tubal ligation) and low testosterone in men.

"Major respiratory infections are frequently unrelenting because the immune system is overactive and poorly functioning. Because of the change of blood flow to the nose, chronic nasal congestion is very common and so is sinusitis. People get antibiotics for these from their doctors and then they get yeast or candida overgrowth. I say avoid antibiotics if you have chronic fatigue. Zinc lozenges are effective—at least 10 mgs of zinc five to eight times a day during the infection. Vitamin C should be boosted to high levels—anywhere from 5,000 to 10,000 mgs a day. Use nasal rinses—half a teaspoon of salt and a cup of lukewarm water, sniffed maybe an inch up each nostril. Blow your nose so you wash out the infection. Echinacea—about 325 mgs—is more effective than antibiotics. Don't use it for more than three to four weeks at a time because then it stops working.

"Because nutritional deficiencies are rampant with chronic fatigue, magnesium is a key player, but the form of magnesium is important. I would take about 300 mgs a day of magnesium or succinate, aspartate. Malic acid: 300 mgs four times a day is important for the muscles. Coenzyme Q10 100: mgs a day. NADA: five mgs twice a day, and potassium magnesium aspartate 1000: mgs maybe one to two times a day. These help the energy factories a lot.

"These things are simple, cheap, nontoxic and if you do them and cut out the sugar and coffee, for a lot of people suffering from fatigue, sometimes that's all it takes.

"People with chronic fatigue commonly suffer from chemical sensitivities because the immune system is over- active, it's non directed, it attacks everything. I find that when I treat the candida, the underactive adrenal gland and the yeast, often these sensitivities go away or diminish quite a bit."

As Dr. Allan Spreen tells us, "Physical and emotional fatigue go hand-in-hand. Fatigue tends to affect mental functioning, so that a person suffering from fatigue feels that his or her memory is not as good as it once was. I consider that type of fatigue biochemically based. I'm sure it's in the genes that some people wear out faster than others.

"Because food sensitivities often manifest themselves as cravings, we try to get people off the foods they crave. Chances are they may be sensitive to these foods, such that their sensitivity can manifest itself as fatigue and mental states tied to fatigue, such as irritability or frustration.

"Depression is another common reaction to fatigue. People think they're getting old or sick, or that they're dying, because they don't have the energy they once had. And depression causes a domino effect. Once people are depressed, they don't care to do anything. If they don't do anything, their self-worth decreases. They feel worse and worse.

"We try to take a complete approach. We find that as digestion improves, with proper foods and supplemental digestive enzymes, fatigue tends to diminish. Subsequently, energy levels and clarity of mind improve. People can concentrate better. The patient can remember things better because his or her mind isn't experiencing brain fog from all of the toxic junk floating around in the body.

"We ask people to give us two weeks. We want them to stop eating the foods they crave the most. If there is anything they feel the day just isn't complete without, we tell them that that's what they need to give up first. Once they give that up, if their fatigue worsens for the next two or three days—if they become more irritable, pick fights with family members, their self-worth diminishes, feel like they're not getting anywhere, have more intestinal problems—I can almost guarantee that that food is a major part of their problem.

"Once they get past that hump, which I call withdrawal—the signs of withdrawal described above confirm the presence of a food sensitivity, or allergy, to craved food in question—they tend to feel much better and everything seems to improve. Their peace of mind improves; they are less fatigued; their depression tends to decrease, if it's not true clinical depression from some other cause; their energy level increases; sleep improves; and the quality of their relationships improves. Their state of mind seems to dominate the other way where everything becomes better. It's not a panacea but it's a place to start."

Dr. Spreen outlines a nutritional approach to regaining energy: "Our efforts here are to optimize a person's biochemical intake nutritionally so that he or she can make the best use of whatever genetic disposition they have and overcome fatigue. Of course, there's always the possibility that fatigue represents the onset of something serious like cancer or something else. Our approach to treatment is to consult on a nutritional basis, complementing whatever diagnosis a patient might have from their primary physician. We don't seek to replace a primary physician.

"Normally I start by taking the known stressors out of the diet. The first three are sugar, sugar, and sugar. When people eat a lot of refined sugar, the body tries to bring the sugar level down. Their sugar levels bounce up and down, up and down. They're getting highs and lows, which make their mind fog up and prevent clear thinking and memory.

"This is a frustrating situation. When people get frustrated they get irritated. When they get irritated they pick fights or get depressed. Their self-worth goes down or they hit their wife or smack their kids when they really don't mean to. Sugary items alone are usually a major part of most people's diets and a hard thing to stop.

"After we've taken the refined sugar out of the diet, we do other simple things. We ask people to eat foods in their natural state, not processed foods. If a person stays on junk all the time—eats 12 candy bars a day, three soft drinks or more (with seven teaspoons of sugar in each soft drink), and smokes and drinks and gets stimulants in other bad foods—taking a multivitamin just isn't going to do the trick.

"I try to get people off caffeine. I give them vitamins and supplements which, hopefully, their bodies will absorb. If their absorption is not good, they may require digestive enzymes, additional acidophilus, or hydrochloric acid supplements."

Finally, Dr. Spreen emphasizes two naturally occurring substances as being of particular importance in the treatment of chronic fatigue: Like other practioners, he recommends starting with a B12 shot, "the old 'quack' remedy that most doctors consider a placebo and don't even like to talk about. I'm batting about three out of four that just with a B12 shot, you'll feel more energy within a day. And B complex, needed today more than ever before because of the American diet. The B vitamins work together, predominantly to help with the assimilation of carbohydrates. When complex carbohydrates are removed from the diet, people use up the B complex stores in the body, which are somewhat limited, being water-soluble. If people consumed more unrefined foods, they would have what is required in food for the assimilation of that food. So I give both B complex in a supplement and extra B12 if fatigue is a problem. Plus I try to get people off refined sugar, refined white flour, refined pasta, and anything else that might stress the body.

"I'm not an herbalist, but I'm using herbs more and more in my practice. To boost mental function, I use ginkgo biloba, probably the number-two herb after ginseng. We'll give a trial of that to people who say they don't remember things the way they used to, and to children with learning disorders. We'll try the herb for about six weeks. If the person doesn't feel a noticeable difference in that time, it probably doesn't work for them. The nice thing about this type of remedy is that it's harmless. If it doesn't work, you've only lost a few dollars; it hasn't done any harm. I think that herbs with a 2,000-year history have done people some good, that herbalists, dating back to the Indian medicine men and ancient Chinese herbalists, knew what they were doing.

"If we can help a person sleep, we can help him or her to think and feel better when awake. Valerian is an herb that has been used for years to help with sleep. Sometimes we mix that with taurine, which is not an herb but an amino acid. These two agents together tend to help people relax, although this does not work all the time.

"Some botanicals that worry us are at the opposite end of the spectrum. We want to get these substances out of the body. Nonherbal teas and coffee are artificial stimulants. They make people feel good momentarily, but harm them in the long run. We compare it to the difference between feeding a horse right and whipping a horse. You can make a horse work harder for awhile with the whip, but you'd better feed him or he won't continue to work. We try to get the whips out of there and enhance nutrition instead."

Dr. Singh Khalsa also encourages exercise in his patients with fibromyalgia. "Because they're in pain," he says, "they avoid it, and I don't blame them. Nevertheless, researchers believe that fibromyalgia involves a brain chemical imbalance. Therefore, whether the exercise is cardiovascular, yoga or meditation, this can help re-balance endorphins and serotonin, which makes the brain function more effectively. Re-balancing the brain this way often relieves many of the painful physical and emotional symptoms of the illness, which include insomnia and depression. Most important, exercise can help fibromyalgia patients enjoy a good night's sleep, which most of them so desperately need."

Patients who are too weak or impoverished to follow Dr. Kalsa's guidelines can still benefit from sustained sessions of long, slow, deep breathing, "even if it's only for five minutes," he says. "Careful, deep, measured breathing helps oxygenate the body and increase blood flow to the brain. And even if you're confined to a bed, you can do this several times over the course of a day to exercise your mind and body. You'll not only feel better physically, but you'll feel a sense of accomplishment because you're doing something really positive and beneficial for yourself."

Dr. Ken Korins explains how homeopathy works, specifically for chronic fatigue. "Homeopathy," he says, "is a type of energy or vibrational medicine. It works by stimulating the person's innate healing forces. In some traditions, for instance Chinese medicine, that's called the chi. In homeopathy, we call it the vital force. It relates to chronic fatigue because chronic fatigue, as well as many other conditions, represents a dis-balance in the person's system, particularly on their energy level. When that is corrected, many things fall into place.

"I treat chronic fatigue and candida together, since many of their symptoms overlap. Although the cause of chronic fatigue is not known, the Epstein Barr virus, a member of the herpes virus group, is often involved. The symptoms may persist for months or years. All these viruses have one thing in common—they establish a lifelong latent infection in the host. In fact, by the end of adulthood most adults do demonstrate antibodies against the Epstein Barr virus, indicating a past infection. Those with the most serious symptoms generally have the highest antibody levels to Epstein Barr. This may actually indicate that the chronic fatigue syndrome is a problem of decreased immune function and not just a disorder caused by a specific virus.

"Susceptibility is a very important issue because the presence of the virus is not enough to cause the syndrome. The terrain must be fertile to enable the virus to propagate and cause disruption to the organism. Any condition that compromises immune function such as AIDS, cancer, chronic kidney failure, rheumatoid arthritis or other primary, or secondary immuno-deficient states.

"In addressing chronic fatigue syndrome it's important to look at detoxification of external toxins such as chemicals and drugs as well as internal toxins such as candida and free radicals. Stimulation of the elimination organs, such as the bowel, liver, kidney, lymph nodes and skin are extremely important. The immune system must also be addressed. There are many nutrients that can help address this but at least people should be on a good multi-vitamin, with carotenes, vitamin C, and zinc; this is extremely important for the immune system and also for the glandular system. Glandular extract such as thymus, spleen, and liver can be very beneficial, as well as certain botanical support such as goldenseal, echinacea, licorice, astragalus, or aloe vera, to name a few.

"The homeopathic remedies are based on the symptoms, not on the diagnosis. There is a lot of overlap between remedies that are used for candida and for chronic fatigue syndrome. Homeopathy works by stimulating the body's innate healing potential and the goal is to be curative, not just to suppress the symptoms.

"The trick is to find the right remedy. I suggest you pick two or three symptoms that are most disturbing, even though you might have a list of 20 or 30, and then find the remedy. If the indicated remedy does not seem to be working, try using what we call a nosode, the homeopathic remedy for Epstein barr virus or candida. This can be very effective in and of itself.

"Gelsemium is a major remedy for chronic fatigue syndrome. It is good for patients who get extremely tired with the least exertion. They may always want to be in bed. Their limbs tremble with exhaustion; there is a lot of muscular soreness; the eyelids may feel heavy to the point where they droop. Blurring of vision and double vision is not uncommon when gelsemium is indicated. Gelsemium is also a remedy for acute flu. It is a good remedy for people that have never been well since the flu. It reduces the thirst that often accompanies fever.

"Phosphoric acid is a remedy for weakness and debility, usually starting in the mental realm and then becoming physical. The phosphoric acid condition seems to result from loss of bodily fluids, particularly sexual bodily fluids. If you've had a very promiscuous period, feel drained sexually and are chronically tired and fatigued, phosphoric acid can be particularly helpful. People who respond to this remedy are usually mentally apathetic and indifferent, and have tearing pains in their joints, as if the bones were scraped. They are better with short naps. There is a craving for sodas and carbonated drinks. Phosphoric acid is also a major remedy in diabetes.

"Arsenicum album is good for people who have anxiety and restlessness with their exhaustion, who fear death and disease and despair of recovery. The sensations often revolve around burning pains in the stomach, hay fever symptoms with excretions that are thin, watery and burning. They have other gastronomical, intestinal symptoms, such as weight loss, and chronic conditions with a lot of diarrhea, especially after eating watery fruits. Shortness of breath with exertion is very common. The skin tends to be dry, rough and scaly. Arsenicum is also indicated during acute Epstein Barr virus or flu-like symptoms especially when there is great thirst.

"Kali phosphorica is related to arsenicum because of anxiety. Both remedies help with anxiety and fear, but kaliphosphricum has a lot more effect on brain fog. People who need this cannot recall names or words. They have problems with memory.

"Baryt carbonica brings focus and helps with slow mental grasp, a lot of confusion, difficulty learning. People in this state often have an enlarged tonsil. The glands are enlarged almost to the point of touching each other and they get colds very easily.

"Anacardium is another remedy for brain fog, for people who are very forgetful and have developed a tendency to use foul language after the development of chronic fatigue. They also tend to have a lot of fixed ideas. There is an obsessive component to the anacardium syndrome.

"Lycopodium is a very important remedy for brain fog with weak memory, confused thoughts, dyslexia, loss of words. There are abdominal symptoms with noisy flatulence, especially after eating and a lot of bloating. They desire sweets, are excessively hungry, have sensitivities of the liver and sore throats that begin on the right side and spread to the left.

"Noxvomica is another remedy that has a lot to do with impaired liver function It is good for problems after eating, like the sensation that the food is stuck in the stomach like a rock and just sits there for hours. Also irritable bowel-like symptoms like constipation alternating with diarrhea.

"The idea is that homeopathy is very specific. It is important to remove the obstacles to the cure. Diet, stress and toxins must be addressed in order for the homeopathic remedies to work most effectively. When we look at health from this mind set, we can help the body to heal and re-balance. With this approach, it is less important to address a particular virus, bacteria or fungi because the immune system is strong and can heal most of these things, including ones yet to be identified."

Dr. Alan Pressman believes that glutathione may be the key to chronic fatigue. First, he explains how the liver works to de-toxify the body: "When our body has to combat environmental pollution and free radical damage, the major organ responsible is your liver, the largest organ of the body. One of the liver's major jobs is to keep you clean, to remove and destroy tremendous amounts of some of the five trillion pounds of chemicals that we are exposed to every year.

"The liver does this in two separate phases. The toxin will come into your system and into your liver and will then be oxidized. We call that activation. That is the phase in which the toxin is being made ready to be taken out of your body in your feces and in your urine and perhaps in your saliva and your perspiration. Mostly in your feces and urine. The second phase—this is a crucial phase—is the removal of this toxin out of your body. If you do not remove it, it builds up and creates problems. When a toxin is made ready to be eliminated from the body, it is actually bio-activated, meaning that it becomes more toxic that it was before. But now it can be packaged in nice little bundles and taken out of the body. That is the responsibility of phase two of liver detox, to take this toxic garbage out of your body.

"Phase 1 and phase 2 must be coordinated. The toxins—mercury, lead, and all the chemicals that accumulate in your system—are taken out of your body through phase 2, which is totally under the control of your levels of glutathione and glutathione enzymes. In order for your body to be clean, to be pure, to be detoxified, you have to have a high level of glutathione in your liver at all times. Glutathione gets used up, so you have to keep replacing it with supplementation.

"If you do not, you can wind up with symptoms ranging from Parkinson's disease to Alzheimer's disease to neuro-toxicity of a number of different brain pathways, all the way down to chronic fatigue syndrome and fibromyalgia. There is new proof in the research on nitric oxide, that in all cases of fibromyalgia and chronic fatigue syndrome, there is a marked deficiency and depletion of glutathione, lypoic acid, and n-acetyl cysteine. If you are suffering from brain fog, if you are mentally confused, if you are disoriented, if you have body pain, if you have frequent illnesses, if your energy is gone, if your zip is gone, if you are having trouble learning, trouble concentrating, having constipation or diarrhea or gastrointestinal discomfort, even cardiac arrhythmia—all this could be related to abnormal detoxification in Phase 2 by the liver.

"If that's the case, it's very inexpensive to discover. A functional liver detoxification profile measures glutathione activity in the liver through urine and saliva. We basically challenge you by having you take a prescribed amount of caffeine, of aspirin and acetaminophen and we watch the urine and saliva to see how successful you are at detoxifying those three substances. From that, we can tell you exactly how your glutathione is functioning. The foods high in glutathione are avocado, asparagus, watermelon, squash, potato, and vegetables like spinach and parsley."

Dr. Andrew Gentile explains that people suffering from chronic fatigue have, "along with the symptom of debilitating exhaustion, cognitive impairment. Intellectual functioning wanes. People say, 'I go from one room to another and I just don't remember why I went into the first room' or 'I see a colleague I have worked with for a number of years and I'm quite embarrassed because I can't remember their first name.' There is also simply an inability to respond to physical and emotional stress. So many patients say, 'I seem to be feeling better and then as soon as I take a brisk walk or go swimming, within 72 hours, I begin to experience what seems like a flu—chills, sore throats, fevers. I get exhausted and go into a relapse and I don't feel well for anywhere from a week or two to months on end.'

"Fatigue is usually a symptom of depression. Because there is no known cause of chronic fatigue, you might see your general practitioner and complain of a list of symptoms and he would diagnose depression. But we now know that chronic fatigue simply is not depression.

"Almost everyone of every age gets this disorder. It was a misnomer when it was called yuppie flu. Age clusters however, do tend to be around the mid 30s, with women getting it twice as much as men do. It is worldwide—in Japan, they call it 'low natural killer syndrome.' Some believe that the number of affected people could be as high as 5 million. The prevalence rates vary depending on the study—at first it was 2 to 7 out of 100,000, but we now know it is much higher, more like 1 out of 100.

"There appears to be a higher percentage of physicians, nurses, and teachers who get it. I myself contracted this disorder in the late '70s, early '80s. I was a clinical psychologist working in a group home with many disadvantaged, multiply handicapped children. Most of the other workers experienced a nondescript, flu-like illness and then would pick up and seem to feel well. I also experienced that and then I took a vacation down south and did a lot of running. I was an avid runner and swimmer and I got a flu. This is what most people say, they got a flu and they just simply never recovered. It took me several years to recover.

"I think of chronic fatigue as an endpoint on a continuum. There are a lot of points along the continuum where people feel tired, they know something is not right, they're not sleeping right, yet we couldn't technically diagnose them as having chronic fatigue. None the less, it's very important to look at what's going on for them so they can get to re-balancing.

"Traditional medicine searches for a single cause—in this case they were looking for single viral agents or several viral agents that cause the whole body to lose it's functional capabilities. In the early '80s, researchers were in a flurry looking for a connection to the Epstein Barr virus. This turned out to be a wild goose chase, as all such simplistic single agent studies will be, because Epstein Barr is widely distributed in the normal population by about age 8. Eighty-five to ninety percent of the population has caught Epstein Barr and recovered and therefore it could not be the causative agent or else why wouldn't everybody being coming down with the syndrome? Human Herpes Virus 6 fell upon a similar fate. It is widely distributed in the normal population and therefore could not be the distinguishing virus. Nobody is now thinking that a single viral agent or a combination of viruses really explain all the data. We are beginning to think that viruses are just a small part of this. I would like us to think about multi-causal arrangements such as allergy, environmental toxicity, candida, stress, attitudes, some behavior such as rushing and too great involvement and being non-self rejuvenating.

"A naturopath would look at everything in a person's life—their stress levels, behaviors that cause stress, a slightly compromised immune system, foods causing allergies, a higher toxic load. They work with a computer—one wonders why they get a headache 3 or 4 hours later? They keep complaining about stale air and everybody in that office is complaining about the same stale air. We look at the long standing nature of these factors. The body tries to meet all these demands, tries to manage the total toxic load on the immune system as if it were a rain barrel. Water was filling up in the rain barrel and it got to the brim and then the slightest drop overflowed the barrel. That's the point at which a person begins to show some real signs of illness.

"The point where one drop in the rain barrel let it overflow is the proverbial straw that broke the camel's back. Traditional medicine will spend millions of dollars investigating the straw. They will not look at the fact that the camel walked for 100 miles with a 100 pounds on its back, which is where the answers are. If we were to carefully investigate an individual who has come down with chronic fatigue, we would find the unique things about that individual's life—they were drinking alcohol and had a lot of marital stress and at the same time, they were doing a lot of running. There were a lot of things suppressing their immune system. They had lost the connection with the general harmony.

"Many of my patients frequently tell me, 'I go to Arizona and I feel different, I come back and I get sick again. I go to Colorado and I can bicycle, I come back here and I can barely walk from my chronic fatigue.' It's not just that they took vacations. We need to look at illness in its total ecological environmental sense—that illness could be seen as a disharmony or disconnection with one's environment.

"We are talking about this on a level of disconnection. The person's own response to their illness, once contracted, that's disconnected if they cannot develop higher ways of understanding how their life has lead them to this point of illness. If they view their illness as the outside superimposed in—"I caught a germ"—that's typical disconnected, linear, analytic thinking, very much the way our medical sciences approach problems. They're on to traditional medicine, doing lots of tests and finding nothing. If they switch thinking and begin to say 'my organism became imbalanced in some way, it could no longer meet the total toxic load and that has to do with the way I live my life,' they could take a different path. They could tie themselves back into the loop of life and make more lifestyle changes, which lead to healthier patterns in living and shorter remediation of their illness and shorter relapses.

"What I believe has been missed with this particular illness is predisposing factors. People say, 'For years before I became diagnosed, I had a problem with sleep' or 'I have always been pushing it.' There are a lot of personality variables here that need to be researched.

"When you begin to look at the body's inability to meet the total toxic load, you notice that the cytokines—a messenger cell in the immune system which carries instructions to other cells—seem quite high for this group. The cytokines themselves may be responsible for causing a lot of the neurologic symptoms, the inability to think clearly. We know that the bowel has certain receptors for these cytokines and high numbers of people with chronic fatigue have bowel symptoms. It's as though the immune system designed to take care of this total lifestyle/viral/bacteriologic load has turned on itself. There were so many demands made on it from the way the person lived, just from sheer external toxicity, that the system could not keep up those levels. The immune system is designed to say, 'this is an alien, let's attack it and get rid of it' and 'this is part of a normal cell in my body, so let's not attack it.' You get into disturbances when this detection is not accurate any longer. You have a perfect metaphor for the body maiming the self.

"Some things are energy depleting and some things are energy rejuvenating. What we know in terms of the mind/body connection from Hans Sele, a landmark physician and researcher in stress, is that the body tries to support energy expenditures by reorganizing itself. It gets much more economical about distributing cholesterol, distributing blood to vital parts of the body and so forth. It continues to do this in a step wise fashion as long as you continue to make the demands. In those early studies, the more demands that were placed on animals, the more they thrived. Researchers scratched their heads and said 'what's the limit? These animals are being placed in challenging if not untoward levels of demand and they are doing better and better.' As soon as they stopped the experiment, the animals started to die. Autopsies showed swollen spleens, shrunken thymus, and enlarged adrenal glands.

"The explanation is in the interface between the hormonal system and the immune system. This is a whole new field of psychoneuroimmunology. Your body tries to meet the demands you put on it and continue to meet them. After the stress has terminated, the body tries to go back to its original level, its homeostasis and it cannot do it. This is virtually what happens when a person gets chronic fatigue.

"There is a way of being with our experience and not losing our own functional integrity, the boundaries where we end and something else begins. It's like singing in a chorus. The product is the sum total of all the voices. The unique contribution you are making needs to be maintained, but you are also in larger harmony with others. It is much what a cell has to learn in order to stay healthy in its environment. It needs to learn how much to take in and only what it truly needs. If it becomes too permeable, it takes in too much toxicity that it can't break down and it will die. If it closes off too much, it will not get what it needs and it will die. That's a metaphor for a way of being with something without losing your own functional integrity. There are situations in which the emotional discharge into what you are doing is depleting and it's not going to be replenished. Your body will actually forget how to self rejuvenate. In chronic fatigue, I see this all the time."

21
HORMONE IMBALANCE

Patient Story: Mrs. X

A 40-year-old woman was having marital difficulties and had been seeing a counselor for a couple of years. While she did need to straighten out her relationship, that wasn't causing her physical and emotional problems. She was deficient in adrenal hormone. She was tired and irritable and couldn't get through the day. She couldn't manage the children. They would get on her nerves and she'd lash out at her husband. I tested her blood level of DHEA and found that it was more than two standard deviations below the mean. I put her on a very minimal dose of DHEA, and within two or three months she had discharged all of her counselors and her husband called me to tell me what saviors we were. These are some of the miracles we see.

Emphasizing the importance of having access to good testing facilities, Dr. Ray Wunderlich, who treated Mrs. X, cites the importance of hormone imbalances among the illnesses that are often misdiagnosed as mental disease. "When we assess people's hormones and glandular functions with good chemistry, we can help make them less sensitive to the toxic assaults of the environment.

"While there are no such things as panaceas in medicine and we want to be aware of unwarranted enthusiasm and zeal," Dr. Wunderlich continues, "the hormone DHEA is probably the closest thing to a panacea in medicine that we have found as of yet. It is the so-called 'mother hormone' of the adrenal gland, an antidepressant that seems to be able to counter a lot of the allergic reactions that we see in people who are accumulating toxic insults as they age, decade after decade. This adrenal hormone declines from the age of 20 to death, due to illness and aging. By intervening with appropriate doses of the adrenal hormone DHEA, we can reverse many of the allergies and immune susceptibilities that we see in people over 25 years of age.

"Mental functioning is also impaired in people who are low in the adrenal hormones, especially in DHEA. When these hormones are down, people become chronically fatigued. They have difficulty getting into mental gear, making decisions, seeing options, and fighting off the chemical assaults found in their environment. We can measure adrenal function in the saliva and the blood, and we can show that it increases with DHEA supplementation.

"Not every case is going to be a miracle cure. But some cases of chronic depression, irritability, and premenstrual syndrome are related to adrenal dysfunction, with low levels of the mother hormone of the adrenal gland. This is particularly so in people with low-blood-sugar symptoms.

"We believe that this DHEA is kind of a baseline hormone. It feeds all the other systems, including the ones that regulate the sugar balance in the body. It can also serve as a precursor to the sex hormones—both female and male—as well as to the electrolytes, the salt and water hormones of the adrenals. It is highly individual in its response, but it is a major reactor that we didn't know about some years ago. The effects of DHEA have been well-researched; it has an anti-cancer, anti-viral, and anti-depressive effect in animals. People have improved through the use of herbs, vitamins, and minerals, which have probably been supporting the functioning of this hormone in the body, among other effects.

"People who are tired when they get up in the morning, who have reactions to sugar, who have to eat frequent meals, who have family histories of low blood sugar, diabetes, or alcoholism, and those with stubborn allergies," Dr. Wunderlich concluded, "frequently have low adrenal function. Vitamins and herbs that help support the adrenal function and the precursors of the adrenal function are vitamin C, pantothenic acid, B-complex, licorice, and Siberian ginseng."

Dr. Joseph Debe believes that on the subject of diet and its effect on moods and emotions, it is interesting that estrogen levels fluctuate tremendously in response to dietary intake. "Unfortunately, a lot of women are being given hormone replacement therapy when it's not necessary. A lot of women reach menopause and are automatically put onto hormone replacement, usually estrogen and progesterone. Upon appropriate testing, which is actually done with salvia samples, it is found that a lot of these women don't actually need hormone replacement. If they are given estrogen when their bodies are still producing adequate quantities, which is not unusual at the beginning of menopause, there are adverse consequences. Not only can a woman be predisposed to increased cancers, such as breast and uterine cancer, but it also has an impact on the brain and the mind. Excess estrogen, also found in pre-menopausal women with PMS, usually results in anxiety, mood swings, and irritability.

"There are so many things that influence our estrogen levels which men also produce. One very important factor is meat intake. If a woman is eating a lot of meat, her body produces more estrogen levels. One way this works is seen in the connection between our diet and the bacteria that live within the intestinal tract. Each of us has about a 100 trillion organisms within the intestinal tract. Most medical doctors don't consider the intestinal flora, but they have metabolic activity on par with the liver. The metabolic bi-products are absorbed into the blood stream partially and influence all aspects of our physiology, including the brain. There are bacteria in the intestinal tract that cause estrogen to be recirculated into the blood stream instead of eliminated. These bacteria feed on meat. So if we are eating a lot of meat, we have more of these bacteria and we have more estrogen returning to circulation.

"Another thing that raises estrogen levels is constipation. If food is in the intestinal tract longer, there is more time for these bacteria to work on the estrogen and re-circulate it into the blood stream. Another thing that raises estrogen levels is a low fiber diet. Not only does low fiber cause constipation, but fiber finds the estrogen and drags it out of the body.

"A woman can effectively lower the active estrogen in her body by consuming flax seeds, ground flax seeds. Flax seeds contain compounds called lignins, which increase binding proteins that take active estrogen out of circulation. Estrogen exists in the circulation in protein-bound form, which is inactive and in free form, which is the active hormone. One way to effectively lower the biological estrogen is to increase protein that binds it and that is done by consuming ground flax seeds.

"Another thing that influences estrogen activity and its effect on the brain is soy. Soy contains estrogen-like compounds that compete with the body's own estrogen for binding to receptor sites. If we have a lot of these isoflavones, as they are called, in circulation, they compete with the body's estrogen and reduce the estrogen stimulation of the brain. Because these isoflavones are weaker, they can normalize estrogen activity.

"Women who are not producing enough estrogen can raise estrogen activity without taking hormones, which carry risk. If they are vegetarian, they can consider adding some animal products to their diet. If that goes against their beliefs, there are other options. Licorice contains compounds that allow the body to retain more estrogen in circulation longer. So do soy isoflavones—the soy substitutes for the woman's inadequate estrogen. Soy has been found to have the same impact on neurotransmitters within the brain as the body's own estrogen does."

Dr. Debe recommends that women consider being tested with the female hormonal panel, "a salivary test that uses eleven salivary samples over the course of a month to measure fluctuations in estrogen and progesterone. When you go to your doctor and he takes a single blood sample for estrogen or progesterone, that tells you nothing about what is going on with your cycle over the course of a month. With eleven salvia samples on different days, we can determine if your estrogen is too low at a particular time in the cycle, progestogen is too high at another part of the cycle and have therapy that is much more specific and we can take steps to re-balance the hormones with that detailed information.

"For example, hormonal balance is influenced by dietary choices. This is something that even most doctors don't appreciate. The way that our hormones respond to dietary choices is really amazing. If we take a look at the stress hormones, these are epinephrine which is commonly known as adrenalin, cortisol and DEHA. Epinephrine is a short acting hormone. That is the hormone that is released in the fight or flight reaction. For example if we are almost involved in a car accident our heart starts pounding, racing and we feel shaky. This is from the release of a lot of adrenaline. Cortisol and DHEA are long-acting stress hormones which are released over a longer period of time and they all have slightly different effects on the body.

"Now as far as diet goes there are a number of ways that diet can cause imbalance in these hormones. One very common way for Americans is by eating too much refined carbohydrate, which can be a problem when the carbohydrate is refined, when the fiber is removed and we are eating convenience foods because we don't want to spend a lot of time on eating because we are always in a hurry, then we are getting unnatural food. We are getting a big burst of sugar in the blood stream. When you eat pasta, cookies, cakes, there is an unnatural spike in blood sugar that results from this. The body is not meant to be exposed to such a sugar load all at once. What happens is the blood sugar spikes, the body tries to control it by releasing insulin and often the body releases too much insulin, the blood sugar dips too low and this has all kinds of consequences.

"A drop in blood sugar causes confusion, mood swings, irritability, anxiety, lightheadedness, head aches, blurred vision. Glucose is a primary fuel source of the brain. It's critical that the brain has a steady supply of glucose so when we are eating excessive convenience foods or refined carbohydrates we have a seesaw of blood sugar. That has a direct impact on the brain but then it further imbalances the stress hormone that I was mentioning. With regard to adrenaline, the blood sugar drops, the adrenaline goes up, and it's interesting that adrenaline when over-secreted over a period of time reduces the brain's production of dopamine. Dopamine is one of the neurotransmitters that has been found to be low in children with ADHD.

"Low blood sugar also causes the body to secrete too much cortisol. Cortisol is a long-acting stress hormone. Cortisol damages the brain in a number of ways. It literally causes brain damage when it is over-secreted for long periods of time. Studies done with rats have found that injecting the animal with cortisol causes them to be unable to find their way through a familiar maze. Upon autopsy, they were found to have physical signs of brain damage.

"Cortisol, specifically, damages part of the brain called the hippocampus, the part of the brain that is involved in Alzheimer's disease. And indeed people with Alzheimer's disease have been found to have high cortisol and low DHEA levels. And one of the causes of high cortisol and low DHEA is eating refined carbohydrates on a regular basis.

"People addicted to eating carbohydrates who don't want to make any drastic change right off can start by not eating the carbohydrate by itself. If you eat several cookies, that is pretty much pure carbohydrates and will cause a big swing in blood sugar. If you have some protein with the cookies—let's say instead of having the cookies between meals, you have them immediately after consuming a balanced meal that has protein (fish, poultry, eggs, legumes, lentils)—the negative effects on the body are much less. The protein causes the body to release another hormone called glucogen, which helps to balance out the blood sugar. We don't have that big seesaw in blood sugar that is detrimental in itself and also causes imbalance in the stress hormones."

22

NUTRIENT IMBALANCES IN THE BODY AND BRAIN

D r. Priscilla Slagle has made a unique and important contribution in her medical practice using amino acid supplements to help patients control their mood illnesses by correcting nutrient imbalances in the body and brain. "I have had a lot of clinical experience controlling moods by using amino acids. Right now, I am quite concerned about the current effort by the FDA to ban amino acids, which takes away the right of individuals to help themselves. In a sense, it's like banning proteins, which is to say, ludicrous. So I hope that people will fight this reactionary effort on the part of our government to make amino acids available only through physicians—which would cost a person far more.

"I have treated patients with amino acids for almost 20 years to control moods, for depression, anxiety, memory loss, and other health problems. I continue to be amazed at their efficacy. I usually use them in combination with proper diagnosis and treatment of other conditions.

"The first step I take with my patients is to make the correct diagnosis. Usually, by the time people get to me, they have already been many places and tried many drugs, and I am the end of the road for them. So these patients don't have simple, straightforward kinds of problems. They usually have multiple-symptom problems, for instance, chemical sensitivities, viruses, food sensitivities, auto-immune problems, parasite problems, fungus problems, and so on.

"So first I find out what is going on. When a patient comes to me, I often do an amino acid panel so that I can measure 42 different aspects of amino acids in their body. There are 22 amino acids, but I am also measuring metabolic breakdown products. Their patterns suggest connective tissue or auto-immune disease, chronic viruses, chemical or food sensitivities, or candida. While it is an extensive diagnostic process, it does seem to find the root cause of some very puzzling complex physical and mental problems which patients are experiencing.

"Then I remove the offending agents, such as chemicals or candida- or yeast-inducing foods, or drugs (many people have drug-induced auto-immune problems). We have to clarify and clean up their environments and their diets.

"For depression, I use tyrosine, which is an amino acid that raises norepinephrine, a major brain chemical that maintains good mood, drive, motivation, and concentration. Glutamine makes glutamic acid, one of the two major brain fuels, and is important for memory, focus, and concentration. I use these two amino acids to treat depression. They must be combined with the active form of B6, which controls the absorption, metabolism, and conversion of amino acids into all their various end products, such as neurotransmitters, antibodies, digestive enzymes, muscles, and tissues in the body.

"I also give my depressed patients a basic multivitamin with minerals. Many depressed people are magnesium-deficient, so I've been using a relatively large amount of magnesium in my practice. I've also incorporated a fair amount of potassium for chronic fatigue syndrome patients. Many of them have potassium problems that are not necessarily picked up by a standard blood test. I check cellular potassium levels rather than the regular blood tests. I use some homeopathic cortisone with certain people with auto-immune disease.

"Some other amino acids that I use are taurine and cysteine. Taurine is a neuro-inhibitory neurotransmitter which has a calming effect. It also controls heart rate and helps with fat metabolism. Many of the people who have chemical sensitivities and yeast problems (probably 90 percent of the ones I see) have a reduced taurine as well as a reduced cysteine level. Cysteine, like taurine, is an amino acid that helps the body to detoxify.

"In many people with chemical sensitivities, the detoxification processes in their bodies has broken down due to overload, or deficiencies of various nutrients, or a liver dysfunction. So they aren't able to handle the same kind of toxic load that other people might handle who aren't dealing with the same variables. I use large doses of vitamin C and multi-amino acids, as well as certain other products which support detoxification pathways.

"At the risk of sounding fanatical, I believe we are poisoning this earth. Many people with chemical sensitivities, auto-immune disorders, and immune deficiency problems are early victims of what is happening to the planet, harbingers of what may later grow into a more serious and more obviously recognized problem. I have begun to see in my practice a vast number of auto-immune problems that I feel are environmentally or chemically induced. This problem is significant and deserves to receive national and international attention. I really appreciate the work that Dr. Rodgers has done and I recommend that people, particularly those with chemical sensitivities, read her books."

Dr. Sidney Baker emphasizes magnesium deficiency in his clinical practice when treating nutrient imbalances that manifest as mental disease. "I presented a paper on magnesium at a conference in La Jolla, California, a few years ago. At this colloquium, there were magnesium experts from all over, mostly academic people, and mostly people who had jobs like running an intensive care unit or a cardiac care unit, or a department of immunology or obstetrics and gynecology. Everyone there from every medical specialty was saying, 'Isn't it amazing that our colleagues are not aware of the very lengthy published information on the prevalence of magnesium deficiency in America, and its very widespread picture in clinical practice?' Any ordinary person would have come away from the conference saying, 'Well, how come this problem is being overlooked?' The cynical answer may be the truth: Magnesium deficiency research has no corporate sponsor.

"I've become convinced that magnesium deficiency is a major epidemic, one that we are experiencing right now in North America. Magnesium deficiency is widespread in its pattern of symptoms. It affects cardiovascular disease, allergies, tension, panic attacks, premenstrual syndrome, and hyperactivity in children, to name just some of the conditions. The underlying theme behind many of the symptoms is what you might call being 'uptight.'

"Both magnesium and yeast problems probably began around 1950. The magnesium problem probably has its roots in the widespread use in agriculture of fertilizers containing potassium. The yeast problem probably arose because of the widespread use of antibiotics in the population, which began around 1950.

"Many people come to see me specifically because they think that I am a yeast specialist, and so perhaps I see these patients in disproportionate numbers. But I think that this epidemic, which is being disregarded by many people in mainstream medicine, is simply overwhelming in its prevalence in the United States. Many people's medical histories show a quite obvious yeast problem. They started getting sick soon after they started taking antibiotics; they have bloating and difficulty concentrating; they have intolerances to foods, gastrointestinal disturbances, and recurring vaginitis. Unfortunately, when they seek help from most doctors, they are told, 'Gee, we're very skeptical about this whole yeast idea; it isn't proven and so therefore we won't put you on simple remedies to see if you might have it.' The dogma has overcome the simple observation of nature.

"As a practitioner, I have a worm's-eye view of the world. I see things very close to nature and hear from my patients directly about what is going on with their health. I have formed strong opinions that these epidemics—magnesium deficiency, problems with fatty acids or yeast, calcium and trace mineral deficiencies—are keys to people's health and well-being, both in terms of finding good preventive measures and in terms of finding cures. It is very dangerous when people who are intelligent and strong-willed get themselves into positions of authority within the medical bureaucracy, and feel quite justified in dictating what they consider to be the truth, rather than letting the truth grow, in an organic way, from the experience of those of us who are seeing patients."

Dr. Lendon Smith has also confirmed the importance of the magnesium factor, both in his clinical practice and in research studies in both animals and humans. "I've been working with a chemist out of Spokane, Washington, whose name is John Kitkoski. He started doing experiments with horses by taking blood samples and then testing for mineral and other nutrient deficiencies. He discovered that some of these horses were low in calcium, or magnesium, for example. So he would put standard feed out in the corral, and then he would put standard feed plus calcium, or magnesium, or zinc, and let the animals go out and freely eat. They would smell everything and eat only what they needed. If they were low in calcium, they would eat just the calcium-supplemented feed, and then when they had had enough he noticed that they would come back to the standard feed. He would take a blood test and find out that their body chemistry had returned to normal. He figured out that the reason why the nose is placed in front of the mouth is to tell us 'don't eat that' or 'do eat this.' The sense of smell, along with taste, is a monitoring system.

"With hundreds of hours of data to verify his hypothesis, Mr. Kitkoski and I have found that people who are low in magnesium are more likely to have emotional problems—to experience anxiety and tension, to be upset, and to be unable to relax in sleep—and that leads to secondary factors. If the body chemistry is balanced, then the body can handle almost any kind of stress or stressors that come along. If it is not, then stress can exacerbate the problem.

"Mr. Kitkoski also noticed that 80 percent of the people living in North America—and he has enough data to verify this—are somewhat alkaline. If the body is alkaline, then minerals are not soluble enough to make the enzymes do their job.

"The way to determine the levels of chemicals in your body is to have blood tests done. If the GGT level is low, a person is low in magnesium because it's a magnesium-run enzyme. If a person has high levels of GGT, they often have too much magnesium. Mr. Kitkoski uses the standard 0 to 40 to 50 on the testing, going by the deviation from the mean. If somebody has around 20 on their GGT, then they are probably alright. But if they are low, and they have signs of anxiety and tension, if they can't relax, get spooked by people, and can't seem to handle the stresses of the world, then magnesium will help."

23

PREMENSTRUAL SYNDROME (PMS)

In the 21st century, PMS has finally been recognized by most orthodox physicians as a legitimate disease, not "just something in a woman's mind" for which she needs a tranquilizer. We now know that women with PMS are often allergic to their own progesterone hormone. We also know that overgrowth of yeast is a big contributor.

Women with PMS need to build themselves up nutritionally. They can do this with magnesium (800 to 1200 milligrams), vitamin B6 (from 25 to 50 milligrams), and vitamin E (400 to 800 units). It is best to take these nutrients in the higher quantity during the second half of the menstrual cycle.

In addition, women can help to alleviate PMS by participating in aerobic exercises. Whether it is power walking, jogging, bicycling, swimming, a lot of people feel the symptoms of their PMS subside. They are improving their immune systems. Also, their central nervous system functions are changing.

Dr. Hyla Cass emphasizes how often biochemical imbalances and psychological problems coexist. In her practice, she combines her work as a holistic psychiatrist with her awareness of and use of naturally occurring substances to restore biochemical balance. A good example of how this approach can work is in the treatment of premenstrual syndrome. Dr. Cass describes a typical case: "A 30-year-old woman came to see me recently, two months after she had broken up with her boyfriend. She was depressed. She'd gained weight. She was exhausted. She had trouble keeping up with her work as a secretary. Psychotherapy wasn't helping. I asked her what she was eating and it turned out that there were a number of dietary patterns that were contributing to her emotional state.

"I took a careful history which revealed that, while she wasn't overeating, she had developed the habit of drinking coffee and eating sweets to counter fatigue. Not only did this cause her to gain weight, but the coffee and sweets induced a hypoglycemic cycle. Her blood sugar levels were irregular, and this caused her to feel anxious. It was as though at a certain time of the day she was going into a withdrawal phase and the caffeine and sugar would help bring her back up.

"So the first part of her problem was this hypoglycemic cycle. Her other problem was PMS, which had grown worse over the past few months. Her symptoms included mood swings, irritability, water retention, craving sweets, and weight gain. She had always thought that PMS was normal, that this was what women (and their hapless partners) had to live with—a misconception held by too many women.

"Her lab work revealed that she did have a fairly low fasting blood sugar level. To handle the hypoglycemia, I prescribed a specific diet and supplement program. For the PMS, I recommended the following regiment: For the first two weeks of her cycle, a dong quai herbal combination; then for the second two weeks, a specific PMS combination containing extra vitamin B6, magnesium, and ingredients that detoxify the liver, an important component in treating PMS. (The specific ZAND herbal formulas are particularly effective.) I also recommended regular exercise.

"After a month on this regimen, she was feeling much, much better. She started to feel like she had some control over the break-up with her boyfriend and over her work problems. She was able to take control of her problems rather than allowing these factors in her life to control her.

"This was one case of depression where psychotherapy alone simply was not enough. What she really needed was psychotherapy plus the combination of herbal and natural remedies, diet, and exercise.

"In cases where this nutritional regimen is not sufficient, I prescribe natural progesterone cream from day 14 until day 28 of the menstrual cycle. The kind of progesterone I recommend is a natural progesterone, not the progesterone that's in the regular pharmaceutical birth control pills or the hormones that are administered by prescription. It's a derivative from the wild Mexican yam and is available in health food stores. It's also useful for menopausal symptoms. It is applied topically to the skin on fatty areas of the body, where it can be easily absorbed." Hormonal imbalance can be corrected naturally. The following case, also from Dr. Hyla Cass, is another example.

"Not long ago, a 48-year-old woman came in to see me complaining that her life 'just wasn't working.' She was a very successful professional. She had a great marriage. Her children were grown and in college and they were doing well. Her husband was successful. She really had a very good life, and yet she was unhappy. Now you could simply call this a mid-life crisis, and do psychotherapy.

"However, when I took a psychological history, aware that this was a time of life for her to start looking inward, to evaluate her life, at the same time I asked her about her menstrual cycles. She said she was still menstruating. Her periods were changing in frequency and amount, but with no other symptoms. I sent her to the lab and it turned out she was very low in progesterone, low in estrogen, but particularly low in progesterone.

"I prescribed the natural progesterone cream, which helped to alleviate most of her psychological symptoms. Her irritability went way down. She realized that her uneasiness was metabolically based. It wasn't simply a personal psychological issue. She was peri-menopausal.

"Hormonal changes occur subtly over time, and peri-menopausal women will often think that their problems are purely psychological in origin. They will not think to look at what's going on biochemically in the body. Aside from the progesterone cream, I also prescribed the herbal formulas, which improved her condition even further."

Dr. Cass concludes: "Even though people do have psychological issues—and it is important to deal with them—it's equally important to look at and treat the underlying chemistry. Often the psychological problems will lessen in severity or even disappear with treatment of biochemical imbalances."

Dr. Doris Rapp emphasizes the part food cravings can play in the development of premenstrual syndrome. "The foods that you crave premenstrually are the foods that could be causing you to feel sick. I know one mother whose premenstrual chocolate cravings were so powerful that she would put the chocolate bars in the freezer to at least slow down the pace at which she would eat them when she was premenstrual. If you are a chocoholic and you can't manage without eating chocolate, it's a good bet that chocolate is a food that is causing you a problem."

24
$\mathscr{T}$HYROID DISORDERS

Personal Accounts of Thyroiditis:
"Jenny"

I first followed the conventional route in medical treatment. In 1988, I was in my fifth year of infertility treatments, had taken multiple infertility drugs, and wound up severely depressed. I'd lost 35 pounds in two months. I couldn't sleep, I had panic attacks. Doctors put me on the conventional Xanax treatment for three years. I had hair loss, skin problems, nail-biting problems and aches all over my body, especially in my legs.

Dr. Spreen got me on a vitamin regimen, which made me feel somewhat better. Then, last summer, he put me on very low doses of thyroid and immediately —within two to three weeks—all the problems were gone. I'd had thyroid checks three times while I was being treated for infertility, and the blood tests had always come up negative. But I knew that my family had thyroid problems. At least six members that I can think of have thyroid disorders, but mine just never showed up on tests.

After taking very low doses of thyroid, my skin problem cleared up, I stopped biting my nails, and my legs stopped aching. The mild depression I was still suffering from vanished. I felt great. I slept like a normal person again. I had energy. People started commenting on how I seemed to be like my old self.

I feel rather fed up with the original doctors. They treated me like I was an hysterical woman who needed to get a grip on things. I have never told them about my recovery using alternative methods because I don't think they'd be receptive to it. I did tell my therapist who has been very receptive to these new treatments and is most interested in the thyroid treatments. But I'd say that the medical community is not open-minded about alternative treatments at all.

"Helen"

I had hives, some kind of an allergic response, about five years ago and it progressed to the point where I had hives on my vocal chords. It was a pretty serious allergic reaction, for which I was treated with antihistamines. Later, I was treated with prednisone. When small doses of prednisone given every other day didn't help, my doctor began increasing the dosage until I was taking 70 mg every day. After about six weeks, I started declining physically from taking this tremendous dose. I gained about 50 pounds. I had conjunctivitis in both eyes. I had open sores. I was so weak that I was almost bedridden.

I found another doctor, who slowly weaned me off of the prednisone. But, my immune system had been damaged. I had a lot of viral illnesses that are usually associated with chronic fatigue syndrome. I could scarcely get out of bed, and I couldn't lose all the weight I had gained. I went from doctor to doctor. Many of them said, "Your metabolic system has been altered by prednisone. Too bad, but you will never lose that weight. Too bad, but your immune system has been damaged." No one could offer me any help at all.

Dr. Atkins finally was a lot of help to me. I learned about dental amalgams, because when your immune system is depleted, you are much more susceptible to any kind of toxins, including mercury leaching from mercury amalgam fillings. It was causing me a great deal of trouble and I did have those removed.

Then I moved to California. I had heard about Dr. Slagle and her work with depression and had referred friends to her. They'd had miraculous cures after two weeks of taking B-complex and amino acids. But I didn't think of going to her myself because I thought of her as someone who only treated depression. In fact, like many alternative physicians, she treats the whole person.

She had worked with fatigue a lot, and she first tested me thoroughly and found that my thyroid and my whole endocrine syste were was not functioning properly—most likelya result of prednisone. She picked up subtleties in the test that other doctor shad ignored. She believes that a body should be healthy and whole. She doesn't need unusual test results to say something is wrong here. So she discovered a rather unusual problem in my thyroid and was able to treat it.

When I began seeing her I still had very limited energy and I still didn't feel normal. In one day, I could either go to the grocery store or go to a doctor's appointment. That was all. The remainder of the day I had to rest. After Dr. Slagle began treating my thyroid, I had a leap of improvement. I regained my energy.

She gave me amino acids, which heightened my mood. Even though I hadn't thought I was depressed—and still don't think I was—the amino acids made me feel healthier. And while I don't have the energy of a lot of people around me, I can pretty much function normally, which is a miracle. It has been a five-year struggle and I'm finally living practically a normal life.

I have learned from my experience that you simply cannot go to a traditional physician and allow that doctor to treat your symptoms with drugs. I learned to use tremendous caution when entrusting my body to someone. If you're going to trust your body to someone, you should know whether that physician treats the whole person and sees you as more than an allergy or a gallbladder.

The thyroid gland is a very important component of the immune system. It is, as Dr. Hyla Cass describes it, "the energy-generating gland located below the Adam's apple in the neck." Thyroiditis is a root cause of a variety of emotional and physical problems, but it is difficult to convince sceptical conventional physicians that this is so.

Dr. Cass explains that "when the thyroid isn't working properly, the immune system is impaired, and this sets up a vicious cycle. You have a person whose immune system is depleted and who is anxious; they're told by regular doctors that the problem is all in their head, that there's nothing physically wrong with them. So then they feel worse. I recently saw a young woman who came in depressed, tired, unable to get up on the morning, and feeling overwhelmed by her work responsibilities. Her history revealed that she was often cold, especially in her hands and feet (she even wore socks to bed), had thinning hair, dry skin, constipation, and was losing the outer part of her eyebrows. I suspected an imbalance in her thyroid. When I asked about thyroid disease, she said that it had been suspected before, but her tests had been normal. I checked her thyroid hormones, including thyroid antibody levels.

"Often despite 'normal' blood tests, there is an underactive thyroid. Dr. Broda Barnes's technique of monitoring thyroid function through body temperature is used by many alternative practitioners. Although this patient's thyroid hormone blood levels were normal, she did, in fact, have antithyroid antibodies, confirming a diagnosis of Hashimoto's thyroiditis. This is an auto-immune disease, treatable with thyroid hormone, antioxidants, and adrenal support. Her signs were those of hypothyroidism, indicating that the circulating hormone was being rendered ineffective. With Hashimoto's thyroiditis, there are often also intermittent signs of hyperthyroidism, or overactive thyroid, such as irritability or heart palpitations.

"I prescribed thyroid hormone from natural (animal) sources, and asked her to monitor her body temperature, so I could adjust the dosage. She asked whether this supplementation would suppress her own thyroid function, and whether she would be taking it for the rest of her life. The answer was 'no' on both counts. The treatment actually supported her own gland, allowing it to heal. Within ten days of starting the program she was feeling alive again.

"A surprisingly large number of patients that I see have thyroiditis. I really can't emphasize the importance of this problem enough because thyroiditis often accompanies the mixed infection syndrome, which can consist of any combination of the following: parasites, candida, and the viral syndromes—including the Epstein-Barr virus and the cytomegalo virus. Psychological components include depression, anxiety and even panic attacks. To treat thyroiditis, I've done nutritional consults on people that were under the care of other physicians. When I suggested that they had thyroiditis and that it was to be treated with low doses of thyroid hormones, I was met with skepticism from the other doctors. "When people have these long-standing chronic conditions, they can become extremely depressed. They feel like they can't go on anymore, particularly when their body has been so wracked by the continuing illness. Also, some of the mixed infection of thyroiditis and the parasites or other viruses can actually affect the brain directly. Thyroiditis and its accompanying infections affect the central nervous system along with every other organ of the body. So people come in extremely depressed, both as a reaction to their prolonged illness and as a primary symptom of the illness—and this is usually totally overlooked. That's why it's crucial to do a good medical work-up on a patient whose disorder may at first appear purely psychological in origin," Dr. Cass concludes.

Dr. Stephen Langer asserts that "many people come into my office with an organic kind of illness that has been misdiagnosed as being either psychosomatic or primarily psychological. Very rarely do I see a patient who comes in with complaints that are primarily psychological in cause. Very often, their complaints have some organic basis which, if taken care of, allows them to resolve much more easily whatever psychological problems they do have.

"The thyroid gland puts out a teaspoon of hormone a year which affects the metabolism and acts as a cellular carburetor for every cell in the body—from our hair follicles down to our toenails. As such, the thyroid can be implicated in just about any kind of condition you can think of. As for its relationship to psychological disorders, since it plays a role in the metabolism of the nervous system, people who have thyroid disorders have conditions like depression, anxiety, panic attacks, and bipolar disorders.

"If a person's metabolism is hypo-functioning, everything is going to be slow. In a book I wrote called *Solve the Riddle of Illness,* I explain why upwards of 40 percent of the population may have subclinical hypothyroidism and not detect it by the traditional blood chemistry work that's done at their general practitioner's office. The symptoms of low thyroid include weakness, dry coarse skin, slow speech, coarse hair, hair loss, weight gain, difficulty breathing, problems with menstruation, nervousness, heart palpitations, brittle nails, and severe chronic fatigue and depression.

"Now if you get somebody with a constellation of symptoms like that they're going to be sick and tired of feeling sick and tired. Plus they're going to feel depressed all the time because they're going from one doctor to another, sometimes with two or three or four pages worth of complaints, and the doctors tell them it's all in their head, or that they should go home and learn to live with it. Obviously you're going to see depression. Now not everything that I see is hypothyroidism by any means. But hypothyroidism is so easy to identify and so ubiquitous in the population, and it can be treated so well and so rapidly for so little money, that it's become a primary interest of mine.

"To treat someone with hypothyroidism, I put them on as little as a quarter of a grain, which is a newborn-infant dose, and this produces a radical change in the way the person functions. Of course, for someone who has low thyroid function, I also use orthomolecular nutrition and a lot of clinical ecology techniques along with treating the thyroid gland.

"Recently I treated a patient who was the wife of a doctor and the mother of two young children. She basically came in and told me that she didn't want to go on living. She was so tired all the time, and so depressed, that she couldn't keep her head off the pillow after two o'clock in the afternoon. If she didn't go to bed, she would just fall apart. I did a history and physical on her and we made some dietary changes, but basically this woman was profoundly hypothyroid. We put her on a quarter of a grain of thyroid, which is what I start my patients with before building them up very gradually. A quarter of a grain is the smallest dose available. It's such a small quantity that most pharmacies don't even carry it, because when doctors order thyroid they don't even think to order so small a dose. But a quarter of a grain of thyroid was enough. Within a three-week period, this woman not only regained her mental health, but she was out taking tennis lessons, which was shocking even to me because although the treatment usually works it usually takes a longer period of time. So, just that amount of metabolic support was enough to turn this person's life around.

"Another person I treated was a 62-year-old woman who was a member of the Catholic clergy. She had been a nun for at least 30 years when I met her and I will never forget this woman. She came in bloated, profoundly depressed, and fatigued. The only thing that kept her going was basically overworking her adrenal glands. She came in and told me that when she was 12 years old, she went under a dark cloud. When I saw her it was 50 years later, and by that time she had been through 30 or 40 different doctors, including internists, endocrinologists, psychiatrists, and psychologists of various sorts. One of the first things that showed up in her—which I thought was a very positive sign—was that she was freezing all the time. When we did a basal body temperature on her, it never went above 95 degrees. Basal body temperature is a person's resting temperature when she wakes up in the morning. However, when I did a blood work-up on her, all her thyroid hormone levels were within normal limits. I empirically placed her on a dose of thyroid that we gradually built up to about four grains a day, which is quite a high dosage. She's one of the few people I've treated who has needed that high an amount. Within three months her depression of 50 years duration was totally gone. Now, obviously she was bitter and angry that she had been suffering for all that time. But the organic feeling that she had of overwhelming fatigue totally disappeared within a three-month period of time, and I've seen that response in thousands of patients over the years. A small dose of thyroid, combined with things like nutritional support and eliminating food allergies, can really turn a person's life around.

"Very often people who are thyroid deficient will have tests that show up normal. It's become apparent, particularly over the past ten years, that some people with thyroid conditions have normal thyroid hormone levels and are suffering from another condition known as Hashimoto's disease, or auto-immune thyroiditis. There is a very precise blood test that any doctor can order called the auto-immune thyroid antibody test, and most of the people who I suspect have thyroid conditions and have normal thyroid hormone levels will have an elevation in their anti-thyroid antibodies. If they have an elevated anti-thyroid antibody level, they have the symptoms that go along with low thyroid, which can be any one of 125 symptoms that we enumerate in *Solve the Riddle of Illness.*

"A lot of the symptoms of thyroiditis are psychological symptoms, such as profound depression. With thyroiditis people get anxiety attacks and panic attacks for no apparent reason. They could be sitting and reading a book. All of a sudden they will develop a cascade of heart palpitations and fearfulness. I've had a number of patients who have been ushed, almost on a monthly basis, to the emergency room to be worked up by cardiologists because their heart was pounding over 200 beats a minute. Cardiologists would do EKGs and echocardiograms and tell them to go see a psychiatrist who would work them up, not find anything, and then put them on an antidepressant or a tranquilizer, and actually make the condition worse. When you have an undiscovered organic basis for a psychological problem, being put on psychotropic medication is like sitting on a thumbtack and being put on pain pills for the rest of your life. It has about the same effect. It wears the system down, and as a result the patient's condition not only does not improve but will in fact deteriorate, because the underlying cause is not being treated.

"To treat patients with thyroiditis, I put them on a trial dose of thyroid and continue to monitor their thyroid hormone levels. Most of these people wind up taking between one and two grains of thyroid a day and their thyroid hormone levels still stay normal despite the fact that their levels were supposedly normal to begin with. More importantly, they get a complete remission of symptoms, many of which manifest themselves as psychological symptoms.

"One woman I treated became a pioneer in the holistic health movement up in northern California. She was in her late 30s and she had exactly the same symptoms that I enumerated above. She had a relatively good job, a stable marriage, and children in school who were no problem, but she was having problems periodically with palpitations and fearfulness, ranging from anxiety to full-blown panic attacks. This woman would call her husband, who was an executive in a large corporation, at least twice a month to tell him that she was having one of the attacks, and he would have to drop everything, come home, and take her to the hospital where she was worked up by psychiatrists and cardiologists who could never find anything. She was, in fact, on a number of different psychotropic medications when she came to see me, in desperation, after reading my book.

"I did a full blood work-up on this woman, and all of her lab tests, with the exception of her anti-thyroid antibodies, were within normal limits. It turned out she did have severe auto-immune thyroiditis. Since her thyroid turned out to be enlarged, we did another test called a thyroid scan, a test that tracks iodine uptake over a 24-hour period and is administered by a radiologist at the hospital. It turned out that her thyroid condition was so severe that she required an operation to remove part of her thyroid—a procedure that is very drastic and is rarely ever indicated. As soon as the operation was done and this woman was placed on a therapeutic diet with the proper nutritional support and a small amount of thyroid, she never had the psychological symptoms again. She went on to become an advocate for holistic and environmental health and founded an organization called the Environmental Health Network which now has thousands of members, including many prominent clinicians. This is an example of how turning one person's life around can affect the lives of many other people.

"The constellation of problems associated with thyroid disorders occurs not only in middle-aged people but also in young people, and not only in women, but also in men. While thyroid disease, particularly auto-immune thyroiditis, is classically considered to be primarily a disease of women, this is just not true. I have seen as many men as women who are suffering from auto-immune thyroiditis and, I might add, from hypothyroidism. Men are really given short shrift and aren't even given the requisite diagnostic tests in many instances to rule out thyroid disease because the medical profession thinks that this is strictly a woman's disorder. Moreover, I have seen teenagers and children who are acting out, who are written off as hyperactive, when they may be suffering from a thyroid disorder. Very young children or teenagers express their emotions differently from adults. Sometimes they get written off as being mentally retarded or having minimal brain dysfunction. Then they're given any one of a number of different drugs and placed in special classes. Many times, these young people have thyroid disorders that can be easily treated. But because thyroid dysfunction often leads to frequent infections, these kids are placed on antibiotics. Then they wind up with an overgrowth of yeast in their gut that in turn causes a low-grade inflammation in their gastrointestinal system. As a result, they don't adequately digest their food, so the body starts regarding the food as a foreign invader and puts out antibodies to the food. The child starts exhibiting the classic symptoms of food allergies, which are psychiatric complaints: anxiety attacks, depression, forgetfulness, inability to concentrate, even full-blown panic attacks. In a lot of these cases, you can actually isolate and eliminate the foods that cause an anxiety attack, but merely removing the food is not enough to get to the underlying cause of the disorder. Frequently patients have food allergies because of a pre-existing condition in their digestive systems which has to be addressed. The presence of such a pre-existing condition can cause immune system alterations which result in auto-immune dysfunction. So this is a vicious circle. One of the chief target organs of auto-immune dysfunction is the thyroid gland. You get auto-immune thyroiditis.

"The question for holistic clinicians to ask themselves, regarding each individual patient, is where they're going to intervene. Different physicians will intervene at different places, depending upon their background and interests. I try, to the best of my ability, to get to the root cause of what's going on. If I am having difficulty figuring out the cause, then I try to intervene at a point in a person's imbalance that will cause the least disruption to their lifestyle and give them the best results for the least amount of money in the quickest period of time. Frequently, that turns out to be treating with small doses of thyroid and altering eating habits. In my clinical experience, I have found that with the thyroid and nutritional support, very often a person will get better. The thyroid is not a lifetime treatment and can be removed after the person's condition has been stabilized. Thyroid treatment is inexpensive, works rapidly, and when done properly it is absolutely nontoxic.

"There is one more connection to be drawn between depression and the thyroid dysfunction," Dr. Langer adds: "Poor libido. One of the classic symptoms of depression is a loss of interest in sex. Those people who in the past were sexually active, but who all of a sudden or gradually started to lose interest in sex, will be diagnosed as being depressed right away. Men come into my office by the score—many of them young—who have potency problems, and they can't figure it out because they have no apparent organic illness. As a result, they get performance anxiety, and if that continues long enough, they wind up getting severely depressed. But I have found that if you go to the root cause of their depression, very often it's the thyroid that's malfunctioning.

"If a person develops an acute depression that leads to a sexual dysfunction—which it frequently does—a doctor would be remiss if he or she didn't look for an imbalance in the thyroid. Patients have got to start taking their health destinies into their own hands and demanding that doctors do thyroid testing and look for auto-immune thyroid disorders and nutritional imbalances, which are frequently the underlying causes of sexual dysfunction and depression. Sleep disturbances are very common with auto-immune thyroiditis. Most people with thyroiditis spend an overwhelming portion of the day in a condition somewhat like low thyroid, which means they're very, very sluggish. The symptoms of thyroiditis include: profound fatigue, memory loss manifested by problems with recent memory and concentration, depression, and nervousness ranging from mild anxiety to full-blown panic attacks. What's really going on is that these people are swinging from low thyroid to high thyroid.

"What triggers an auto-immune response? Imagine auto-immune thyroiditis to be like rheumatoid arthritis of the thyroid gland. A person can have rheumatoid arthritis, which is an auto-immune condition where the body puts out antibodies to the joints. Frequently people with rheumatoid arthritis stay in long periods of remission. When they are under a great deal of stress, the body puts out antibodies to the joints and all their joints swell up. Similarly with the thyroid, if a person gets stressed out for any reason whatsoever, the body can start pumping out antibodies to the thyroid gland. The thyroid becomes acutely inflamed and the hormone which should not be in the system starts escaping. The clinical term for the gland is an 'escaping gland.' The hormone escapes from the gland and it's almost like pumping speed into your system. For some reason (possibly having to do with the cyclical variations in hormone output called diurnal variations), it happens very frequently that people with thyroiditis have an auto-immune reaction at night, making the body put out antibodies, and these people will wake up with their minds racing, their hearts pounding, and feeling anxious and nervous. The problem is often written off as just a sleep disorder—sleep apnea or some sleep problem of unknown cause—when in fact its cause can be detected and corrected," Dr. Langer concludes.

Dr. Allan Spreen reminds us that while thyroid supplementation is an important modality, it is not fail-safe. "I'd love to say that correcting thyroid function is a panacea. While it doesn't work 100 percent of the time, if a patient comes in complaining of fatigue and depression that is linked with the physical findings of foods not digesting well, and cold extremities, then an underactive thyroid may be the root cause. People come and say, 'Oh, my husband says, Don't touch me with your feet at night because they're just ice cold.' These are the same people who are comfortable in a room when everybody else is boiling and they're freezing in a room when everybody else is comfortable. Their thinking seems to have slowed down, they just don't seem to be able to concentrate like they used to, and they don't remember lists the way they used to.

"In this kind of a situation, once I find that their blood levels of thyroid are normal, I go back to the old school of Broda Barnes, who, 40 or 50 years ago, did axillary temperature testing. I ask my patients to keep a record of their early morning basal body temperature. If their basal metabolic rate based on early-morning body temperatures is really low, then I consider them to be candidates for thyroid supplementation. In axillary testing, Broda Barnes talked about temperature ranges between 97.8 and 98.2 degrees Fahrenheit, which is lower than the 98.6 people think of as normal. But the axillary temperature is taken in the armpit first thing in the morning, using a mercury thermometer that stays there for ten minutes before they get up. If their temperature is, much of the time, down in the 96.8, 96.7, 96.5 range, I at least consider the possibility that the person needs low doses of natural thyroid, which is still available.

"Thyroid is a prescription drug, but it can be broken down into very low doses. Some doctors who use this type of testing use synthetic thyroid. I prefer to prescribe natural thyroid in very low doses. If a person responds—either their temperature rises or their symptoms lift —then I retest them to see if their blood levels of thyroid have changed. Many times a person with this profile of symptoms who takes thyroid will feel better, and their blood tests will have remained unchanged, including their thyroid stimulating hormone and their actual thyroid hormone levels. So the blood testing has missed the diagnosis, and yet the person feels well with the increased, but undetectable dose of thyroid hormone."

A

ℛESOURCES

Biographies and Addresses

DR. RICHARD ASH, M.D., went to the Medical College of Pennsylvania in Philadelphia. He has been in private practice since then, specializing in internal medicine, and alternative and complementary therapies. He also founded the Ash Center for Comprehensive Medicine. He has a radio show every Sunday in New York.

Ash Center for Comprehensive Medicine
800A Fifth Avenue
New York NY 10021
Tel: (212) 758-3200

ROBERT C. ATKINS, M.D., graduated from Cornell University Medical College and has hospital affiliations with both Columbia and Rochester Universities. He is the founder and Executive Medical Director of the Atkins Centers for Complementary Medicine, established in 1970, and President of the Foundation for the Advancement of Innovative Medicine. He specializes in treating a wide variety of disorders, including asthma, cancer, chronic fatigue, hypoglycemia and immune system disorders.

152 E. 55th Street
New York NY 10022
Tel: (212) 758-2110
www.atkinscenter.com

SIDNEY M. BAKER, M.D., is a practicing physician with an interest in nutritional, biochemical and environmental aspects of chronic illness in adults and children. Since leaving the full time faculty in Medical Computer Sciences at Yale Medical School in 1971, he has specialized in computer applications that help the clinician maintain accurate, detailed, structured medical records to enhance the ability of doctors to make clinical portraits of patients both as individuals and as groups.

FRED BAUGHMAN, JR., M.D., is a pediatric neurologist in La Mesa, California, and medical advisor for the National Right to Read Foundation and a Fellow of the American Academy of Neurology.

SYD BAUMEL is a graduate student in physiology at Manitoba Graduate School, specializing in natural health and medicine.

ROBERT BERNSTEIN is an educational therapist with a private practice in Dobbs Ferry, New York. He has a masters degree in special education from Teacher's College of Columbia University. He goes to schools and other institutions to give presentations on education, and is a consultant to the Putnam New York chapter of the National Council on Alcohol and other Drug Dependencies.

191 Woodlands Avenue
White Plains NY 10607
Tel: (914) 478-4868
E-mail: RobEDU@aol.com

MARY ANN BLOCK, M.D., founded the Block Center in Dallas, Texas, and has written several books on health and nutrition.

Tel: (817) 280-9933

NEIL BLOCK, M.D., is a board-certified specialist in family practice, preventive nutrition, and ortho-molecular body-brain imbalances. He has certificates in homeopathy, naturopathy, herbal medicine, bach flower remedies, and sports performance and training. His special interests include fatigue syndrome, endocrine disturbances, holistic healing, ADD, sleep-mood disorders, and respiratory diseases.

60 Dutch Hill Road
Orangeburg NY 10962
Tel: (914) 359-3300

PETER R. BREGGIN, M.D., graduated from Harvard College and attended Case Western Reserve School of Medicine. Since 1968, he has been in full-time private practice with individuals, families, and children, with a focus on the adverse effects of psychiatric treatments and medical-legal issues. He is the founder and director of the International Center for the Study of Psychiatry and Psychology, which publishes a peer-reviewed journal and a newsletter and holds national conferences.

4628 Chestnut Street
Bethesda MD 20814
Tel: (301) 652-5580

Fax: (301) 652-5924
www.breggin.com

HAROLD BUTTRAM, M.D., specializes
in family practice, environmental
medicine, nutrition-based
modalities, and the treatment of
allergies.

5724 Clymer Road
Quakertown PA 18951
Tel: (215) 536-1890

CHRISTOPHER CALAPAI, M.D., is an
osteopathic physician board certified
in family practice. He specializes in
a variety of treatment modalities,
including the use of intravenous
vitamin therapy, chelation therapy
and reconstructive nerve therapy.

1900 Hempstead Turnpike
E. Meadow NY 11554
Tel: (516) 794-0404
or
18 E. 53rd Street, 3rd Floor
New York NY 10022
Tel: (212) 838-9100

DR. PAULA CAPLAN, PH.D., is a
Radcliffe-Harvard graduate and
Affiliated Scholar at Brown
University's Pembroke Center. She is
the author of ten books, including
*They Say You're Crazy: How the
World's Most Powerful Psychiatrists
Decide Who's Normal*; *Don't Blame
Mother: Mending the Mother-
Daughter Relationship*; and *The
Myth of Women's Masochism*.

Pembroke Center
Brown University
Box 1958
Providence RI 02912

CATHERINE CARRIGAN, a graduate
of Brown University, spent three
years researching depression at the
Emory University Medical Library in
Atlanta, Georgia.

Tel: (770) 590-7282

HYLA CASS, M.D., is a holistic
psychiatrist who integrates
psychotherapy and nutritional
medicine in her Santa Monica–based
practice. In addition to being a media
and corporate consultant, speaker, and
seminar leader, she is an assistant
clinical professor of psychiatry at
UCLA School of Medicine.

2730 Wilshire Boulevard, #301
Santa Monica CA 90403
Tel: (310) 459-9866
Fax: (310) 459-9466
E-mail: HCassMD@wirkdbet.att.bet
www.doctorcass.com

ALAN COHEN, M.D., graduated from
SUNY Stonybrook School of
Medicine, and is board-certified in
family practice and homeopathy. He
has a private practice, where he
treats entire families, from newborns
to seniors, by integrating both
conventional and alternative
approaches.

67 Cherry Street
Milford CT 06460
Tel: (203) 877-1936

TY COLBERT, PH.D., is a licensed
clinical psychologist who is currently
in the process of setting up the
Center for Psychological
Alternatives to Biopsychiatry, a
publishing and website venture for
practioners and patients looking for
information and resources. He is an
active member of the National
Association for Rights, Protection
and Advocacy and is on the advisory
council for the Center for the Study
of Psychiatry.

P.O. Box 178
Tuston CA 92781
Tel: (714) 838-9771
www.pab2000.org

GABRIEL COUSENS, M.D., is a holistic
medical doctor, a psychiatrist and
family therapist, and a licensed
homepathic physician in the state of
Arizona.

Tree of Life Rejuvenation Center
Padagonia AZ 85624
Tel: (520) 394-2520

WILLIAM CROOK, M.D., received his
medical education and training at
the University of Virginia, the
Pennsylvania Hospital, Vanderbilt,
and John Hopkins. He is the author
of numerous reports published in
peer review journals and ten books.

International Health Foundation
P.O. Box 3494
Jackson TN 38303
www.candida-yeast.com

DR. JOSEPH DEBE has a doctor of
chiropractics degree from the Los
Angeles College of Chiropractics,
received his CCST (Certified
Chiropractic Sports Practitioner) at
New York Chiropractic College.
Board-certified in nutrition, he
currently manages three private
practices around the tristate area.

North Shore Fitness
38 Great Neck Road
Great Neck NY 11021
Tel: (516) 829-1515
www.drdebe.com
E-mail: Inquiry@drdebe.com

JERRY DORSMAN is a certified
addiction counselor working in
Elton, Maryland.

P.O. Box 71
Elk Mills MD 21920
Tel: (410) 392-9685
www.self-renewal.com

JOHN EADES is a counselor in
Chemical Dependency Services for
the Singer River Hospital in
Mississippi. He has a twenty-year
history of working in the field of
addictive diseases and chemical
dependencies with major hospitals.

DR. SAMUEL DUNKELL is director of
the Insomnia Medical Services in

New York City, former director of Payne Whitney's Insomnia Clinic, and assistant professor of psychiatry at Cornell University Medical College.

1065 Lexington Avenue
New York NY 10021
Tel: (212) 628-2236

EVA EDELMAN, N.D., holds a B.A. in psychology from SUNY Binghamton and an N.D. from Washington, D.C. She has worked twenty-five years in the field of natural health, specializing in mental health. She works as a nutritional consultant at SAFE, a drop-in center run by and for people with mental disorders.

PMB 188
3762 W. 11th Avenue
Eugene OR 97402
Tel: (541) 683-8720
E-mail: edelman@boragebooks.com

LEANDER T. ELLIS, M.D., is a board-certified psychiatrist who has, for more than twenty-five years, studied the effect of allergies, infections, nutrition, and other physical factors on emotional conditions such as anxiety, depression, autism, and auto-immune diseases.

LYNNE FREEMAN, PH.D., has her doctorate in counseling and psychology and is the director of the Open Doors Institute in Los Angeles, California.

KENDALL GERDES, M.D., is board certified in both internal medicine and allergy/immunology. He was an early student of Theron Randolph, the father of environmental medicine. Dr. Gerdes is a past president of the American Academy of Environmental Medicine. He has been in private practice since 1979.

1617 Vine Street
Denver CO 80206
Tel: (303) 377-8837

WILLIAM J. GOLDWAG, M.D., is the medical director of the Center for Preventive/Holistic Medicine in Southern California, and is on the board of directors of the American Holistic Medical Association. He has been one of the pioneers in the use of chelation therapy and other nutritional and complementary medical therapies for the treatment of chronic health disorders.

7499 Cerritos Avenue
Stanton CA 90680
Tel: (714) 827-5180

JAMES S. GORDON, M.D., a graduate of the Harvard Medical School, was a research psychiatrist at the National Institute of Mental Health for ten years. Founder and director of the Center for Mind-Body Medicine, he is also a clinical professor in the departments of psychiatry and family medicine at the Georgetown University School of Medicine. Dr.

Gordon served as the first Chair of the Program Advisory Council of the National Institutes of Health's Office of Alternative Medicine. He integrates relaxation therapies, hypnosis, meditation, acupuncture, nutrition, herbalism, musculoskeletal manipulation, dance, yoga, and physical exercise in his own practice of medicine and psychiatry.

Center for Mind-Body Medicine
5225 Connecticut Avenue, NW
Suite 414
Washington DC 20015
Tel: (202) 966-7338
Fax: (202) 966-2589
E-mail: cmbm@mindspring.com
www.cmbm.org

JAN GAGNON, M.D., is a naturopathic physician in Seattle, Washington. She spent many years working at the Tufts Mental Health Center in Massachusetts and the Virginia Mason Hospital in Seattle, and regularly integrates mind, body, healing into her practice.

JANE GUILTINAN, N.D., studied naturopathic medicine at Bastyr University in Seattle, Washington, and is currently Dean of Clinical Affairs there. She is responsible for the outpatient training clinic at the University, which sees about 30,000 patients a year. She also has a private practice, with a focus on women's health.

1307 North 45th Street, Suite 300
Seattle WA 98103

LETHA HADADY, D. AC., received her Diplomate of Acupuncture from the Tri-State Institute for Traditional Chinese Medicine and also did special studies in China. Besides being in private practice for nearly twenty years, she also consults and holds rejuvenation workshops. She teaches doctors at the Botanical Medicine in Modern Clinical Practice Conference at Columbia's Rosenthal Center every year. She is adjunct faculty for the New York Botanical gardens. She is an author and internet columnist for seniors.com and eastearthtrade.com. She has a regular Q&A at www.winghopfung.com, and can be contacted through the site.

PHILIP JAY HODES, Ed.D., has spent three decades learning about holistic health, detoxification, and orthomolecular nutritional therapies to rectify and prevent various conditions. He is a researcher, writer, speaker, and educator, as well as a health care practitioner.

144 Keer Avenue
Newark NJ 07112-1915

ABRAM HOFFER, M.D., Ph.D., received his Ph.D. from the University of Minnesota and his M.D. from the University of Toronto. He was director of psychiatric research for the Province of Saskatchewan from 1950 to 1967. In private practice since 1967 specializing in the treatment of schizophrenia and cancer, he helped introduce orthomolecular medicine, in which vitamins are used as a primary treatment modality.

2727 Quadra Street, Suite 3-A
Victoria BC V8T 4E5
Canada
Tel: (250) 386-8756

DHARMA SINGH KHALSA, M.D., is a graduate of Creighton University of Medicine in Omaha, Nebraska, and was trained at the University of California and Harvard Medical School. Since 1981, he has been an American Sikh. He is board certified by the American Academy of Anti Aging Medicine, of which he is also the founding member. Currently he is the president and medical director of the Alzheimer's Prevention Foundation. He has written numerous articles and is the author of two books.

2420 N. Pantano Road
Tuscon AZ 85715
Tel: (520) 749-8374
www.brain-longevity.com

DR. PARRIS KIDD, PH.D., is a nutrition educator and dietary supplement developer. He received his Ph.D. in cell biology from the University of California at Berkeley. Dr. Kidd is internationally recognized for his expertise in brain nutraceuticals.

Fax: (570) 526-6114

KEN KORINS, M.D.
200 West 57th Street
New York NY 10019
Tel: (212) 246-5122
E-mail: kskorinsmd@email.msn.com

RICHARD A. KUNIN, M.D., is a founder and past president of the Orthomolecular Medical Society. He is in private practice, specializing in orthomolecular ecology medicine, in San Francisco.

2698 Pacific Avenue
San Francisco CA 94115
Tel: (415) 346-2500

STEPHEN LANGER, M.D., practices preventive medicine in Berkeley, California, specializing in the treatment of chronic fatigue, among other illnesses. He is the president of the American Nutritional Medical Association.

3031 Telegraph Avenue, #230
Berkeley CA 94705
Tel: (510) 548-7384

MICHAEL LAPCHICK is the author of *The Label Reader's Pocket Dictionary of Food Additives*. He is a Philadelphia-based health and nutrition writer.

Tel: (215) 533 0598

WARREN M. LEVIN, M.D., is currently celebrating his twentieth anniversary as an orthomolecular physician. He is board certified in family practice, environmental medicine, and chelation therapy.

24 W. 57th Street, Suite 701
New York NY 10019
Tel: (212) 397-5900

JOAN MATTHEWS-LARSON, Ph.D., holds a doctorate in nutrition and is the founder and executive director of the Health Recovery Center in Minneapolis. She writes and speaks on psycho-biological approaches to treating addiction.

www.healthrecovery.com

JAY LOMBARD, M.D., is the chief of neurology of Westchester Square Medical Center and the clinical assistant professor of neurology at Cornell University Medical College. Board certified in neurology, he is in private practice in New York City. Dr. Lombard has published in several peer reviewed journals and is the author of *The Brain Wellness Plan*.

Tel: (718) 597-6925

MICHAEL NORDEN, M.D., is a psychiatrist and Clinical Associate Professor at the University of Washington.

JAMES PEARL, Ph.D., is a member of the Sleep Panel at the Presbyterian St. Luke Medical Center in Denver, Colorado, and is in private practice as a psychologist.

DORIS J. RAPP, M.D., is a board-certified pediatric allergist and specialist in environmental medicine. She has written and presented her videos of children's responses to treatment to physicians and the public in many countries. Videotapes of patients' responses to treatment can be obtained by calling 1-800-787-8780.

8179 East Del Cuarzo Drive
Scotsdale AZ 85258
E-mail: drrappmd@aol.com
www.drrapp.com

JUDYTH REICHENBERG-ULLMAN is a board-certified diplomate of the Homeopathic Academy of Naturopathic Physicians. She is a graduate of Bastyr University in Seattle, Washington, and received her master's degree in Psychiatric Social Work from the University of Washington. She has had more than fifteen years of clinical experience as a naturopathic and homeopathic physician.

JOEL ROBERTSON, M.D., is the director of the Robertson Institute, which provides neurochemical evaluations and treatment techniques for individuals in the mental health field and those who feel they need it.

SHERRY ROGERS, M.D., is the author of *Depression: Cured at Last* and other books on health.

Tel: (941) 349-7127

JUDITH SACHS has taught stress management at the College of New Jersey and conducts workshops on stress, mid-life, and menopause and sexuality, throughout the tristate area.

404 Burd Streer
Pennington NJ 08534
Tel: (609) 737-8310

RAY SAHELIAN, M.D., obtained a B.Sc. in nutrition from Drexel University and completed his training at Thomas Jefferson Medical School, both in Philadelphia. He is certified by the American Board of Family Practice, is the author of books on leading edge nutrients and hormones, and is editor of *Longevity Research Update*.

www.raysahelian.com

MICHAEL B. SCHACHTER, M.D., is a graduate of Columbia University's College of Physicians and Surgeons and a board-certified psychiatrist. He has been practicing ortho-molecular medicine and psychiatry since 1974. Dr. Schachter directs a health care facility in Suffern, New York, using nutritional medicine, chelation therapy, homeopathy, and other complementary treatment methods.

2 Executive Boulevard, Suite 202
Suffern NY 10901
Tel: (914) 368-4700
E-mail: office@mbschachter.com
www.mbschachter.com

ALEXANDER SCHAUSS, Ph.D., is a research psychologist and mental health therapist, and holds associate professorships at colleges of naturopathic medcine in Oregon and Arizona. He is the research director of the life sciences division at the American Institute for Biosocial Research, and is the author of *The Health Benefits of Cat's Claw: Its Role in Treating Cancer, Arthritis, Prostate Problems, Asthma, and Many Other Chronic Conditions*.

Tel: (206) 922-0448

PRISCILLA ANNE SLAGLE, M.D., has private practices in Los Angeles and Palm Springs. Specializing in nutritional medicine and psychiatry, she treats most illnesses from the perspective of diet change, nutritional supplementation, and natural hormones as needed.

16542 Ventura Boulevard, Suite 306
Encino CA 91436
Tel: (310) 826-0175

LENDON H. SMITH, M.D., a graduate

of the University of Oregon Medical School, practiced psychiatry in the U.S. Army from 1947 to 1949, then returned to civilian life in general practice/pediatrics. He has specialized in nutrition-based therapies since 1975.

2129 NE 13th Avenue, Apt. 2
Portland OR 97212
Tel: (503) 493-7429
E-mail: Lsmith13@uswest.net
Smithsez.com

ALLAN N. SPREEN, M.D., is a general practitioner in Jacksonville, Florida, with a specialization in nutrition-based medicine.

WALT STOLL, M.D., A.B.F.P., is a board-certified family practitioner with more than thirty years of experience, the last seventeen of which were spent as a holistic physician. During those seventeen years he has combined his traditional Western (allopathic) training with fifteen other healing philosophies, practiced by trained professionals in his Holistic Medical Centre in Lexington, Kentucky. On November 17, 1994, after fourteen years of harassment by the Kentucky Medical Licensing Board, his license to practice medicine was revoked.

415 South Bonita Avenue
Panama City FL 32401-3963
Tel: (904) 747-8669
Fax: (904) 769-1436

RICARDO B. TAN, M.D., practices holistic and preventive medicine, including nutrition-based modalities, chelation therapy, acupuncture, sclerotherapy, and homeopathy.

3220 North Freeway
Fort Worth TX 76111
Tel: (817) 626-1993

JACOB TEITELBAUM, M.D., is the author of *From Fatigued to Fantastic*. He received his medical degree at Ohio State University, where he lost a year when he contracted chronic fatigue syndrome. For more than a decade he has worked with chronic fatigue and fibromyalgia patients.

Tel: (408) 372-1234

LINDA TOTH, Ph.D., received a doctorate in communications from UCLA. She is a senior staff writer for the *Journal of Longevity Research* and the author of *Why Can't I Remember?*

Tel: (310) 475-3139

JOSEPH TRACHTMAN, M.D., received his doctorate of optometry degree from Pennsylvania College of Optometry, a masters in education from Johns Hopkins University, masters in vision science from State University in New York. He also has a Ph.D. in experimental psychology from Yeshiva University. During the past twenty years, Dr. Trachtman has developed instruments and computer software to improve vision disorders using biofeedback techniques.

Tel: (718) 852-0625

AUBREY M. WORRELL, JR., M.D., is a board certified allergist/immunologist with special interests in clinical ecology, environmental medicine, and nutrition.

RAY C. WUNDERLICH, JR., M.D., is a graduate of Columbia University's College of Physicians and Surgeons. He practices nutritional and preventive medicine.

666 6th Street South
St. Petersburg FL 33701-4845
Tel: (813) 822-3612

JOSÉ A. YARYURA-TOBIAS, M.D., is the medical director at the Institute for Bio-Behavioral Therapy and Research. He has worked extensively on OCD and schizophrenia, and is a visiting professor at the University of Cuyo in Argentina.

935 Northern Boulevard
Great Neck NY 11021
Tel: (516) 487-7116
E-mail: Yaryura1@aol.com

GARRY M. VICKAR, M.D., F.R.C.P. (C.), is a psychiatrist who specializes in acutely ill patients. With an active full-time private practice, Dr. Vickar is board certified by the Royal College of Physicians and Surgeons of Canada and the American Board of Psychiatry and Neurology. He is the chairman of the department of psychiatry at Christian Hospital Northeast, where he is the medical director of the schizophrenia treatment and education programs. He is a Fellow of the American Psychiatric Association.

1245 Graham Road, Suite 506
St. Louis MO 63031
Tel: (314) 837-4900
Fax: (314) 837-5646

BRUCE WEISMAN, national president of the Citizens' Commission on Human Rights, holds a graduate degree from California State University, San Jose. A former chairman of the department of history at John F. Kennedy University, he has been a human rights advocate and an outspoken critic of damaging psychiatric abuses for more than twenty years.

Citizens Committee on Human Rights
6362 Hollywood Boulevard, Suite B
Los Angeles CA 90028
Tel: (727) 723-2176

ALFRED V. ZAMM, M.D., is a diplomate of both the American Board of Dermatology and the American Board of Environmental Medicine. In addition to his private practice based in Kingston, New York, he is a consultant to five hospitals in the Hudson Valley.

111 Maiden Lane
Kingston NY 12401-4597
Tel: (914) 338-7766

MARCIA ZIMMERMAN is a certified nutritionist, specializing in ADHD. She has been in practice for twenty-five years.

Clinical Studies

Scientific Article Summaries, by Subject

The following are capsule descriptions of just some of the recent scientific articles that demonstrate the connection between nutritional factors and mental illness. The articles are all from respected peer-reviewed journals. They were assembled through a computer search, then selected and edited at a cost of thousands of dollars to myself and my publisher.

Physicians reading this book will want to use this appendix as a matchless resource guide. It will lead them to the original scientific research, which in turn will bolster and substantiate the ideas and clinical strategies expounded in this book. I encourage you to follow this lead and have your secretary or assistant request reprints of individual articles that address your area of specialization directly from the medical journals themselves. You may find yourself more open to the practice of orthomolecular psychiatry than you ever expected.

For the general reader, you too will find that just reading the short summaries of some of the articles listed below will help strengthen your resolve. There is solid medical research to support many of the claims our contributing physicians have been making in earlier chapters.

Aging

[Effects of L-acetylcarnitine on Mental Deterioration in the Aged: Initial Results.] Cipolli C; Chiari G. *Clin Ter*, 1990 March 31, 132(6 Suppl):479-510.

Results of this double-blind, placebo-controlled study indicated that the administration of 1500 mg per day of acetyl-L-carnitine to elderly patients with mild mental impairments proved to be beneficial against cognitive and emotional-affective mental impairment.

L-acetylcarnitine Treatment of Mental Decline in the Elderly. Salvioli G; Neri M. *Drugs Exp Clin Res*, 1994, 20(4): 169-176.

This single-blind, placebo-controlled study examined the effects of 1500 mg per day of acetyl-L-carnitine for 90 days on elderly subjects with mild mental impairment. Results showed the treatment to be effective with respect to improvements on cognitive performance, and behavioral measures.

Effect of Acetyl-L-carnitine on Geriatric Patients Suffering from Dysthymic Disorders. Bella R; et al. *International Journal of Clinical Pharmacology Research*, 1990, 10(6):355-360.

Results of this double-blind, placebo-controlled study showed that the administration of 3 g per day of acetyl-L-carnitine for 30-60 days significantly reduced the severity of symptoms associated with depression relative to controls in senile subjects between the ages of 60-80.

Acetyl-L-carnitine in the Treatment of Mildly Demented Elderly Patients. Passeri M; et al. *International Journal of Clinical Pharmacology Research*, 1990, 10(1-2):75-79.

Results of this double-blind, placebo-controlled study showed that the administration of 2 g per day of acetyl-L-carnitine for three months led to significant improvements in elderly patients suffering from mental impairment.

Acetyl-L-carnitine Affects Aged Brain Receptorial System in Rodents. Castorina M; Ferraris L. *Life Science*, 1994, 54(17):1205-1214.

This review article cites studies supporting the efficacy of acetyl-L-carnitine in counteracting negative age-induced effects on physiological and pathological brain modifications in rats.

Acetyl-L-carnitine Affects Aged Brain Receptorial System in Rodents. Castorina M; Ferraris L. *Life Science*, 1994, 54(17):1205-1214.

This review article notes that studies have confirmed acetyl-L-carnitine's ability to counteract the age-dependent reduction of several receptors in rodent central nervous systems.

Oral Choline Alfoscerate Counteracts Age-Dependent Loss of Mossy Fibres in the Rat Hippocampus. Ricci A; et al. *Mech Aging*, 1992, 66(1):81-91.

Results of this study showed that treatment with choline alfoscerate treatment counteracted various anatomical changes of the rat hippocampus associated with aging.

Possible Role of Pineal Melatonin in the Mechanisms of Aging. Sandyk R. *International Journal of Neuroscience*, 1990 May, 52(1-2):85-92.

This article reviews recent findings concerning the role of melatonin in aging. Evidence is cited indicating melatonin may delay the effects of aging by attenuating negative effects associated with free radical–induced neuronal damage.

Effects of Long-term Administration of Melatonin and a Putative Antagonist on the Aging Rat. Oaknin-Bendahan S; et al. *Neuroreport*, 1995 March 27, 6(5):785-8.

Results of this study showed that melatonin attenuated decreases in survival rates, testosterone and brain 125I-melatonin binding sites associated with aging in rats.

[Treatment of Cerebral Aging Disorders with Ginkgo Biloba Extract. A Longtitudinal Multicenter Double-Blind Drug vs. Placebo Study.] Taillandier J; et al. *Presse Med*, 1986 September 25, 15(31):1583-7.

Results of this double-blind, placebo-controlled study found that Ginkgo biloba extract proved efective against aging-induced cerebral disorders in humans.

[Treatment of the Disorders of Aging with Ginkgo Biloba Extract. From Pharmacology to Clinical Medicine.] Allard M. *Presse Med*, 1986 September 25, 15(31):1540-5.

This review article cite numerous studies supporting the use of Ginkgo biloba in the treatment of various conditions associated with cerebral aging.

The Morphology of Lipopigment in Rat Purkinje Neurons after Chronic Acetyl-L-carnitine Administration: The Effect of Acetyl-L-carnitine Administration. Dowson JH; et al. *Biol Psychiatry*, 1992 July 15, 32(2):179-87.

This study examined the effects of acetyl-L-carnitine administration for 37 weeks on lipopigment in the

Purkinje neurons of rats. Results showed acetyl-L-carnitine to have prophylactive effects against adverse effects of cerebral aging.

Acetyl-L-carnitine in the treatment of midly demented elderly patients. Passeri M; Cucinotta D; Bonati PA; Iannuccelli M; Parnetti L; Senin U. *International Journal of Clinical Pharmacology Research*, 1990, 10 (1-2):75-9.

In a double-blind study, acetyl-L-carnitine, which acts to alleviate defects in nerve signals, was shown to help mildly demented elderly patients in the areas of behavior, memory, attention, and verbal fluency.

Immunological Parameters in Aging: Studies on Natural Immunomodulatory and Immunoprotective Substances. Franceschi C; et al. *International Journal of Clinical Pharmacology Research*, 1990, 10 (1-2):53-7.

This study examined the effects of L-carnitine and acetyl-L-carnitine on cell proliferation in peripheral blood lymphocytes from donors varying in age. Results found that phytohaemagglutinin-induced peripheral blood lymphocyte proliferation increased significantly in L-carnitine- or acetyl-L-carnitine-preloaded lymphocytes from subjects of all ages, but with the strongest increases seen in older subjects.

Aggression

A neuropsychopharmacological profile of "Cinkara," a polyherbal preparation. Sakina MR; Khan EA; Hamdard ME; Dandiya PC. *Indian Journal of Physiology and Pharmacology*, 1989 Jan-Mar, 33(1):43-6.

In rats, the herbal preparation known as Cinkara appears to stimulate the central nervous system, but, unlike other such stimulants, it lowers aggressive behavior.

Acute and chronic effects of ginseng saponins on maternal aggression in mice. Yoshimura H; Watanabe K; Ogawa N. *European Journal of Pharmacology*, 1988 Jun 10, 150(3):319-24.

Ginseng root contains an ingredient that suppresses maternal aggression in mice, without impairing their movement abilities.

Aminergic studies and cerebrospinal fluid actions in suicide. Banki CM; Arato M; Kilts CD. *Annals of the New York Academy of Sciences*, 1986, 487:221-30.

Suicidal psychiatric patients were shown to have significantly lower levels of magnesium in their cerebrospinal fluid than did a control group.

Anxiolytic activity of Panax ginseng roots: an experimental study.

Bhattacharya SK; Mitra SK. *Journal of Ethnopharmacology*, 1991 Aug, 34(1):87-92.

Ginseng root was shown to be effective in reducing anxiety and aggression in rats and mice, when given over a period of 5 days (as opposed to single-dose administration, which had little effect). Ginseng's effectiveness was comparable to that of diazepam (Valium).

Cerebrospinal fluid magnesium and calcium related to amine metabolites, diagnosis, and suicide attempts. Banki CM; Vojnik M; Papp Z; Balla KZ; Arato M. *Biological Psychiatry*, 1985 Feb, 20(2):163-71.

Suicidal female psychiatric patients suffering from depression, schizophrenia, or adjustment disorder had decreased levels of magnesium in their cerebrospinal fluid.

Lithium in scalp hair of adults, students, and violent criminals. Effects of supplementation and evidence for interactions of lithium with vitamin B12 and with other trace elements. Schrauzer GN; Shrestha KP; Flores-Arce MF. *Biological Trace Element Research*, 1992 Aug, 34(2):161-76.

Lithium levels in human hair are low in certain pathological conditions, such as heart disease, and in learning disabled subjects and violent criminals. Hair levels of lithium rise with extradietary supplementation, and it is suggested that lithium may help distribute vitamin B12 in the body. Lithium also interacts with other trace elements.

Magnesium alters the potency of cocaine and haloperidol on mouse aggression. Kantak KM. *Psychopharmacology*, 1989, 99(2):181-8.

Magnesium given to mice was shown to increase the potency of a single dose of cocaine, and a magnesium-deficient diet reduced its potency. With chronic cocaine use, however, magnesium countered cocaine's effects.

Psychotropic effects of ginseng saponins on agonistic behavior between resident and intruder mice. Yoshimura H; Watanabe K; Ogawa N. *European Journal of Pharmacology*, 1988 Feb 9, 146(2-3):291-7.

Crude ginseng saponins and pure ginsenocide given to mice reduce aggressive behavior in certain situations.

Stimulant-like effects of magnesium on aggression in mice. Izenwasser SE; Garcia-Valdez K; Kantak KM. *Pharmacology, Biochemistry and Behavior*, 1986 Dec, 25(6):1195-9.

Low levels of magnesium in mice are linked to reduced aggression, heightened levels to increased aggression, and extremely high levels to reduced aggression. Since magnesium works with the neurotransmitters dopamine, norepinephrine, and serotonin, which affect aggressive behavior, the effects shown may be related to these systems.

Alcoholism

A hypothetical mechanism for fetal alcohol syndrome involving ethanol inhibition of retinoic acid synthesis at the alcohol dehydrogenase step. Duester G. *Alcoholism, Clinical and Experimental Research*, 1991 Jun, 15(3):568-72.

A mechanism is offered to explain how ethanol causes the bodily abnormalities of fetal alcohol syndrome. To develop normally, embryonic tissues require certain levels of retinoic acid-the active form of vitamin A-and ethanol inhibits the enzyme needed to create this essential molecule.

ABC of Nutrition: Nutritional advice for other chronic diseases. Truswell, AS. *Brit Med J. London: British Medical Association.* July 20, 1985, v. 291, 197-200.

Nutritional guidelines are given for preventing various chronic diseases, including cirrhosis of the liver due to alcoholism.

Abnormalities of peripheral nerve conduction in relation to thiamine status in alcoholic patients. D'Amour ML; Bruneau J; Butterworth RF. *Canadian Journal of Neurological Sciences*, 1991 May, 18(2):126-8.

Alcoholic patients were shown to be severely thiamine-deficient, a condition that may contribute to the nervous-system abnormalities seen in alcoholics. (Other factors that may be involved in these abnormalities are deficiencies of other vitamins, as well as the direct effects of alcohol itself.)

Age-related effects of chronic ethanol intake on vitamin A status in Fisher 344 rats. Mobarhan S; Seitz HK; Russell RM; Mehta R; Hupert J; Friedman H; Layden TJ; Meydani M; Langenberg P. *Journal of Nutrition*, 1991 Apr, 121(4):510-7.

In rats, chronic ethanol ingestion alters tissue distribution of vitamin A.

Alcohol and bone disease. Rico H. *Alcohol and Alcoholism*, 1990, 25(4):345-52.

Excessive alcohol consumption leads to decreased bone formation, defective mineralization, and osteoporosis, the latter due possibly to excessive zinc excretion induced by alcohol.

Alcohol, liver, and nutrition. Lieber CS. *Journal of the American College of Nutrition*, 1991 Dec, 10(6): 602-32.

Liver disease in alcoholics used to be attributed mainly to dietary deficiencies, but now more is understood about how alcohol affects the liver directly. It's been shown, for instance, that animals given ethanol, along with vitamin-A-rich diets, had low levels of the vitamin in their livers, and this was especially so when the ethanol was combined with other drugs, mimicking a common circumstance in humans. When supplementing patients with vitamin A, however, it is essential to understand that too much of the vitamin is toxic to the liver-and that this is particularly so in alcoholics-so that the amount given is crucial. This decreased "therapeutic window" for alcoholics taking vitamin A applies to other nutritional supplements as well.

Alcohol-induced bone marrow damage: status before and after a 4-week period of abstinence from alcohol with or without disulfiram. A randomized bone marrow study in alcohol-dependent individuals. Casagrande G; Michot F. *Blut*, 1989 Sep, 59(3):231-6.

Alcohol can induce bone marrow damage, which has been shown to be reversed in patients who totally abstain. However, patients who detoxified while taking the drug disulfiram (Antabuse) continued to have bone marrow pathology.

Alcoholism in the elderly. How to spot and treat a problem the patient wants to hide. Tobias CR; Lippmann S; Pary R; Oropilla T; Embry CK. *Postgraduate Medicine*, 1989 Sep 15, 86(4):67-70, 75-9.

Increased awareness of alcoholism by physicians, with early diagnosis and treatment, can reduce its damaging effects. Especially in the elderly, all medications used should be monitored, and nonessential ones should be discontinued. Also suggested are treating withdrawal symptoms with thiamine, multivitamins, and perhaps sedatives; treating any underlying psychiatric disorder; psychosocial support; and possibly the use of disulfiram (Antabuse).

Anemia in alcoholics. Savage D; Lindenbaum J. *Medicine*, 1986 Sep, 65(5):322-38.

A deficiency of folic acid in alcoholics is a factor in anemia in these patients. A diagnostic approach to anemia in alcoholics was developed, as were suggestions for therapy.

Ascorbic acid chronic alcohol consumption in the guinea pig. Susick RL Jr; Abrams GD; Zurawski CA; Zannoni VG. *Toxicology and*

Applied Pharmacology, 1986 Jun 30, 84(2):329-35.

Protection against the toxic effects of chronic alcohol consumption was observed in guinea pigs maintained on a high-ascorbic-acid diet, as opposed to those on a low-ascorbic-acid diet.

Assessment of nutritional status and in vivo immune responses in a disease. Mills PR; Shenkin A; Anthony, RS; McLelland, AS; Alistair NH; MacSween RNM; Russell RI. *Am. J. Clin. Nutr.*, Bethesda, Md.: American Society for Clinical Nutrition 1983. v.38(6):849-859.

High alcohol intake resulted in metabolic and cellular changes, including the depletion of potassium, magnesium, and phosphate in the blood.

Blood thiamine and thiamine phosphate concentrations in excessive drinkers with or without peripheral neuropathy. Poupon RE; Gervaise G; Riant P; Houin G; Tillement JP. *Alcohol and Alcoholism*, 1990, 25(6):605-11.

Thiamine phosphate (but not free thiamine) was found to be at low levels in groups of excessive drinkers with and without peripheral nerve damage.

Bone and mineral metabolism and chronic alcohol abuse. Lalor BC; France MW; Powell D; Adams PH; Counihan TB. *Quarterly Journal of Medicine*, 1986 May, 59(229):497-511.

Significant changes in bone structure and mass appear to be common among heavy drinkers. In a group of alcoholic patients with varying degrees of liver damage, but with no clinical evidence of metabolic bone disease, osteoporosis and osteo-malacia were found, and related to various factors, including magnesium deficiency, low blood levels of calcitriol, the state of liver function, and the type of alcohol consumed.

Calcium status and calcium-regulating hormones in alcoholics. Bjorneboe GE; Bjorneboe A. Johnsen J; Skylv N; Oftebro H; Gautvik KM; Hoiseth A; Morland J; Drevon CA. *Alcoholism, Clinical and Experimental Research*, 1988 Apr, 12(2):229-32.

Vitamin D3 levels were shown to be lower in alcoholics than in a control group, during the winter season. Dietary intake of the vitamin did not differ significantly between the groups, and so it seems that the activities of enzymes crucial in vitamin D3 metabolism may be altered in alcoholics, resulting in low calcium levels.

Carotenoids and liposoluble vitamins in liver cirrhosis. Rocchi E; Borghi A; Paolillo F; Pradelli M;

Casalgrandi G. *Journal of Laboratory and Clinical Medicine*, 1991 Aug, 118(2):176-85.

The role of carotenoids, retinol, and tocopherol in quenching oxidative cellular damage and combatting tumor growth is well documented; this research looked at their activity in human liver cirrhosis. In patients with this disease, significantly reduced blood levels were found of alpha- and beta-carotene and several other vitamin factors. Improved diet for patients with liver cirrhosis is discussed.

Changes in the activation of red blood cell transketolase of alcoholic patients during treatment. Jeyasingham MD; Pratt OE; Shaw GK; Thomson AD. *Alcohol and Alcoholism*, 1987, 22(4):359-65.

An enzyme test can monitor the effectiveness of thiamin therapy used in alcohol detoxification.

Chronic administration of ethanol with high vitamin A supplementation in a liquid diet to rats does not cause liver fibrosis. 1. Morphological observations. Bosma A; Seifert WF; Wilson JH; Roholl PJ; Brouwer A; Knook DL. *Journal of Hepatology*, 1991 Sep, 13(2):240-8.

Rats fed a high-ethanol diet supplemented with vitamin A did not develop liver fibrosis, suggesting that the main effects of chronic ethanol consumption to the liver may be secondary to interference with host resistance to infections.

Chronic administration of ethanol with high vitamin A supplementation in a liquid diet to rats does not cause liver fibrosis. 2. Biochemical observations. Seifert WF; Bosma A; Hendriks HF; Blaner WS; van Leeuwen RE; van Thiel-de Ruiter GC; Wilson JH; Knook DL; Brouwer A. *Journal of Hepatology*, 1991 Sep, 13(2):249-55.

The inability of a high-alcohol, high-vitamin-A diet to induce liver fibrosis in rats (see abstract above) was further evaluated. The hypothesis that interaction between alcohol and retinoids is a major factor in alcoholic liver disease needs to be reconsidered.

Chronic alcohol treatment results in disturbed vitamin D metabolism and skeletal abnormalities in rats. Turner RT; Aloia RC; Segel LD; Hannon KS; Bell NH. *Alcoholism, Clinical and Experimental Research*, 1988 Feb, 12(1):159-62.

Rats on a high-alcohol diet, when compared to a control group, had low blood levels of magnesium and of substances metabolized from vitamin D.

Chronic ethanol feeding and acute ethanol exposure in vitro: effect on intestinal transport of biotin. Said HM; Sharifian A; Bagherzadeh A; Mock D. *American Journal of Clinical Nutrition,* 1990 Dec, 52(6):1083-6.

Alcohol-fed rats showed lowered biotin levels in their blood, as well as lowered ability to absorb biotin from the intestine.

Concentrations of zinc and copper in pregnant problem drinkers and infants. Halmesmaki E; Ylikorkala, O; Alfthan G. *Brit. Med. J.* London: British Medical Association, 1985 Nov 23, 291:1470-1471.

Reduced zinc levels were found in infants of mothers who were problem drinkers.

Current progress toward the prevention of the Wernicke-Korsakoff syndrome. Bishai DM; Bozzetti LP. *Alcohol and Alcoholism,* 1986, 21(4):315-23.

Wernicke-Korsakoff syndrome, a neurological disorder seen mainly in alcoholics, may be prevented by supplementing alcoholic beverages with thiamin. Also relevant to the disease are folate and magnesium levels.

Decreased serum selenium in alcoholics as related to liver structure and function. Korpela H; Kumpulainen J; Luoma PV; Arranto AJ. *Am. J. Clin. Nutr.,* Bethesda, Md.: American Society for Clinical Nutrition, 1985, 42(1):147-151.

A group of alcoholic patients showed low blood levels of selenium, with those patients having the most damaged livers showing the lowest levels. Inadequate dietary selenium intake, as well as alcohol-caused changes in liver structure and function, are probable factors.

Depressed selenium and vitamin E levels in an alcoholic population. Possible relationship to hepatic injury through increased lipid peroxidation. Tanner AR; Bantock I; Hinks L; Lloyd B; Turner NR; Wright R. *Digestive Diseases and Sciences,* 1986 Dec, 31(12):1307-12.

Blood levels of both selenium and vitamin E were shown to be significantly depressed in alcoholics, with selenium more markedly depressed in those with established liver disease. Depressed selenium correlated closely with poor nutritional status, and liver disease activity was more markedly abnormal in subjects with combined vitamin E and selenium deficiency.

Diminished serum concentration of vitamin E in alcoholics. Bjorneboe GE; Johnsen J; Bjorneboe A; Bache-Wiig JE; Morland J; Drevon CA. *Annals of Nutrition and Metabolism,* 1988, 32(2):56-61.

A group of alcoholic subjects showed low blood levels of vitamin E when compared with a control group, and it was reported as well that their estimated dietary intake of this vitamin was significantly lower than that of the controls. Selenium was also lower in the alcoholics, and the reduced levels of these substances may affect cell structure and function, and contribute to development of diseases frequently observed in alcoholics.

Discovery and importance of zinc in human nutrition. Prasad AS. *Fed. Proc. Fed. Am. Soc. Exp. Biol.*, Bethesda, Md.: The Federation, 1984 Oct, 13:2829-2834.

Zinc appears to be involved in many biological functions; its roles in enzymatic functions, cell membranes, and immunity have been well established. Cases of deficiency of this trace element can be traced to several causes, and alcoholism is a predisposing factor.

Disorders of divalent ions and vitamin D metabolism in chronic alcoholism. Pitts TO; Van Thiel DH. *Recent Developments in Alcoholism*, 1986, 4:357-77.

Deficient vitamin D metabolism in alcoholics can result from liver problems, lack of sun exposure, poor diet, and malabsorption. Low vitamin D may contribute to calcium and phosphate deficiencies, and to osteoporosis. Alcoholics should be screened for vitamin D deficiency and given supplements if needed.

Effect of abstinence from alcohol on the depressin of glutathione peroxidase activity and selenium and vitamin E levels in chronic alcoholic patients. Girre C; Hispard E; Therond P; Guedj S.; Bourdon R; Dally S. *Alcoholism, Clinical and Experimental Research*, 1990 Dec, 14(6):909-12.

Chronic alcoholics without severe liver disease were shown to have deficiencies in their antioxidant defense systems. Blood factors indicating this were seen to normalize during 14 days of alcohol abstinence.

Effect of alcohol consumption on serum concentration of 25-hydroxyvitamin D3, retinol, and retinol-binding protein. Bjorneboe GE; Johnsen J; Bjorneboe A; Rousseau B; Pederson JI; Norum KR; Morland J; Drevon CA. *American Journal of Clinical Nutrition*, 1986 Nov, 44(5):678-82.

Chronic alcohol consumers had significantly lower levels of vitamin D in their blood than did a control group, even though the two groups seemed to have similar dietary intake of the nutrient. The alcoholics also had lower calcium levels.

Effect of chronic consumption of ethanol and vitamin E on fatty acid composition and lipid peroxidation in rat heart tissue. Pirozhkov SV; Eskelson CD; Watson RR; Hunter GC; Piotrowski JJ; Bernhard V. *Alcohol*, 1992 Jul-Aug, 9(4):329-34.

Rats were given large amounts of ethanol and vitamin E, and the latter was shown to have a stabilizing effect on phospholipids in the heart, by preventing their deterioration.

Effect of chronic ethanol administration on thiamine transport in microvillous vesicles of rat small intestine. Gastaldi G; Casirola D; Ferrari G; Rindi G. *Alcohol and Alcoholism*, 1989, 24(2):83-9.

Intestinal absorption of thiamine was markedly lower in rats that had been administered ethanol over a period of time than in nonalcoholic rats.

Effect of free radical scavengers on superoxide dismutase (SOD) enzyme in patients with alcoholic cirrhosis. Feher J; Lang I; Nekam K; Muzes G; Deak G. *Acta Medica Hungarica*, 1988, 45(3-4):265-76.

Silymarin and other antioxidants have an effect protective of the liver in alcoholics.

Effect of heavy alcohol consumption on serum concentrations of fat-soluble vitamins and selenium. Bjorneboe GA; Johnsen J; Bjorneboe A; Morland J; Drevon CA. *Alcohol and Alcoholism*, 1987, Suppl 1:533-7.

A group of alcoholics showed blood levels of vitamin E and selenium that were significantly lower than those of a control group, and it is noted that these antioxidants protect against cell damage. Also lower in the alcoholics was vitamin D; this may be a factor-through disturbance of calcium and phosphate metabolism-in the high frequency of bone fractures and osteomalacia in alcoholics.

Effect of silibinin on the activity and expression of superoxide dismutase in lymphocytes from patients with chronic alcoholic liver disease. Feher J; Lang I; Nekam K; Csomos G; Muzes G; Deak G. *Free Radical Research Communications*, 1987, 3(6):373-7.

Silibinin acts to protect the liver, possibly through antioxidant activity.

Effects of acute ethanol on urinary excretion of 5-methyltetrahydrofolic acid and folate derivatives in the rat. Eisenga BH; Collins TD; McMartin KE. *Journal of Nutrition*, 1989 Oct, 119(10):1498-505.

Ethanol-treated rats were shown to excrete more folic acid in their urine than did a control group. This effect has been implicated in the deficiency of this vitamin often seen in alcoholics.

Ethanol and fetal nutrition: effect of chronic ethanol exposure on rat placental growth and membrane-associated folic acid receptor binding activity. Fisher SE; Inselman LS; Duffy L; Atkinson M; Spencer H; Chang B. *Journal of Pediatric Gastroenterology and Nutrition*, 1985 Aug, 4(4):645-9.

Rat fetuses whose mothers were fed alcohol were smaller than those of control-group mothers, and their placentas were less able to process folic acid.

Folate absorption in alcoholic pigs: in vitro hydrolysis and transport at the intestinal brush border membrane. Naughton CA; Chandler CJ; Duplantier RB; Halsted CH. *American Journal of Clinical Nutrition*, 1989 Dec, 50(6):1436-41.

An enzymatic process required for intestinal absorption of folic acid was seen, in the miniature pig, to be impeded by chronic consumption of alcohol.

Food and nutrient intake of alcoholic laborers. Chhabra KB; Ramesh P; Mehta U. *Ecol. Food Nutr.*, London: Gordon & Breach Science Publishers, 1991, 2:51-57.

Fifty subjects-30 alcoholics and 20 nonalcoholics-were selected from an industrial area of Ludhiana City, Punjab, India, and their dietary intake was assessed. Although both groups consumed about the same number of calories, the nutrient intake of the alcoholics was lower, resulting in deficiencies.

Hypothesis: prenatal ethanol-induced birth defects and retinoic acid. Pullarkat RK. *Alcoholism, Clinical and Experimental Research*, 1991 Jun, 15(3):565-7.

Prenatal exposure to alcohol causes birth defects in humans and animals, specifically, central nervous system and limb abnormalities. It is hypothesized that this comes about as a result of ethanol's inhibitory effect of the formation of retinoic acid from retinol. Retinoic acid is important in the development of the central nervous system, and of limbs.

Inhibitory effect of maternal alcohol ingestion on rat pup hepatic 25-hydroxyvitamin D production. Milne M; Baran DT. *Pediatric Research*, 1985 Jan, 19(1):102-4.

Eighteen days of alcohol consumption had no effect on liver synthesis of vitamin D in pregnant rats, but did inhibit fetal production of the vitamin.

Interaction of alcohol with other drugs and nutrients. Implication for the therapy of alcoholic liver disease. Lieber CS. *Drugs*, 1990, 40 Suppl 3:23-44.

New understanding of how alcohol damages the liver has led to more successful therapy with drugs and nutritional factors, such as vitamin A. Vitamin A is depleted in the alcoholic, but excess vitamin A is extra-toxic in the alcoholic.

Interaction of niacin and zinc metabolism in patients with alcoholic pellagra. Vannucchi H; Moreno FS. *American Journal of Clinical Nutrition*, 1989 Aug, 50(2):364-9.

In patients with alcoholic pellagra, zinc interacts with niacin metabolism, through a probable mediation by vitamin B6.

Intestinal absorption, liver uptake, and excretion of 3H-folic acid in folic acid-deficient, alcohol-consuming nonhuman primates. Blocker DE; Thenen SW. *American Journal of Clinical Nutrition*, 1987 Sep, 46(3):503-10.

Chronic alcohol ingestion in nonhuman primates impaired folic acid utilization.

Iron uptake from transferrin and asialotransferrin by hepatocytes from chronically alcohol-fed rats. Potter BJ; McHugh TA; Beloqui O. *Alcoholism, Clinical and Experimental Research*, 1992 Aug, 16(4):810-5.

Alcohol-fed rats showed impaired ability to use iron.

Lipoprotein cholesterol, vitamin A, and vitamin E in an alcoholic population. D'Antonio JA; LaPorte RE; Dai WS; Hom DL; Wozniczak M; Kuller LH. *Cancer*, 1986 May 1, 57(9):1798-802.

Elevated alcohol consumption is associated with increased cancer risk, due possibly to altered vitamin A, vitamin E, and cholesterol metabolism in alcoholics.

Liver cell protection in toxic liver lesion. Feher J; Cornides A; Pal J; Lang I; Csomos G. *Acta Physiologica Hungarica*, 1989, 73(2-3):285-91.

In animal experiments, silymarin, silibinin, and Aica-P were shown to have liver-protecting effects related to their actions as free-radical scavengers.

Metabolism of vitamin D in patients with primary biliary cirrhosis and alcoholic liver disease. Mawer EB; Klass HJ; Warnes TW; Berry JL. *Clinical Science*, 1985 Nov, 69(5):561-70.

Alcoholism may lead to impairment of the liver's function in processing vitamin D.

Nutrition and alcoholic encephalopathies. Thomson AD; Jeyasingham MD; Pratt OE; Shaw GK. *Acta Medica Scandinavica*, Suppl., 1987, 717:55-65.

Chronic alcoholism may cause vitamin B deficiencies due to impaired uptake of thiamin as well as disruption of thiamin metabolism. This may subsequently cause brain damage.

Plasma amino acid patterns in alcoholic pellagra patients. Vannucchi H; Moreno FS; Amarante AR; de Oliveira JE; Marchini JS. *Alcohol and Alcoholism*, 1991, 26(4):431-6.

Alcoholics with pellagra (a disease resulting from lack of B complex vitamins) showed lowered levels for 11 amino acids in the blood.

Plasma osteocalcin levels in liver cirrhosis. Capra F; Casaril M; Gabrielli GB; Stanzial A; Ferrari S; Gandini G; Falezza G; Corrocher R. *Italian Journal of Gastroenterology*, 1991 Mar-Apr, 23(3):124-7.

Cirrhosis of the liver results in lowered levels of osteocalcin, and therefore a lowered ability to replace bone. The low osteocalcin levels may be due to low vitamin D and blood calcium levels.

Prenatal ethanol exposure decreases hippocampal mossy fiber zinc in 45-day-old rats. Savage DD; Montano CY; Paxton LL; Kasarskis EJ. *Alcoholism, Clinical and Experimental Research*, 1989 Aug, 13(4):588-93.

In rats, a brain region important in the process of memory consolidation is affected by prenatal exposure to alcohol. Pregnant rats on an alcohol diet had offspring with lower than normal zinc levels in the hippocampal formation.

Randomized controlled trial of silymarin treatment in patients with cirrhosis of the liver. Ferenci P; Dragosics B; Dittrich H; Frank H; Benda L; Lochs H; Meryn S; Base W; Schneider B. *Journal of Hepatology*, 1989 Jul, 9(1):105-13.

Silymarin, the active principle of the milk thistle, Silybum marianum, protects experimental animals against various substances toxic to the liver. In a double-blind study of human patients with cirrhosis, silymarin was shown to have an effect protective of the liver.

Reduced concentration of hepatic alpha-tocopherol in patients with alcoholic liver cirrhosis. Bell H; Bjorneboe A; Eidsvoll B; Norum KR; Raknerud N; Try K; Thomassen Y; Drevon CA. *Alcohol and Alcoholism*, 1992 Jan, 27(1):39-46.

The vitamin E content in the liver was significantly lower in patients with alcoholic cirrhosis compared with patients with normal livers.

Role of acetyl-L-carnitine in the treatment of cognitive deficit in chronic alcoholism. Tempesta E; Troncon R; Janiri L; Colusso L; Riscica P; Saraceni G; Gesmundo E; Calvani M; Benedetti N; Pola P. *International Journal of Clinical Pharmacology Research*, 1990, 10(1-2):101-7.

Acetyl-L-carnitine can be a useful and safe therapeutic agent in ameliorating the cognitive disturbances of chronic alcoholics. Fifty-five one-month-abstinent alcoholics were put in a double-blind placebo-controlled study to assess the effects of the substance, which did help the group that took it perform better or regain performance abilities faster than those who did not. Memory, logic, and constructional abilities were among those improved.

Selenium status in patients with liver cirrhosis and alcoholism. Johansson U; Johnsson F; Joelsson B; Berglund M; Akesson B. *British Journal of Nutrition*, 1986 Mar, 55(2):227-33.

Blood levels of selenium and vitamins A and E were shown to be reduced in patients with alcoholic cirrhosis.

Some aspects of antioxidant status in blood from alcoholics. Bjorneboe GE; Johnsen J; Bjorneboe A; Marklund SL; Skylv N; Hoiseth A; Bache-Wiig JE; Morland J; Drevon CA. *Alcoholism, Clinical and Experimental Research*, 1988 Dec, 12(6):806-10.

Blood levels of vitamin E were 30 percent lower in a group of alcoholics compared to a control group of nonalcoholics. After this measurement was taken, half of the alcoholics in the study received vitamin E supplementation, as did half of the nonalcoholics; the other halves of each group were supplemented with placebo capsules. Of the four groups, only the alcoholics receiving the vitamin E supplements showed increased blood levels of the vitamin, showing that reduced levels of vitamin E can be normalized by supplementation.

The Wernicke-Korsakoff syndrome in Queensland, Australia: antecedents and prevention. Price J. *Alcohol and Alcoholism*, 1985, 20(2):233-42.

Wernicke-Korsakoff syndrome may be the end result of thiamine deficiency in alcoholics. To prevent the syndrome, fortification of alcoholic beverages with thiamine has been proposed in Queensland, Australia, and the publicity this suggestion has generated has alerted some heavy drinkers to the need for supplementary B vitamins.

The antioxidant status of patients with either alcohol-induced liver damage or myopathy. Ward RJ;

Peters TJ. *Alcohol and Alcoholism*, 1992 Jul, 27(4):359-65.

Alcoholics showed low blood levels of beta-carotene, zinc, and selenium, and in patients with alcoholic cirrhosis, alpha-tocopherol levels were also low.

The clinical spectrum of alcoholic pellagra encephalopathy. A retrospective analysis of 22 cases studied pathologically. Serdaru M; Hausser-Hauw C; Laplane D; Buge A; Castaigne P; Goulon M; Lhermitte F; Hauw JJ. *Brain*, 1988 Aug, 111 (Pt 4):829-42.

Alcoholic pellagra has often gone unrecognized, and therefore untreated with niacin. Multiple vitamin therapy should be given in the treatment of undiagnosed brain abnormalities in alcoholic patients.

The concentration of thiamin and thiamin phosphate esters in patients with alcoholic liver cirrhosis. Tallaksen CM; Bell H; Bohmer T. *Alcohol and Alcoholism*, 1992 Sep, 27(5):523-30.

Current alcohol misuse was shown to be associated with low thiamin concentrations in the blood.

The effect of vitamin E (alpha-tocopherol) supplementation on hepatic levels of vitamin A and E in ethanol and cod liver oil fed rats. Odeleye OE; Eskelson CD; Alak JI;

Watson RR; Chvapil M; Mufti SI; Earnest D. *International Journal for Vitamin and Nutrition Research*, 1991, 61(2):143-8.

Ethanol consumption in rats resulted in decreased levels of vitamins A and E in their livers, but supplementation with vitamin E restored levels of this vitamin to normal, and restored levels of vitamin A somewhat. Rats consuming cod liver oil along with ethanol also had lowered vitamin A and E levels, although the levels were higher than those of the rats not receiving cod liver oil.

Thiamin deficiency and prevention of the Wernicke-Korsakoff syndrome. A major public health problem. Yellowlees PM. *Medical Journal of Australia*, 1986 Sep 1, 145(5):216-9.

In order to prevent Wernicke-Korsakoff syndrome in Australia, it is recommended that flour and bread, as well as alcoholic beverages, be fortified with thiamin.

Thiamin status and biochemical indices of malnutrition and alcoholism in settled communities of !Kung San. van der Westhuyzen J; Davis RE; Icke GC; Jenkins T. *Journal of Tropical Medicine and Hygiene*, 1987 Dec, 90(6):283-9.

Settled groups of !Kung San in the northern Kalahari Desert of Namibia show a high prevalence of thiamin deficiency, and alcohol abuse seems to be the main factor.

Tissue thiamin levels of hospitalised alcoholics before and after oral or parenteral vitamins. Baines M; Bligh JG; Madden JS. *Alcohol and Alcoholism*, 1988, 23(1):49-52.

Oral supplementation of thiamin is effective for most alcoholics.

Trace element and vitamin deficiency in alcoholic and control subjects. Cook CC; Walden RJ; Graham BR; Gillham C, Davies S; Prichard BN. *Alcohol and Alcoholism*, 1991, 26(5-6):541-8.

A wide range of trace elements and vitamins was studied in alcoholic patients admitted for detoxification and in healthy controls. The alcoholics were found to be deficient relative to the controls in magnesium and vitamin E, but there was also a surprising range of deficiencies in the control group, which points to the prevalence of undetected nutritional deficiency in the general population.

Vitamin A status of alcoholics upon admission and after two weeks of hospitalization. Chapman KM; Prabhudesai M; Erdman JW Jr. *Journal of the American College of Nutrition*, 1993 Feb, 12(1):77-83.

Elevated bilirubin levels seen in alcoholics may indicate low vitamin A levels. Caution in levels of vitamin A therapy in these cases is advised, and consideration should instead be given to beta-carotene supplementation.

Vitamin B12 and folate function in chronic alcoholic men with peripheral neuropathy and encephalopathy. Gimsing P; Melgaard B; Andersen K; Vilstrup H; Hippe E. *Journal of Nutrition*, 1989 Mar, 119(3):416-24.

Folate deficiency may contribute to the development of nerve problems in alcoholics.

Vitamin B6 status in cirrhotic patients in relation to apoenzyme of serum alanine aminotransferase. Ohgi N; Hirayama C. *Clinical Biochemistry*, 1988 Dec, 21(6):367-70.

Alcoholic cirrhotic patients have vitamin B6 deficiency.

Vitamin K deficiency in chronic alcoholic males. Iber FL; Shamszad M; Miller PA; Jacob R. Alcoholism, *Clinical and Experimental Research*, 1986 Dec, 10(6):679-81.

Blood clotting defects are frequently present in alcoholics, suggesting vitamin K deficiency. Alcoholics given vitamin K did show more normal clotting protein in their blood than those not given the vitamin.

Zinc and vitamin A status of alcoholics in a medical unit in Sri Lanka. Atukorala TM; Herath CA; Ramachandran S. *Alcohol and Alcoholism*, 1986, 21(3):269-75.

Alcoholics had lower blood levels of zinc and vitamin A than did controls, with female alcoholics having levels lower than those of males, although they drank less.

Zinc nutrition in fetal alcohol syndrome. Keppen LD; Moore DJ; Cannon DJ. *Neurotoxicology*, 1990 Summer, 11(2):375-80.

Experiments with mice suggest that zinc intake should be optimized during pregnancy; the Recommended Daily Allowance should not be exceeded.

Ethanol, Immune Reponses, and Murine AIDS: The Role of Vitamin E as an Immunostimulant and Antioxidant. Wang Y; Watson RR. *Alcohol*, 1994 March-April, 11(2):75-84.

This review article argues that, based on studies, supporting the positive effects of vitamin E on the numerous immune problems involved with AIDS, vitamin E may also be an effective treatment for alcohol-relate immunosuppression.

[The Use of an Infusion of St. John's Wort in the Combined Treatment of Alcoholics with Peptic Ulcer and Chronic Gastritis.] Krylov AA; Ibatov AN. *Vrach Delo*, 1993 February-March, (2-3):146-8.

In this study, hypericum herbal infusion was used in combination with rational psychotherapy of depressive manifestations in 57 outpatients with alcoholism and concomitant diseases of digestive organs. Results found that two months of daily intake proved to be effective.

Alzheimer's Disease

A histochemical study of iron, transferrin, and ferritin in Alzheimer's diseased brains. Connor JR; Menzies SL; St. Martin SM; Mufson EJ. *Journal of Neuroscience Research*, 1992 Jan, 31(1):75-83.

Iron, and iron-regulating proteins, are abnormally distributed in the brains of Alzheimer's disease patients.

A natural and broad spectrum nootropic substance for treatment of SDAT-the Ginkgo biloba extract. Funfgeld EW. *Progress in Clinical and Biological Research*, 1989, 317:1247-60.

Ginkgo biloba extract was found to be therapeutic, and without side effects, in Parkinson's patients with additional signs of Alzheimer's-type dementia.

A search for longitudinal variations in trace element levels in nails of Alzheimer's disease patients. Vance DE; Ehmann WD; Markesbery WR. *Biological Trace Element Research*, 1990 Jul-Dec, 26-27:461-70.

Progressive changes in trace-element levels occur in the nails of Alzheimer's disease patients, and imbalances are detected even in the earliest stages of the disease. Mercury levels were seen to decrease progressively with the level of the disease and with age, and potassium and zinc to increase with these same factors.

Acetyl-L-carnitine: a drug able to slow the progress of Alzheimer's disease? Carta A; Calvani M. *Annals of the New York Academy of Sciences*, 1991, 640:228-32.

Clinical studies suggest that acetyl-L-carnitine, which has protective effects against aging processes and nerve degeneration, may slow the natural course of Alzheimer's disease.

Changes in calcium homeostasis during aging and Alzheimer's disease. Peterson C; Ratan R; Shelanski M; Goldman J. *Annals of the New York Academy of Sciences*, 1989, 568:262-70.

Alzheimer's disease patients and normal aged patients had altered calcium regulation compared to that of young patients.

Cultured cells as a screen for novel treatments of Alzheimer's disease. Malow BA; Baker AC; Blass JP. *Archives of Neurology*, 1989 Nov. 46(11):1201-3.

L-carnitine normalized two properties normally measured as abnormal in Alzheimer's diseased cells.

Double-blind parallel design pilot study of acetyl levocarnitine in patients with Alzheimer's disease. Sano M; Bell K; Cote L; Dooneief G; Lawton A; Legler L; Marder K; Naini A; Stern Y; Mayeux R. *Archives of Neurology*, 1992 Nov, 49(11):1137-41.

Acetyl levocarnitine shows the ability to retard the deterioration in some cognitive areas in those suffering from Alzheimer's disease.

Effects of free $Ca2_$ on the $[Ca2_ \_ Mg2\_]$-dependent adenosinetriphosphatase (ATPase) of Alzheimer and normal fibroblasts. Rizopoulos E; Chambers JP; Wayner MJ; Martinez AO; Armstrong LS. *Neurobiology of Aging*, 1989 Nov-Dec, 10(6):717-20.

Calcium regulation is different in Alzheimer's disease cells than in normal cells.

Essential fatty acids in Alzheimer's disease. Corrigan FM; Van Rhijn A; Horrobin DF. *Annals of the New York*

Academy of Sciences, 1991, 640: 250-2.

Essential fatty acids are abnormal in Alzheimer's disease patients. Twenty-week treatment with essential fatty acids improved the levels.

Folate, vitamin B12 and cognitive impairment in patients with Alzheimer's disease. Levitt AJ; Karlinsky H. *Acta Psychiatrica Scandinavica*, 1992 Oct, 86(4): 301-5.

An inverse relationship was found between vitamin B12 levels and the severity of cognitive impairment in Alzheimer's disease patients.

Hair aluminium in normal aged and senile dementia of Alzheimer type. Kobayashi S; Fujiwara S; Arimoto S; Koide H; Fukuda J; Shimode K; Yamaguchi S; Okada K; Tsunematsu T. *Progress in Clinical and Biological Research*, 1989, 317:1095-109.

In Alzheimer's disease, decreased calcium and magnesium levels enhance accumulation of aluminum in the brain. In normal aged individuals, cerebral blood flow levels decrease as hair aluminum levels increase, suggesting that aluminum may contribute to aging of the brain.

Hypothesis regarding amyloid and zinc in the pathogenesis of Alzheimer disease: potential for preventive intervention. Constantinidis, J. *Alzheimer Disease and Associated Disorders*, 1991 Spring, 5(1):31-5.

It is suggested that amyloid production in the cerebral cortex causes a zinc deficiency in the brain; toxic metals (such as iron, aluminum, and mercury) then displace the zinc in some enzymes. Application of a zinc complex that crosses the blood-brain barrier may mitigate these effects.

Lipid peroxidation and free radical scavengers in Alzheimer's disease. Jeandel C; Nicolas MB; Dubois F; Nabet-Belleville F; Penin F; Cuny G. *Gerontology*, 1989, 35(5-6):275-82.

The blood of a group of Alzheimer's patients, when compared with that of a group of healthy age-matched controls, showed lower levels of glutathione peroxidase activity in red blood cells, as well as lower levels of vitamins E, C, and A, and zinc.

Long-term acetyl-L-carnitine treatment in Alzheimer's disease. Spagnoli A; Lucca U; Menasce G; Bandera L; Cizza G; Forloni G; Tettamanti M; Frattura L; Tiraboschi P; Comelli M. *Neurology*, 1991 Nov, 41(11):1726-32.

The effects of acetyl-L-carnitine on Alzheimer's patients were assessed in a double-blind, placebo-controlled study over one year. After this period, both the treated and placebo groups worsened, but the treated group showed a slower rate of deterioration in 13 of the 14 outcome measures, with statistically significant results in five of them. No significant side effects were seen.

Low B12 levels related to high activity of platelet MAO in patients with dementia disorders.
A retrospective study. Regland B; Gottfries CG; Oreland L; Svennerholm L. *Acta Psychiatrica Scandinavica*, 1988 Oct, 78(4): 451-7.

Vitamin B12 levels were shown to be reduced in the blood of Alzheimer's patients and patients with confusional states.

Magnesium depletion and pathogenesis of Alzheimer's disease. Durlach J. *Magnesium Research*, 1990 Sep, 3(3):217-8.

Magnesium depletion in a particular region of the brain, along with aluminum incorporation into the brain, is associated with Alzheimer's disease. Further research should seek to control the alterations of albumin, which may induce the magnesium depletion.

Nutrient intakes and energy expenditures of residents with senile Alzheimer's type. Litchford MD; Wakefield LM. *J. Am. Diet Assoc.*, Chicago, Ill.: The Association, Feb 1987. v. 87(2).

In a study conducted over three days, Alzheimer's patients were seen to exhibit lower nutrient intake than did a control group. Significant intake differences were noted for vitamin A, thiamin, niacin, riboflavin, and calcium, as well as for total calories and other factors.

Oxidative damage in Alzheimer's dementia, and the potential etiopathogenic role of aluminosilicates, microglia and micronutrient interactions. Evans PH; Yano E; Klinowski J; Peterhans E. *Exs*, 1992, 62:178-89.

In laboratory experiments, aluminosilicate particles have stimulated the generation of tissue-damaging free radicals in nervous-system cells. Similar aluminosilicate deposits have been found in the brains of Alzheimer's patients, and it is suggested that antioxidant micronutrients and pharmacological agents would be useful in preventing and treating Alzheimer's disease.

Plasma concentrations of vitamins A and E and carotenoids in Alzheimer's disease. Zaman Z; Roche S; Fielden P; Frost PG; Niriella DC; Cayley AC. *Age and Ageing*, 1992 Mar, 21(2):91-4.

Compared to controls, Alzheimer's patients had lower levels of vitamins

E and A, and of beta-carotene, in their blood.

Possible participation of calcium-regulating factors in senile dementia in elderly female subjects. Ogihara T; Miya K; Morimoto S. *Gerontology*, 1990, 36 Suppl 1:25-30.

Calcium and calcium-regulating hormones may play several roles in senile dementia.

Regional distribution of iron and iron-regulatory proteins in the brain in aging and Alzheimer's disease. Connor JR; Snyder BS; Beard JL; Fine RE; Mufson EJ. *Journal of Neuroscience Research*, 1992 Feb, 31(2):327-35.

Levels of blood proteins that regulate the body's use of iron are altered in the aging brain, particularly in Alzheimer's disease. The decreased availability of iron that results could be important in explaining the degenerative changes that occur in the disease.

Specific reduction of calcium-binding protein (28-kilodalton calbindin-D) gene expression in aging and neurodegenerative diseases. Iacopino AM; Christakos S. *Proceedings of the National Academy of Sciences of the United States of America*, 1990 Jun, 87(11):4078-82.

In Alzheimer's disease, and in aging in general, decreased levels of calcium-binding protein have been observed in humans, and in rats. Disturbances in calcium balance within nerves may be responsible for some of the degeneration seen in these conditions.

The hypothesis of zinc deficiency in the pathogenesis of neurofibrillary tangles. Constantinidis J. *Medical Hypotheses*, 1991 Aug, 35(4):319-23.

Functional zinc decreases leading to abnormal metals reaching the brain may be responsible for a number of conditions, including Alzheimer's disease. A nontoxic zinc compound crossing the blood-brain barrier may be useful in treating Alzheimer's, which is associated with decreased levels of zinc and increased brain levels of aluminum and iron.

Thiamine and Alzheimer's disease. A pilot study. Blass JP; Gleason P; Brush D; DiPonte P; Thaler H. *Archives of Neurology*, 1988 Aug, 45(8):833-5.

In a double-blind, placebo-controlled study, Alzheimer's patients showing no signs of thiamine deficiency, but treated with thiamine over three months, showed cognitive improvements.

Vitamin B12 levels in serum and cerebrospinal fluid of people with Alzheimer's disease. Ikeda T; Furukawa Y; Mashimoto S;

Takahaski K; Yamada M. *Acta Psychiatrica Scandinavica*, 1990 Oct, 82(4):327-9.

Low levels of vitamin B12 in the cerebrospinal fluid of Alzheimer's patients are characteristic of the disease.

Vitamin B12-induced reduction of platelet monoamine oxidase activity in patients with dementia and pernicious anaemia. Regland B; Gottfries CG; Oreland L. *European Archives of Psychiatry and Clinical Neuroscience*, 1991, 240(4-5):288-91.

There is a significant connection between vitamin B12 deficiency and Alzheimer's disease. When Alzheimer's patients were treated with B12, their increased platelet monoamine oxidase activity (a characteristic of the disease), was significantly reduced.

Vitamin E and Alzheimer's disease in subjects with Down's syndrome. Jackson CV; Holland AJ; Williams CA; Dickerson JW. *Journal of Mental Deficiency Research*, 1988 Dec, 32 (Pt 6):479-84.

People with Down's syndrome are at high risk of developing Alzheimer's disease; they seem, because of their genetic make-up, to be more susceptible to oxidative damage. Blood levels of vitamin E in 12 Down's syndrome subjects with

Alzheimer's disease were lower than those in 12 Down's subjects without the disease, suggesting an interaction between risk of Alzheimer's and the protective action of vitamin E against oxidative damage.

Pharmacokinetics of IV and Oral Acetyl-L-carnitine in a Multiple Dose Regimen in Patients with Senile Dementia of Alzheimer Type. Parnetti L; et al. *European Journal of Clinical Pharmacology*, 1992, 42(1):89-93.

Results of this study showed that the oral and intravenous administration of acetyl-L-carnitine increased CSF and plasma concentrations in Alzheimer's patients.

Clinical and Neurochemical Effects of Acetyl-L-carnitine in Alzheimer's Disease. Pettegrew JW; et al. *Neurobiol Aging*, 1995 Jan-Feb, 16(1): 1-4.

Results of this double-bind, placebo-controlled study found that patients treated with acetyl-L-carnitine experienced significantly less deterioration in mental status than controls.

Long-term Effects of Phosphati-dylserine, Pyritinol, and Cognitive Training in Alzheimer's Disease. A Neuropsychological, EEG, and PET Investigation. Heiss WD; et al.

Dementia, 1994 March-April, 5(2):88-98.

Results of this study showed that phosphatidylserine administered in doses of 400 mg per day led to significant, short-term neurophysical improvements in patients with Alzheimer's disease relative to controls.

Double-blind Cross-over Study of Phosphatidylserine vs. Placebo in Patients with Early Dementia of the Alzheimer Type. Engel RR; et al. *Eur Neuropsychoparmacol*, 1992 June, 2(2):149-155.

Results of this double-blind, placebo-controlled study showed that the administration of 300 mg per day of phosphatidylserine for 8 weeks led to significant clinical improvements in patients with mild primary degenerative dementia relative to controls.

Effects of Phosphatidylserine in Alzheimer's Disease. Crook T; et al. *Psychopharmacol Bulletin*, 1992, 28(1):61-6.

In this double-blind, placebo-controlled study, Alzheimer's patients received 100 mg per day of bovine cortex phosphatidylserine for 12 weeks. Results showed the treatment improved several cognitive measures relative to controls.

Vitamin E Protects Nerve Cells from Amyloid Beta Protein Toxicity. Behl C; et al. *Biochem Biophys Res Commun*, 1992 July 31, 186(2): 944-50.

This review article notes that vitamin E inhibits amyloid beta protein induced cell death, a key factor in Alzheimer's disease.

Vitamin E and Alzheimer's Disease in Subjects with Down's Syndrome. Jackson CV; et al. *Journal of Mental Deficit Research*, 1988 Dec, 32(Pt 6):479-84.

This article notes that Down's syndrome patients are at high risk for Alzheimer's disease. Vitamin E has been shown to protect against oxidative damage caused by gene coding of superoxide dismutase-/on chromosome 21 resulting in excess activity of the enzyme, thus suggesting its potential as a preventive approach to Alzheimer's.

Alzheimer's and Parkinson's Disease. Brain Levels of Glutathione, Glutathione Disulfide, and Vitamin E. Adams, Jr. JD; et al. *Mol Chem Neuropathol*, 1991 June, 14(3):213-26.

This study found that vitamin E levels were twice as high in the midbrain of Alzheimer's patients and Alzheimer's patients with signs of Parkinson's disease relative to controls. Such findings, the authors argue, suggest that compensatory increases in vitamin E levels occur in such patients after specific regions of the brain have been damaged.

Serum Dehydroepiandrosterone (DHEA) and DHEA-sulfate (DHEA-S) in Alzheimer's Disease and in Cerebrovascular Dementia. Yanase T; et al. *Endocr Journal*, 1996 February, 43(1):119-23.

Results of this study found significantly lower levels of serum DHEA-S in elderly Japanese patients suffering from Alzheimer's and/or cerebrovascular dementia relative to age-matched healthy controls.

[The Significance of Quantified EEG in Alzheimer's Disease. Changes Induced by Piracetam.] Pierlovisi-Lavaivre M; et al. *Neurophysical Clin*, 1991 December, 21(5-6): 411-23.

Results of this placebo-controlled study showed that the administration of 9 g per day to a group of 12 Alzheimer's patients and 2.4 g per day in 16 patients with mild senile dementia led to increases in alertness among patients in both groups.

Anorexia

Evidence of zinc deficiency in anorexia nervosa and bulimia nervosa. Schauss AG; Bryce-Smith D. *Nutrients and brain function*, Essman WB, ed. Basel: Kargel, 1987 (151-162).

A review is presented on the use of zinc in treating anorexia nervosa, and on the zinc taste-test for assessing zinc deficiency, which is frequent in anorexics.

Nutrition in the elderly [clinical conference]. Morley JE; Mooradian AD; Silver AJ; Heber D; Alfin-Slater RB. *Annals of Internal Medicine*, 1988 Dec 1, 109(11):890-904.

Unrecognized depression is a common, and treatable, cause of loss of appetite in the elderly. Lack of vitamin D can be a problem, due to decreased exposure to sunlight, and lack of ability to form this vitamin. Zinc and selenium levels may be low, which can lead to deteriorating vision and increased cancer risk, respectively.

Zinc absorption in anorexia nervosa. Dinsmore, WW; Alderdice, JT; McMaster, D; Adams, CEA; Love, AH. *Lancet*, 1985 May 4, 1(8):1041-1042.

Anorexics have a lower intestinal uptake of zinc than do normal subjects.

Anorexia Nervosa Responding to Zinc Supplementation: A Case Report. Yamaguchi H; et al.

Gastroenterol Jpn, 1992 August, 27(4):554-8.

This article reports on the case of a 16-year-old hospitalized for anorexia, who experienced significant benefits following initial treatment with 40 mumol per day of intravenous zinc for 7 days, which was then reduced to oral intake of 15 mg of elemental zinc per day for 60 days.

Zinc Deficiency in Anorexia Nervosa. Katz RL; et al. *Journal of Adolescent Health Care*, 1987 September, 8(5):400-6.

Results of this study found that zinc deficiency is common among adolescent anorexics and that supplementation with 50 mg per day of elemental zinc improved symptoms of anxiety and depression among such patients.

Anxiety

Effect of a herbal psychotropic preparation, BR-16A (Mentat), on performance of mice on elevated plus-maze. Verma A; Kulkarni SK. *Indian Journal of Experimental Biology*, 1991 Dec, 29(12):1120-3.

In experiments with mice, the herbal preparation BR-16A (Mentat) was shown to reduce anxiety.

Magnesium, schizophrenia and manic-depressive disease. Kirov GK; Tsachev KN. *Neuropsychobiology*, 1990, 23(2):79-81.

Magnesium levels in the blood of schizophrenic and depressed patients were shown to be lower than normal. The levels increased for those schizophrenics achieving clinical remission. It is hypothesized that the high stress level in severely ill psychiatric patients can sometimes lead to magnesium deficiency, which in turn could exacerbate symptoms such as anxiety, fear, hallucinations, weakness, and physical complaints.

Pre-operative anxiety and serum potassium. McCleane GJ; Watters CH. *Anaesthesia*, 1990 Jul, 45(7):583-5.

Two hundred pre-operative patients were assessed for anxiety, and the most anxious ones showed lowered blood potassium levels.

Role of an indigenous drug geriforte on blood levels of biogenic amines and its significance in the treatment of anxiety neurosis. Upadhyaya L; Tiwari AK; Agrawal A; Dubey GP. *Activitas Nervosa Superior*, 1990 Mar, 32(1):1-5.

The herbal preparation Geriforte was found effective in reducing anxiety and stress in neurotic anxiety patients.

The impact of selenium supplementation on mood. Benton D; Cook

R. *Biological Psychiatry*, 1991 Jun 1, 29(11):1092-8.

To look into the possibility that a subclinical deficiency of selenium exists in a sample of the British population, 50 subjects were given either a selenium supplement or a placebo, in a double-blind study over five weeks. The selenium was shown to elevate mood and, in particular, to decrease anxiety, and these effects were more pronounced in those subjects who had lower levels of selenium in their diets to begin with. The results are discussed in terms of the low level of selenium in the food chain in some parts of the world.

Vitamin B12 and folic acid serum levels in obsessive compulsive disorder. Hermesh H; Weizman A; Shahar A; Munitz H. *Acta Psychiatrica Scandinavica*, 1988 Jul, 78(1):8-10.

Vitamin B12 deficiency was shown to be associated with a subgroup of patients with obsessive compulsive disorder.

Vitamin C status in chronic schizo-phrenia. Suboticanec K; Folnegovic-Smalc V; Korbar M; Mestrovic B; Buzina R. *Biological Psychiatry*, 1990 Dec 1, 28(11):959-66.

Schizophrenic patients on the same hospital diet as control group patients showed lower levels of vitamin C in their blood, and even when they were supplemented to normalize their blood levels of the vitamin, levels excreted in their urine remained lower than those of the control group. The results support the view that schizophrenic patients need more vitamin C than the suggested requirement for healthy people.

Effect of a special kava extract in patients with anxiety-, tension-, and excitation states of non-psychotic genesis. Double-blind study with placebos over 4 weeks. (in German) Kinzler E; Kromer J; Lehmann E. *Arzneimittel-Forschung*, 1991 Jun, 41(6):584-8.

In a double-blind study, patients with anxiety syndrome not caused by psychotic disorders were treated with either kava extract or a placebo. A significant, and progressive, anxiety-reducing effect was seen for the kava over a period of four weeks. No side effects were noted.

Psychosomatic dysfunctions in the female climacteric. Clinical effectiveness and tolerance of Kava Extract WS 1490. (in German) Warnecke G. *Fortschritte der Medizin*, 1991 Feb 10, 109(4):119-22.

In a double-blind study, kava extract worked better than a placebo in relieving menopausal symptoms, and was well-tolerated.

Autism

Biotin-responsive infantile encephalopathy: EEG-polygraphic study of a case. Colamaria V; Burlina AB; Gaburro D; Pajno-Ferrara F; Sandubray JM; Merino RG; Dalla Bernardina B. *Epilepsia*, 1989 Sep-Oct, 30(5):573-8.

An infant suffering from autistic-like behavior, progressive lethargy, muscle spasms, generalized seizures, and other symptoms was treated with biotin twice daily and showed dramatic improvement of all symptoms.

Controversies in the treatment of autistic children: vitamin and drug therapy. Rimland B. *Journal of Child Neurology*, 1988, 3 Suppl:S68-72.

A survey of approximately 4000 questionnaires completed by parents of autistic children provided ratings of various treatments. Among the biomedical treatments, the highest-ranking one was the use of high-dosage vitamin B6 and magnesium, with 8.5 parents reporting behavioral improvement to every one reporting behavioral worsening. The most-used drug on the list, thioridazine hydro-chloride (Mellaril), came in fourth, with a helped-worsened ratio of 1.4:1.

The effects of combined pyridoxine plus magnesium administration on the conditioned evoked potentials in children with autistic behavior. Martineau J; Barthelemy C; Roux S; Lelord G. *Curr. Top. Nutr. Dis.*, 1988, 19:357-362.

Vitamin B6 plus magnesium was shown to be effective in the treatment of autistic children.

Nutritional treatments currently under investigation in autism. Coleman M. *Clin. Nutr.*, 1989 Sept/Oct, 8(5):210-212.

Autism has multiple causes, and many types of autism can be treated by nutritional approaches, e.g., the folic acid therapy of the fragile X syndrome, the low-phenylalanine diet of phenylketonuria, the restricted purine diet of purine autism, the high-calcium diet of autism with hypocalcinuria, and the ketogenic diet of autism with lactic acidosis. Such targeted therapies appear to be the future approach to autism.

Vitamin B6 versus fenfluramine: A case-study in medical bias. Rimland B. *J. Nutr. Med.*, 1991, 2(3):321-322.

Vitamin B6 and magnesium-as opposed to the drug fenfluramine-constitute the first-choice treatment in the treatment of autistic children and adults.

Bipolar Disorder

Abnormal intracellular calcium ion concentration in platelets and lymphocytes of bipolar patients. Dubovsky SL; Murphy J; Thomas M; Rademacher J. *American Journal of Psychiatry*, 1992 Jan, 149(1): 118-20.

There seems to be a disturbance in calcium regulation in the systems of patients with bipolar disorder.

Calcium function in affective disorders and healthy controls. Bowden CL; Huang LG; Javors MA; Johnson JM; Seleshi E; McIntyre K; Contreras S; Maas JW. *Biological Psychiatry*, 1988 Feb 15, 23(4): 367-76.

Calcium activity was shown to be abnormal in bipolar depressed and manic patients, and in unipolar patients. Also, unipolar and bipolar patients showed different types of disturbances in calcium metabolism.

Elevated platelet intracellular calcium concentration in bipolar depression. Dubovsky SL; Lee C; Christiano J; Murphy J. *Biological Psychiatry*, 1991 Mar 1, 29(5): 441-50.

It is suggested that untreated bipolar depressed patients had changes in calcium regulation within their cells that were not characteristic of untreated unipolar depressed patients.

Folate concentration in Chinese psychiatric outpatients on long-term lithium treatment. Lee S; Chow CC; Shek CC; Wing YK; Chen CN. *Journal of Affective Disorders*, 1992 Apr, 24(4):265-70.

While folate deficiency is uncommon among Chinese psychiatric patients, it was shown that patients with a good response to lithium treatment over one year had a higher folate level in their blood than those showing an unsatisfactory response. This supports recent evidence that folate at high concentrations enhances the benefits of lithium.

Folic acid enhances lithium prophylaxis. Coppen A; Chaudhry S; Swade C. *Journal of Affective Disorders*, 1986 Jan-Feb, 10(1):9-13.

In a double-blind study of patients on lithium therapy, those receiving a folic acid supplement showed a significant reduction of their symptoms compared to a group receiving a placebo.

Further studies of vanadium in depressive psychosis. Naylor GJ; Corrigan FM; Smith AH; Connelly P; Ward NI. *British Journal of Psychiatry*, 1987 May, 150:656-61.

Changes in tissue vanadium concentration may explain the changes in sodium transport that occur in depressive psychosis.

Incorporation of inositol into the phosphoinositides of lymphoblastoid cell lines established from bipolar manic-depressive patients. Banks RE; Aiton JF; Cramb G; Naylor GJ. *Journal of Affective Disorders*, 1990 May, 19(1):1-8.

Patients with manic-depressive disorder showed lower uptake of inositol when compared with a control group.

Lithium mechanisms in bipolar illness and altered intracellular calcium functions. Meltzer HL. *Biological Psychiatry*, 1986 May, 21(5-6):492-510.

Calcium acts between cells in a variety of ways by activating a wide range of enzymes. Since lithium seems to alter many calcium-dependent processes, it may be that bipolar illness is a result of disturbances in calcium-regulated functions.

Long-term lithium treatment. Some clinical, psychological and biological aspects. Smigan L. *Acta Psychiatrica Scandinavica*, 1985 Feb, 71(2): 160-70.

Patients with affective disorders who responded favorably to lithium treatment showed a rise in calcium levels in their blood during the first four months of treatment. Those who did not respond to lithium showed unaltered calcium levels.

Red cell folate concentrations in psychiatric patients. Carney MW; Chary TK; Laundy M; Bottiglieri T; Chanarin I; Reynolds EH; Toone B. *Journal of Affective Disorders*, 1990 Jul, 19(3):207-13.

Depressed patients were found to have low folate levels.

The calcium second messenger system in bipolar disorders: data supporting new research directions. Dubovsky SL; Murphy J; Christiano J; Lee C. *Journal of Neuropsychiatry and Clinical Neurosciences*, 1992 Winter, 4(1):3-14.

Irregularities in calcium's signal-sending actions within cells may explain bipolar disorders. Lithium and other mood-stabilizing treatments seem to work by regulating calcium ion hyperactivity.

The use of sodium and potassium to reduce toxicity and toxic side effects from lithium. Cater RE. *Medical Hypotheses*, 1986 Aug, 20(4):359-83.

In rats, toxic side effects of lithium were prevented by feeding sodium and potassium. While sodium alone has been used to reduce side effects in humans, it can reduce lithium's benefits. Evidence suggests that using both sodium and potassium together would be better because the lithium dose could be slightly raised without adverse effect.

Trace elements and the electroencephalogram during long-term lithium treatment. Harvey NS: Jarratt J; Ward NI. *British Journal of Psychiatry*, 1992 May, 160:654-8.

Raised bromine levels have been found in patients during lithium treatment, and it is suggested that bromine may aid the therapeutic effect of lithium.

Vanadium and other trace elements in patients taking lithium. Campbell CA; Peet M; Ward NI. *Biological Psychiatry*, 1988 Nov, 24(7):775-81.

Compared to controls, patients on lithium had lower levels of vanadium and cobalt in their blood, and higher levels of aluminum.

Vitamin B12 and folate status in acute geropsychiatric inpatients: affective and cognitive characteristics of a vitamin nondeficient population. Bell IR; Edman JS; Marby DW; Satlin A; Dreier T; Liptzin B; Cole JO. *Biological Psychiatry*, 1990 Jan 15, 27(2):125-37.

A study was done of geriatric patients admitted to a psychiatric hospital. Although they were not generally vitamin-deficient, those with below-median values of vitamin B12 and folate had more severe psychiatric problems than those with higher levels of one or both vitamins. It is suggested that biochemically interrelated vitamins such as B12 and folate may exert both a separate and combined influence on mental state, and that poorer vitamin status may contribute to some psychiatric disorders in the elderly.

Vitamin B6 in clinical neurology. Bernstein AL. *Annals of the New York Academy of Sciences*, 1990, 585:250-60.

Vitamin B6 supplementation may be useful in treating a number of conditions. For instance, headache, chronic pain, and depression, all associated with serotonin deficiency, have, in some studies, been shown to have been helped by B6, which raises serotonin levels. In addition, B6 may reverse the effects of toxic substances associated with hyperactivity and aggressive behavior.

Brain Function/Injury

Pharmacological Treatment with Phosphatidyl Serine of 40 Ambulatory Patients with Senile Dementia Syndrome. Lomardi GF. *Minerva Med.*, 1989 June, 80(6): 599-602.

Results of this study showed that patients suffering from chronic cerebral decomponensation experienced improvements in mnesic and neuropsychic symptomatology following phosphatidylserine administration for 60 days.

Chronic Treatment with Phosphatidylserine Restores Muscarinic Cholinergic Receptor Deficits in the Aged Mouse Brain. Gelbmann CM; Muller WE. *Neurobiol Aging*, 1992 Jan-Feb, 13(1):45-50.

Results of this study showed that the administration of phosphatidylserine for 21 days led to partial restoration of decreased density of muscarinic cholinergic receptors in age mouse brains in a dose-dependent manner.

Effects of Phosphatidylserine in Age-associated memory Impairment. Crook TH; et al. *Neurology*, 1991 May, 41(5):644-9.

Results of this double-blind, placebo-controlled study showed that age-associated memory impairment patients treated with 100 mg of phosphatidylserine for 12 weeks experienced clinical improvement relevant to controls.

Double-Blind Randomized Controlled Study of Phosphatidylserine in Senile Demented Patients. Delwaide PJ; et al. *Acta Neurol. Scand.*, 1986 Feb, 73(2):136-40.

This double-blind, placebo-controlled study examined the effects of 3 x 100 mg of phosphatidylserine on patients hospitalized with dementia. Results showed a significant improvement in the patients receiving phosphatidylserine relative to controls.

Effects of Phosphatidylserine Therapy in Geriatric Patients with Depressive Disorders. Maggioni M; et al. *Acta Psychiatr. Scand.*, 1990 March, 81(3):265-70.

This double-blind, placebo-controlled study examined the effects of 300 mg per day of phosphatidylserine for 30 days on cognitive, affective, and behavioral symptoms of elderly women with depressive disorders. Results showed that patients receiving phosphatidylserine experienced improvements with respect to memory, behavior, and depressive symptoms relative to controls.

Cognitive Decline in the Elderly: A Double-blind, Placebo-controlled Multicenter Study on Efficacy of Phosphatidylserine Administration. Cenacchi T; et al. *Aging*, 1993 April, 5(2):123-33.

This double-blind, placebo-controlled study examined the effects of 300 mg per day of phosphatidylserine in cognitive impaired geriatric patients. Results showed the treatment had significant positive cognitive and behavioral effects relative to controls.

Age-related Alterations of NMDA-receptor Properties in the Mouse

Forebrain: Partial Restoration by Chronic Phosphatidylserine Treatment. Cohen SA; Muller WE. *Brain*, 1992 July 3, 584(1-2):174-80.

Results of this study found that the aged mice treated with 20 mg/kg ip per day of phosphatidylserine over a period of three weeks totally normalized enhanced efficacy and affinity of L-glutamate and glycine and elevated NMDA receptor density by approximately 25 percent.

Pharmacological Effects of Phosphatidylserine Enzymatically Synthesized from Soybean Lecithin on Brain Functions in Rodents. Sakai M; et al. *Journal of Nutr Sci Vitaminol*, 1996 Feb, 42(1):47-54.

Results of this study indicated that the oral administration of 300 mg per day of soybean transphosphatidylated phosphatidylserine can improve and/or prevent senile dementia in humans.

Activity of Phosphatidylserine on Memory Retrieval and on Exploration in Mice. Valzelli L; et al. *Methods Find Exp Clin Pharmacol*, 1987 Oct, 9(10):657-60.

Results of this study showed definite improvements in memory performance in mice treated with bovine brain phosphatidylserine relative to controls.

Phosphatidylserine Administration During Postnatal Development Improves Memory in Adult Mice. Fagioli S; et al. *Neurosci Letters*, 1989 June 19, 101(2):229-33.

Results of this study showed that the postnatal administration of an aqueous suspension of phosphatidylserine led to improvements of memory processes in mice.

Chronic Phosphatidylserine Treatment Improves Spatial Memory and Passive Avoidance in Aged Rats. Zanotti A; et al. *Psychopharmacology*, 1989, 99(3):316-21.

Results of this study showed that oral administration of 50 mg/kg per day of phosphatidylserine for 12 weeks improved spatial memory and passive avoidance retention of aged impaired rats.

Ginkgo Biloba Extract Facilitates Recovery from Penetrating Brain Injury in Adult Male Rats. Attella MJ; et al. *Exp Neurol*, 1989 July, 105(1):62-71.

Results of this study found that rats suffering from brain lesions which received treatment with 100 mg/kg Ginkgo biloba extract (GBE) intraperitoneally for 30 days experienced less impairment and a reduction in brain swellings induced by lesions than rats treated with saline or sham controls.

[Evidence for a Therapeutic Effect of Ginkgo Biloba Special Extract. Meta-analysis of 11 Clinical Studies in Patients with Cerebrovascular Insufficiency in Old Age.] Hopfenmuller W. *Arzneimittelforschung*, 1994 September, 44(9):1005-13.

Results of this meta-analysis incoving 7 double-blind, placebo-controlled clinical trials found Ginkgo biloba extract (mean dose of 150 mg per day) significantly effective in reducing clinical sumptoms associated with cerebrovascular insufficiency in old age.

Ginkgo Biloba for Cerebral Insufficiency. Kleijnen J; Knipschild P. *Clin Ther*, 1993 May-June, 15(3):549-558.

Results of this double-blind, placebo-controlled study found that elderly subjects with age-related memory impairment experienced significant improvement in the speed of information processing following treatment with either 320 mg or 600 mg of Ginkgo biloba extract 1 hour prior to performing a dual-code test.

A Double-blind, Placebo-controlled Study of Ginkgo Biloba Extract ("tanakan") in Elderly Outpatients with Mild to Moderate Memory Impairment. Rai GS; et al. *Curr Med Res Opin*, 1991, 12(6):350-5.

In this double-blind, placebo-controlled study, patients over 50 with some level of memory impairment received treatment with oral doses of 120 mg of Ginkgo biloba per day. Results found that Ginkgo biloba had significant beneficial effects on cognitive function at both 12 and 24 weeks.

Influence of an Extract of Ginkgo Biloba on Cerebral Blood Flow and Metabolism. Krieglstein J; et al. *Life Sci*, 1986 December 15, 39(24):2327-34.

This study examined the effects of Ginkgo biloba eztract on the levels of blood glucose, local cerebral blood flow, and cerebral glucose concentration and consumption. Results found the extract reduced the concentration of cortical glucose and did not changing other substrate levels, indicating Ginkgo biloba can inhibit glucose and may play a role in its capacity to protect brain tissue from hypoxic or ischemic damage.

[Clinical Psychopharmacology of Ginkgo Biloba Extract.] Warburton DM. *Presse Med*, 1986 September 25, 15(31):1595-1604.

The authors of this extensive review article on the clinical psycho-pharmacology of Ginkgo biloba extract concluded that the extract appears to be effective in treating vascular disorders, dementia, and cognitive disorders secondary to depression. The authors also suggest that there are no risks associated with taking the frug in doses well above its recommended levels.

[Ginkgo—Myth and Reality.] Z'Brun A. *Schweiz Rundsch Med Prax*, 1995 January 3, 84(1):1-6.

This review article cites clinical studies supporting efficacy of Ginkgo biloba extracts in the treatment of cerebral insufficiency and athero-sclerotic disease of the peripheral arteries.

Bulimia

Plasma and cerebrospinal fluid measures of arginine vasopressin secretion in patients with bulimia nervosa and in healthy subjects. Demitrack MA; Kalogeras KT; Altemus M; Pigott TA; Listwak SJ; Gold PW. *Journal of Clinical Endocrinology and Metabolism*, 1992 Jun, 74(6):1277-83.

Normal-weight female bulimic patients who had abstained from binge eating and purging for at least a month were studied. It was shown that they had irregularities in the hormonal process that regulates fluid volume in the body, a fact that may be relevant to their behavior.

The effect of bulimia upon diet, body fat, bone density, and blood components. Howat PM; Varner LM; Hegsted M; Brewer MM; Mills GQ. *Journal of the American Dietetic Association*, 1989 Jul, 89(7):929-34.

Bulimic subjects were compared with controls, and it was found that the bulimics' folacin intake was significantly lower than that of the controls. Also, the bulimics consumed lower quantities of vitamin/mineral supplements, and their bone mineral densities and hemoglobin levels were lower.

Zinc deficiency and eating disorders. Humphries L; Vivian B; Stuart M; McClain CJ. *Journal of Clinical Psychiatry*, 1989 Dec, 50(12):456-9.

Zinc status was evaluated in bulimic and anorexic patients, many of whom were found to be deficient in the mineral. This is due to a variety of reasons-lower dietary intake of zinc, impaired absorption, vomiting, diarrhea, and binging on low-zinc foods. Since zinc deficiency results in decreased food intake, the acquired zinc deficiency of bulimics and anorexics could exacerbate their altered eating behavior.

Zinc status before and after zinc supplementation of eating disorder patients. McClain CJ; Stuart MA; Vivian B; McClain M; Talwalker R; Snelling L; Humphries L. *Journal of the American College of Nutrition*, 1992 Dec, 11(6):694-700.

Since reduced food intake results from zinc deficiency, the acquired zinc deficiency of eating disorder patients may act as a sustaining factor for their abnormal eating behavior. Hospitalized bulimics and anorexics were shown to be deficient in the mineral, and to benefit from supplementation.

Candida

Allium sativum (garlic) inhibits lipid synthesis by Candida albicans. Adetumbi M; Javor GT; Lau BH. *Antimicrobial Agents and Chemotherapy*, 1986 Sep, 30(3): 499-501.

Garlic extract was shown to inhibit the proliferation of the Candida albicans fungus.

Carrot phytoalexin alters the membrane permeability of Candida albicans and multilamellar liposomes. Amin M; Kurosaki F; Nishi A. *Journal of General Microbiology*, 1988 Jan, 134 (Pt 1):241-6.

Carrots have an ingredient that inhibits the candida organism by damaging its cell membranes.

Effect of calcium ion uptake on Candida albicans morphology. Holmes AR; Cannon RD; Shepherd MG. *Fems Microbiology Letters*, 1991 Jan 15, 61(2-3):187-93.

Calcium was shown to inhibit the growth of Candida albicans yeast cells.

Inhibition of Candida adhesion to buccal epithelial cells by an aqueous extract of Allium sativum (garlic). Ghannoum MA. *Journal of Applied Bacteriology*, 1990 Feb, 68(2):163-9.

Garlic extract inhibits the adhesion of candida cells to human cells taken from the inside of the cheek.

Respiratory burst and candidacidal activity of peritoneal macrophages are impaired in copper-deficient rats. Babu U; Failla ML. *Journal of Nutrition*, 1990 Dec, 120(12): 1692-9.

In rats, a copper-deficient diet resulted in reduced resistance to candida cells. Rats fed a diet with adequate copper, by contrast, had better systemic defenses against candida.

Studies on the anticandidal mode af action of Allium sativum (garlic). Ghannoum MA. *Journal of General Microbiology*, 1988 Nov, 134 (Pt 11):2917-24.

Garlic extract slows the growth of Candida albicans by affecting the outer surface of the cells and reducing their oxygen consumption, among other means.

Cognitive Function

Ramdomized Study of Cognitive Effects of Iron Supplementation in Non-anaemic Iron-deficient Adolescent Girls. Bruner AB; et al. *Lancet*, 1996 October 12, 348(9033):992-6.

This double-blind, placebo-controlled study examined the effects of 13 mg per day of supplemental iron for 8 weeks on cognitive function in adolescent girls with non-anaemic iron deficiency. Results showed that girls receiving iron scored higher on verbal learning and memory tests relative to controls.

Aged Garlic Extract Prolongs Longevity and Improves Spatial Memory Deficit in Senescence-Accelerated Mouse. Moriguchi T; et al. *Biol Pharm Bull*, 1996 February, 19(2):305-7.

Results of this study showed that the chronic dietary administration of aged garlic extract improved spatial learning in senescence-accelerated mice.

Prolongation of Life Span and Improved Learning in the Senescence –Accelerated Mouse Produced by Aged Garlic Extract. Moriguchi T; et al. *Biol Pharm Bull*, 1994 December, 17(12):1589-94.

Results of this study showed that the chronic dietary administration of aged garlic extract improved memory retention in senescence-accelerated mice.

Ginseng Root Prevents Learning Disability and Neuronal Loss in Gerbils with 5-minute Forebrain Ischemia. Wen TC; et al. *Acta Neuropathol*, 1996, 91(1):15-22.

This study examined the neuroprotective effects of ginseng roots in 5-minute ischemic gerbils. Red ginseng powder, crude ginseng saponin, crude ginseng non-saponin, and pure ginsenosides Rb1, Rg1 and Ro were administered 7 days prior to ischemia. Results showed that red ginseng and crude ginseng saponin prevented delayed neuronal death.

An Herbal Prescription, S-113m, Consisting of Biota, Ginseng, and Schizandra, Improves Learning Performance in Senescence Accelerated Mouse. Nishiyama N; et al. *Biol Pharm Bull*, 1996 March, 19(3):388-93.

Results of this study showed that the ginseng containing herbal prescription improved memory retention disorder in the senescence accelerated mouse on a passive avoidance test, increased conditioned avoidance rate in lever press test.

Panax Ginseng Extract Improves the Performance of Aged Fischer 344 Rats in Radial Maze Task but Not in

Operant Brightness Discrimination Task. Nitta H; et al. *Biol Pharm Bull*, 1995 September, 18(9):1286-8.

Results of this study showed that the administration of 8g/kg per day of a Panax ginseng extract over a period of 12-33 days reduced impairment of learning performance on a radial maze task in aged rats.

[Effects of Chinese Ginseng Root and Stem-leaf Saponins on Learning, Memory, and Biogenic Monoamines of Brain in Rats.] Wang A; et al. *Chung Kuo Chung Yao Tsa Chih*, 1995 August, 20(8):493-5.

Results of this study found that 50 mg/kg x 7d of ginseng root saponins enhanced the memory and learning of male rats. The same dosage of ginseng stem-leaf saponins had even stronger effects on antielectroconvulsive shock-induced memory impairment.

Effects of Ginseng Stem-leaves Saponins on One-way Avoidance Behavior in Rats. Ma TC; et al. *Chung Kuo Yao Li Hsueh Pao*, 1991 September, 12(5):403-6.

Results of this study showed that repeated administrations of ginseng stem-leaves saponins to rats facilitated learning and memory acquisition in rats.

Memory Effects of Standardized Extracts of Panax Ginseng (G115), Ginkgo Biloba (GK 501) and Their Combination Gincosan (PHL-00701). Petkov VD; et al. *Planta Med*, 1993 April, 59(2), 106-114.

Results of this study showed that the oral adminstration standardized extracts of Panax ginseng, Gonkgo biloba, and their combination Gincosan exhibited positive effects on learning and memory in young and old rats.

DHEA Administration Increases Rapid Eye Movement Sleep and EEG Power in the Sigma Frequency Range. Friess E; et al. *American Journal of Physiol*, 1995 January, 268(1 Pt 1):E107-13.

This double-blind, placebo-controlled study examined the effects of a 500 mg oral dose of DHEA on the sleep stages, sleep stage-specific electroencephalogram (EEG) power spectra, and concurrent hormone secretion in 10 healthy young male subjects. Results showed that DHES significantly increased REM sleep relative to controls, with no changes seen in the other sleep variables. Previous studies have shown REM sleep to be involved in memory storage, thus these findings point to a benefit of DHEA in age-related dementia.

Piracetam: An Overview of its Pharmacological Properties and a Review of its Therapeutic Use in

Senile Cognitive Disorders. Vernon MW; Sorkin EM. *Drugs Aging*, 1991 January, 1(1):17-35.

This article reviews findings from both animal and human studies supporting the use of piracetam in the treatment of a host of cognitive disorders.

Dementia

Calcium and phosphorus levels in serum and CSF in dementia. Subhash MN; Padmashree TS; Srinivas KN; Subbakrishna DK; Shankar SK. *Neurobiology of Aging*, 1991 Jul-Aug, 12(4):267-9.

There is a significant decrease in levels of calcium and phosphorus in the cerebrospinal fluid of patients with Alzheimer's-type dementia and in dementia caused by blood-vessel disease or stroke. The drops in the levels of these minerals in the patient groups go beyond those associated with normal aging.

Cephaloconiosis: a free radical perspective on the proposed particulate-induced etiopathogenesis of Alzheimer's dementia and related disorders. Evans PH; Klinowski J; Yano E. *Medical Hypotheses*, 1991 Mar, 34(3):209-19.

It is suggested that Alzheimer's dementia and related disorders are caused by fiber-like deposits of inorganic substances in the brain.

Antioxidants-either micronutrients or pharmacological agents-may be therapeutic.

Double-blind, placebo controlled study of acetyl-l-carnitine in patients with Alzheimer's dementia. Rai G; Wright G; Scott L; Beston B; Rest J; Exton-Smith AN. *Current Medical Research and Opinion*, 1990, 11(10):638-47.

Patients with Alzheimer's-type dementia were treated with acetyl-l-carnitine and compared with a control group. The treated group showed less deterioration than did the group receiving placebos, particularly in the area of short-term memory.

Low serum cobalamin levels in primary degenerative dementia. Do some patients harbor atypical cobalamin deficiency states? Karnaze DS; Carmel R. *Archives of Internal Medicine*, 1987 Mar, 147(3):429-31.

Low levels of vitamin B12 in the blood are frequent in cases of primary degenerative dementia.

Treatment of Alzheimer-type dementia with intravenous mecobalamin. Ikeda T; Yamamoto K; Takahashi K; Kaku Y; Uchiyama M; Sugiyama K; Yamada M. *Clinical Therapeutics*, 1992 May-Jun, 14(3):426-37.

Intravenous mecobalamin was seen to be a safe and effective treatment for patients with Alzheimer's-type dementia; it improved intellectual functions, such as memory, as well as emotional functions and communication abilities.

Study of the efficacy and tolerability of L-acetylcarnitine therapy in the senile brain. Bonavita E. *International Journal of Clinical Pharmacology, Therapy, and Toxicology*, 1986 Sep, 24(9):511-6.

A double-blind, placebo-controlled study showed that treatment with L-acetylcarnitine can improve the mental abilities of senile patients.

Neuropsychological changes in demented patients treated with acetyl-L-carnitine. Sinforiani E; Iannuccelli M; Mauri M; Costa A; Merlo P; Bono G; Nappi G. *International Journal of Clinical Pharmacology Research*, 1990, 10(1-2):69-74.

Patients suffering mild to moderate dementia were treated with acetyl-L-carnitine or piracetam. Significant improvement was shown in the acetyl-L-carnitine group-but not in the piracetam group-in the areas of behavior, attention, and psychomotor performance.

Depression

Acute antidepressant effect of lithium is associated with fluctuation of calcium and magnesium in plasma. A double-blind study on the antidepressant effect of lithium and clomipramine. Linder J; Fyro B; Pettersson U; Werner S. *Acta Psychiatrica Scandinavica*, 1989 Jul, 80(1):27-36.

Lithium treatment of patients with major depressive disorder was associated with fluctuations in blood calcium and magnesium levels. These fluctuations were not seen in treatment with the drug clomipramine.

Erythrocyte electrolytes in psychiatric illness. Esche I; Joffe RT; Blank DW. *Acta Psychiatrica Scandinavica*, 1988 Dec, 78(6): 695-7.

Fluctuations in sodium and potassium were found within the red blood cells of patients with psychiatric disorders experiencing changes in mood state. These fluctuations were not found in a healthy control group.

Levels of copper and zinc in depression. Narang RL; Gupta KR: Narang AP; Singh R. *Indian Journal of Physiology and Pharmacology*, 1991 Oct, 35(4):272-4.

Copper levels in depressed patients were significantly higher than those in controls, as well as higher than those in the same patients after they had recovered from depression. Zinc levels in depressed patients were not significantly lower than those of controls, but they were significantly lower than those of the same patients once they had recovered.

Myths about vitamin B12 deficiency. Fine EJ; Soria ED. *Southern Medical Journal*, 1991 Dec, 84(12):1475-81.

Deficiency of vitamin B12 can cause nerve problems, depression, and dementia. Vitamin B12 replacement should be given to patients with borderline levels of the vitamin, since the advantages of doing so outweigh any disadvantages of therapy.

Nutritional aspects of psychiatric disorders. Gray GE; Gray LK. *J. Am. Diet Assoc.*, 1989 Oct, 89(10): 1492-8.

Dietitians have a role as part of a multidisciplinary team in the treatment of psychiatric patients. Psychiatric illnesses may adversely affect food intake and nutritional status. Also, the drugs used to treat the disorders, including antipsychotics, antidepressants, monoamine oxidase inhibitors, and lithium, can affect appetite and gastrointestinal function, and can interact with foods.

The biology of folate in depression: implications for nutritional hypotheses of the psychoses. Abou-

Saleh MT; Coppen A. *Journal of Psychiatric Research*, 1986, 20(2):91-101.

Folate deficiency is common in psychiatric disorders, particularly depression. This deficiency-with or without deficiencies of other nutritional factors-may predispose people to psychiatric disturbances, or may worsen existing conditions.

Zinc in depressive disorder. McLoughlin IJ; Hodge JS. *Acta Psychiatrica Scandinavica*, 1990 Dec, 82(6):451-3.

Levels of zinc in the blood of patients admitted to a hospital for depression were lower than those in a control group. Upon release from the hospital after treatment, the patients' zinc levels had gone up significantly.

Evaluation of the Effects of L-acetylcarnitine on Senile Patients Suffering from Depression. Garzya G; et al. *Drugs Exp. Clin. Res.*, 1990, 16(2):101-6.

Results of this double-blind, placebo-controlled study found that the administration of 1500 mg per day of acetyl-L-carnitine led to significant improvements in patients between the ages of 70 and 80 suffering from symptoms of depression.

Evaluation of the Effects of L-acetylcarnitine on Senile Patients

Suffering from Depression. Garzya G; et al. *Drugs Exp. Clin. Res.*, 1990, 16(2):101-6.

Results of this study showed the administration of acetyl-L-carnitine to be significantly effective relative to controls in reducing depressive symptoms among elderly patients hospitalized for depression.

Double-blind, Controlled Trial of Inositol Treatment of Depression. Levine J; et al. *American Journal of Psychiatry*, 1995 May, 152(5):792-4.

Results of this double-blind, placebo-controlled study found that the administration of 12 g per day of inositol for 4 weeks led to significant improvements in patients suffering from depression.

Inositol Treatment in Psychiatry. Benjamin J; et al. *Psychopharmacol Bulletin*, 1995, 31(1):167-175.

This review article cites findings from double-blind, placebo-controlled studies supporting the efficacy of inositol as a treatment for depression.

Brief Communication. Vitamin B1, B2, and B6 Augmentation of Tricyclic Antidepressant Treatment in Geriatric Depression with Cognitive Dysfunction. Bell IR; et al. *Journal of the American College of Nutrition*, 1992 April, 11(2):159-63.

This double-blind, placebo-controlled study examined the efficacy of augmenting open tricyclic antidepressant treatment with vitamins B1, B2, and B6 a doses of 10 mg each in geriatric depression inpatients. Results showed those taking vitamins exhibited significantly stronger B2 and B6 status on enzyme activity coefficients and trends toward improved depressed and cognitive function scores relative to controls.

Cimicifuga for Depression. Frances D. *Medical Herbalism*, 1995 Spring/Summer, 7(1-2):1-2.

This article reports on the successful use of black cohosh in tincture form as a treatment for depression in 3 different case studies.

St. John's Wort for Depression—an Overview and Meta-analysis of Randomized Clinical Trials. Linde K; et al. *British Medical Journal*, 1996 August 3, 313(7052):253-258.

Results of this meta-analysis involving 23 randomized studies, 15 of which were placebo-controlled, found that hypericum extracts proved significantly effective in the treatment of patients suffering from moderate to mildly severe depression.

[Antidepressive Effect of a Hypericum Extract Standardized to an Active Hypericine Complex. Biochemical and Clinical Studies.] Muldner H; Zoller M. *Arzneimittelforschung*, 1984, 34(8):918-20.

Results of this study showed that the administration of a hypericum extract to middle-aged women suffering from depression led to improvements in anxiety, dysphoric mood, anorexia, hypersomnia, indomnia, loss of interest and feelings of worthlessness.

[Animal Experiments on the Psychotropic Action of a Hypericum Extract.] Okpanyi SN; Weischer ML. *Arzneimittelforschung*, 1987 January, 37(1):10-13.

Results of this study showed that extracts of hypericum perforatum exhibited positive effects on numerous measures of depressive activity in mice.

[Treatment of Depressive Symptoms with a High Concentration Hyper-icum Preparation. A Multicenter Placebo-controlled Double-blind Study.] Witte B; et al. *Fortschr Med*, 1995 October 10, 404-8.

Results of this double-blind, placebo-controlled study involving 97 depression outpatients showed that 100 to 120 mg of hypericum extract led to noticeable improvement in 70 percent of the patients.

Placebo-controlled Double-blind Study Examining the Effectiveness of an Hypericum Preparation in 105 Mildly Depressed Patients. Sommer H; Harrer G. *Journal of Geriatric Psychiatry Neurol*, 1994 October, 7(suppl 1):S9-11.

Results of this double-blind, placebo-controlled study showed that 3 x 300 mg of hypericum extract over a period of 4 weeks led to significant improvements in depression outpatients relative to controls.

Benefits and Risks of the Hypericum Extract LI 160: Drug Monitoring Study with 3250 Patients. Woelk H; et al. *Journal of Geriatr Psychiatry Neuro*, 1994 October, 7(Suppl 1): S34-S38.

This study evaluated the effects of a 4-week treatment program with hypericum extract in 3,250 patients suffering from various levels of depression. Results showed that 30% of the patients experienced improvement while receiving the therapy.

Hypericum in the Treatment of Seasonal Affective Disorder. Martinez B; et al. *Journal of Geriatr Psychiatry Neurol*, 1994 October, 7(Suppl 1):S29-S33.

Results of this study showed that treatment with 900 mg per day of hypericum coupled with two hours of daily light therapy significantly reduced symptoms of depression in patients suffering from seasonal affective disorder.

Multicenter Double-Blind Study Examining the Antidepressant Effectiveness of the Hypericum Extract LI 160. Hansgen KD; et al. *Journal of Geriatr Psychiatry Neurol*, 1994 October, 7(Suppl 1):S15-18.

Results of this double-blind, placebo-controlled study showed that treatment with hypericum extract over a period of four weeks led to significant improvements in patients suffering from depression.

[St. John's Wort as Antidepressive Therapy.] Ernst E. *Fortxchr Med*, 1995 September 10, 113(25):354-55.

This review article notes that recent studies have shown that St. John's Wort is a clinically effective depression treatment equal to standard medication and without its negative side effects.

[St. John's Wort Extract in the Ambulatory Therapy of Depression: Attention and Reaction Ability are Preserved.] Schmidt U; Sommer H. *Fortschr Med*, 1993 July 10, 111(19):339-42.

This placebo-controlled, randomized, double-blind study examined the effects of a St. John's wort extract, LI 160, on patients

suffering from moderately severe depression. Sixty-six percent of those receiving treatment responded positively versus opnly 26.7 percent of the controls.

Therapeutische Aquivalenz Eines Hochdosierten Phytoharmakons mit Amitriptylin bei Angstlich-Depressiven Verstimmugen— Reanalyse einer Randomisierten Studie unter Besonderer Beachtung Biometrischer und Klinischer Aspekte. Hiller KO; Rahlfs V. *Forsch-Komplementarmed*, 1995, 2(3):123-32.
T
his study compared the antidepressive-anxiolytic effects of a Valerian root and St. John's wort extract to amitriptyline. Results showed the herbal extract to be equally as effective as the amitriptyline, prompting the authors to argue for the use of phytomedicines in treating the depression and mood disorders.

Hypericum Treatment of Mild Depression with Somatic Symptoms. Hubner WD; et al. *Journal of Geriatr Psychiatry Neurol*, 1994 October, 7(Suppl):1-S12-4.

In this randomized, double-blind study, placebo-controlled study, 300 mg of the hyperium extract LI 160 was administered to depression patients 3 times daily for 4 weeks. The treatment group showed significant improvement compared to controls, with 70 percent showing no symptoms after 4 weeks.

Psychotropic Effects of Japanese Valerian Root Extract. Sakamoto T; et al. *Chemical Pharmacology Bulletin*, 1992 March, 40(3):758-61.

In this study, the psychotropic effects of "Hokkai-Kisso," i.e., roots of Japanese valerian, were compared with those of diazepam and imipramine. Results showed that valerian extract may be considered an antidepressant due to its action on the central nervous system of mice.

Antidepressant Principles of Valerian Fauriei Roots. Oshima Y; et al. *Chemical Pharm Bulletin*, 1995 January, 43(1):169-70.

Results of this study showed that a methanol extract of the roots of Valerian fauriei exhibited antidepressant activity in mice.

L-tyrosine Cures, Immediate and Long Term, Dopamine-dependent Depressions. Mouret J; et al. *C R Acad Sci III*, 1988, 306(3):93-8.

Results of this study showed that 3200 mg of oral tyrosine per day proved effective in the treatment of dopamine-dependent depression.

DL-phenylalanine as an Antidepressant. Open Study.

Beckmann H; Ludolph E. *Arzneimittelforschung*, 1978, 28(8):1283-4.

Results of this study showed that the administration of 75 200mg per day of DL-phenylalanine over a period of 20 days exhibited antidepressive effects in patients suffering from depression.

L-tryptophan: A Rational Anti-depressant and a Natural Hypnotic?. Boman B. *Aust N Z J Psychiatry*, 1988 March, 22(1):83-97.

This review article notes studies have shown that L-tryptophan may be useful in mild cases of depression and improve the depressed mood of Parkinsonian patients.

A Controlled Study of the Antidepressant Efficacy and Side Effects of (-)-deprenyl. A Selective Monoamine Oxidase Inhibitor. Mann JJ; et al. *Arch Gen Psychiatry*, 1989 January, 46(1):45-50.

Results of this double-blind, placebo-controlled study showed that the administration of 30 mg per day or more of (-)-deprenyl for a minimum of 6 weeks exhibited superior antidepressant effects in depressed outpatients relative to controls.

L-deprenyl Plus L-phenylalanine in the Treatment of Depression. Birkmayer W; et al. *Journal of*

Neural Transmission, 1984, 59(1): 81-7.

This study examined the effects of 5-10 mg per day of L-deprenyl coupled with 250 mg per day of L-phenylalanine in patients suffering from unipolar depression. Results indicated that the oral as well as intravenous administration of both drugs showed beneficial anti-depressive effects in 90 perent of outpatients and 80.5 percent of inpatients.

Dehydroepiandrosterone (DHEA) Treatment of Depression. Wolkowitz OM; et al. *Biol Psychiatry*, 1997 February 1, 41(3):311-8.

In this study, 30-90 mg of DHEA per day was administered to six middle-aged and elderly patients over a period of 4 weeks. Results showed significant improvements in symptoms of depression and memory performance.

S-adenosylmethionine and Affective Disorder. Carney MW; et al. *American Journal of Medicine*, 1987 November 20, 83(5A):104-6.

This review article notes that numerous open and double-blind studies have indicated SAMe may possess antidepressant effects.

Open Trial of S-adenosylmethionine for Treatment of Depression. Lipinski JF; et al. *American Journal of Psychiatry*, 1994 March, 141(3):448-550.

Results of this study showed 7 of 9 patients receiving treatment with SAMe for depression experienced improvement or total remission of symptoms.

Oral S-adenosylmethionine in Depression: A Randomized, Double-blind, Placebo-controlled Trial. Kagan BL; et al. *American Journal Psychiatry*, 1990 May, 147(5):591-5.

Results of this double-blind, placebo-controlled study found that the oral administration of SAMe proved to be an effective and quick-acting antidepressant in patients suffering from major depression.

S-adenosyl-L-methionine (SAMe)as Antidepressant: Meta-analysis of Clinical Studies. Bressa GM. *Acta Neurol Scand Suppl*, 154: 7-14.

Results of this double-blind, placebo-controlled found SAMe, a natural occurring compound to be an effective treatment against depression comparable to tricyclic antidepressant but with relatively fewer side effects.

Rapidity of Onset of the Antidepressant Effect of Parenteral S-adenosyl-L-methionine. Fava M; et al. *Psychiatry Research*, 1995 April 28, 56(3):295-7.

Results of this study found that the parental administration of 400 mg of SAMe over a period of 15 days remitted depressive symptoms in patients suffering from depression.

Eating Disorders

Anorexia nervosa responding to zinc supplementation: a case report. Yamaguchi H; Arita Y; Hara Y; Kimura T; Nawata H. *Gastroenterologia Japonica*, 1992 Aug, 27(4):554-8.

Zinc supplementation may be a therapeutic option in anorexia. In an anorexic patient with a low zinc level, supplementary zinc was given. The patient's digestive symptoms disappeared, and she regained normal weight.

Oral zinc supplementation in anorexia nervosa. Safai-Kutti S. *Acta Psychiatrica Scandinavica*, 1990, Suppl., 361:14-7.

There is evidence to suggest that zinc deficiency is a causative factor in anorexia nervosa. Anorexic patients receiving zinc supplementation showed weight gain. The design of a placebo-controlled study of zinc supplementation in anorexia is described.

Treatment of childhood anorexia with spleen deficiency by Qiang Zhuang Ling. Zou ZW; Li XM. *Journal of Traditional Chinese Medicine*, 1989 Jun, 9(2):100-2.

The traditional Chinese herbal prescription Qiang Zhuang Ling was used to treat a group of patients suffering from childhood anorexia with spleen deficiency. The therapeutic effect of the herbs was significantly greater than that seen in another group of patients treated with a zinc sulphate solution.

Zinc deficiency and childhood-onset anorexia nervosa. Lask B; Fosson A; Rolfe U; Thomas S. *Journal of Clinical Psychiatry*, 1993 Feb, 54(2):63-6.

Zinc deficiency was found to be common in childhood-onset anorexia nervosa.

Zinc status in anorexia nervosa. Varela P; Marcos A; Navarro MP. *Annals of Nutrition and Metabolism*, 1992, 36(4):197-202.

The body's zinc-dependent functions may be impaired in anorexia nervosa as a consequence of zinc unavailability.

General

Effect of Peppermint and Eucaplytus Oil Preparations on Neurophysiological and Experimental Algesimetric Headache Parameters. Gobel H; et al. *Cepahalalgia*, 1994 June, 14(3):228-34.

This double-blind, placebo-controlled study examined the effects of peppermint oil and eucalyptus oil preparations on neurophysiological, psychological and experimental algesimetric parameters 32 healthy subjects. Results showed that combination preparations increased cognitive performance, had a muscle-relaxing and mentally relaxing effect, and had a significant analgesic effect with a reduction in sensitivity to headache.

Evaluation of Some Pharmacological Activities of a Peppermint Extract. Della Loggia R; et al. *Fitoterapia*, 1990, LXI(3):215-21.

Results of this study found that peppermint extract had clear sedative effects when administered to mice in a saline solution.

Hyperkinesis

Developmental effects of vitamin B6 restriction on the locomotor behavior of rats. Guilarte TR; Miceli RC; Moran TH. *Brain Research Bulletin*, 1991 Jun, 26(6):857-61.

Newborn rats on a vitamin-B6-restricted diet were less active than those in a control group. However, when the vitamin-B6-deprived rats got older, they became hyperactive. Long-term B6 deprivation seems to result in damage to the nerve systems associated with locomotor behavior.

Neonatal hyperexcitability in relation to plasma ionized calcium, magnesium, phosphate and glucose. Nelson N; Finnstrom O; Larsson L. *Acta Paediatrica Scandinavica*, 1987 Jul, 76(4):579-84.

Newborn, full-term babies who seemed hyperactive at birth were shown to have low magnesium levels. The levels normalized spontaneously at five days of age.

Vitamin B12 improves cognitive disturbance in rodents fed a choline-deficient diet. Sasaki H; Matsuzaki Y; Meguro K; Ikarashi Y; Maruyama Y; Yamaguchi S; Sekizawa K. *Pharmacology, Biochemistry and Behavior*, 1992 Oct, 43(2):635-9.

Rats on a choline-deficient diet were less able to learn than rats on a choline-enriched diet. However, when the choline-deficient diet was supplemented with vitamin B12, there were no differences in learning ability between the groups.

Subtle abnormalities of gait detected early in vitamin B6 deficiency in aged and weanling rats with hind leg gait analysis. Schaeffer MC; Cochary EF; Sadowski JA. *Journal of the American College of Nutrition*, 1990 Apr, 9(2):120-7.

Motor abnormalities have been observed in every species made vitamin-B6-deficient. In rats, a deficiency of the vitamin is reflected in an abnormal gait at 2-3 weeks of age.

Learning Disorders and Dyslexia

Learning and memory disabilities in young adult rats from mildly zinc deficient dams. Halas ES; Hunt CD; Eberhardt MJ. *Physiology and Behavior*, 1986, 37(3):451-8.

Rats whose mothers had had a mildly zinc-deficient diet during pregnancy and lactation were shown to have a learning deficit in that their short-term memory was impaired.

The effects of acetyl-l-carnitine on experimental models of learning and memory deficits in the old rat. Valerio C; Clementi G; Spadaro F; D'Agata V; Raffaele R; Grassi M; Lauria N; Drago F. *Functional Neurology*, 1989 Oct-Dec, 4(4): 387-90.

Aged rats, which generally have impaired learning and memory capacity, were treated with acetyl-l-carnitine. They showed significant improvement in these areas.

Mania

A Controlled Clinical Trial of L-tryptophan in Acute Mania. Chouinard G; et al. *Biol Psychiatry*, 1985 May, 20(5):546-57.

Results of this double-blind, placebo-controlled study showed

that 12 g per day of L-tryptophan administered over a period of 1 week led to a significant reduction in manic symptoms in newly admitted manic patients.

Memory

The Potent Free Radical Scavenger Alpha-lipoic Acid Improves Memory in Aged Mice. Stoll S; et al. *Pharmacol. Biochem. Behav.*, 1995 Oct-Dec, 111(4): 6-8.

Results of this study showed that alpha-lipoic acid improved memory in aged mice.

Vitamin B6 Supplementation in Elderly Men: Effects on Mood, Memory, Performance, and Mental Effort. Deijen JB; et al. *Psychopharmacology*, 1992, 109(4):489-96.

Results of this double-blind, placebo-controlled study showed that vitamin B6 supplementation improved memory in healthy elderly men when administered in doses of 20 mg pyridoxine HCL per day for 3 months.

Memory-improving Effect of Aqueous Extract of Astragalus Membranaceus (Fisch.) Bge. Hong GX; et al. *Chung Kuo Chung Yap Tsa Chih*, 1994 November, 19(11):687-8.

Results of this study found that an aqueous Astragalus membranaceus extract improved anisodine-induced impairment on memory acquisition and alcohol-induced memory retrieval deficit in step-down behavior of mice.

Menopause

Cimicifuga Racemosa (L) Nutt. (Ranunculaceae). Snow JM. *The Protocol Journal of Botanical Medicine*, 1996 Spring: 17-19.

This review article cites studies supporting the use of black cohosh as an estrogenic agent in the treatment of women suffering from menopausal symptoms.

Neurological Disorders

Reversal of Brain Atrophy with Biotin Treatment in Biotinidase Deficiency. Bousounis DP; et al. *Neuropediatrics*, 1993 Aug, 24(4): 214-7.

This article reports on the cases of two children with biotinidase deficiency that presented with seizures at 2 months of age due to brain atrophy. Biotin supplements produced marked improvement in both.

Obsessive Compulsive Disorder

Inositol Treatment of Obsessive-Compulsive Disorder. Fux M; et al. *American Journal of Psychiatry*, 1996 September, 153(9):1219-21.

Results of this double-blind, placebo-controlled, crossover study found that the administration of 18 g per day of inositol for 6 weeks had significant beneficial effects in patients suffering from obsessive compulsive disorder.

Lithium and Tryptophan Augmentation in Clomipramine-resistant Obsessive-compulsive Disorder. Rasmussen SA. *American Journal of Psychiatry*, 1984 October, 141(10):1283-5.

Results of this study showed that patients suffering from symptoms associated with obsessive-sompulsive disorder that were resistant to clomipramine experienced improvement following treatment with lithium or L-tryptophan.

Organic Mental Disorders

Acetyl-L-carnitine in the treatment of midly demented elderly patients. Passeri M; Cucinotta D; Bonati PA; Iannuccelli M; Parnetti L; Senin U. *International Journal of Clinical Pharmacology Research*, 1990, 10(1-2):75-9.

In a double-blind study, acetyl-L-carnitine, which acts to alleviate defects in nerve signals, was shown to help mildly demented elderly patients in the areas of behavior, memory, attention, and verbal fluency.

Acute organic psychosis caused by thyrotoxicosis and vitamin B12 deficiency: case report. Lassen E; Ewald H. *Journal of Clinical Psychiatry*, 1985 Mar, 46(3):106-7.

A patient developed an acute psychosis due to a deficiency of thyroid hormone and vitamin B12. Replacement of thyroid hormone and B12 corrected the condition.

Alterations in calcium content and biochemical processes in cultured skin fibroblasts from aged and Alzheimer donors. Peterson C; Goldman JE. *Proceedings of the National Academy of Sciences of the United States of America*, 1986 Apr, 83(8):2758-62.

Calcium balance and certain functions within cells are altered in both aging and Alzheimer's disease, but they are altered more in Alzheimer's than in normal aging.

Biological effects of aging on bone and the central nervous system. Fujita T. *Experimental Gerontology*, 1990, 25(3-4):317-21.

The most common diseases of the elderly are osteoporosis and senile dementia. These conditions may be related in that abnormalities of calcium metabolism affect both the skeletal and nervous systems.

Cerebral atrophy and hypoperfusion improve during treatment of

Wernicke-Korsakoff syndrome. Meyer JS; Tanahashi N; Ishikawa Y; Hata T; Velez M; Fann WE; Kandula P; Mortel KF; Rogers RL. *Journal of Cerebral Blood Flow and Metabolism*, 1985 Sep, 5(3):376-85.

Early recognition and treatment of Wernicke-Korsakoff syndrome improves patients' cognitive and neurological impairments rapidly. Treatment includes alcohol withdrawal, nutritious diet, and thiamine supplements.

Clinical signs in the Wernicke-Korsakoff complex: a retrospective analysis of 131 cases diagnosed at necropsy. Harper CG: Giles M; Finlay-Jones R. *Journal of Neurology, Neurosurgery and Psychiatry*, 1986 Apr, 49(4):341-5.

Alcoholics are at risk of Wernicke-Korsakoff syndrome, which often goes undiagnosed. Repeated episodes of vitamin B1 deficiency may be the cause of the syndrome, and alcoholics should be monitored for this.

Cytosolic free calcium and cell spreading decrease in fibroblasts from aged and Alzheimer donors. Peterson C; Ratan RR; Shelanski ML; Goldman JE. *Proceedings of the National Academy of Sciences of the United States of America*, 1986 Oct, 83(20):7999-8001.

At the cellular level, Alzheimer's disease is not just a cerebral disease, but a systemic one: Alterations in calcium regulation are found throughout the body. These alterations are found in normal elderly people as well, but not to the same extent as in Alzheimer's patients. Some of the cellular changes in Alzheimer's patients can be partially reversed by treatment with a form of calcium.

Disappearance of high-incidence amyotrophic lateral sclerosis and parkinsonism-dementia on Guam. Garruto RM; Yanagihara R; Gajdusek DC. *Neurology*, 1985 Feb, 35(2):193-8.

Nutritional deficiences of calcium and magnesium, with resultant deposition of calcium and aluminum in neurons, may have been factors in the high rates of amyotrophic lateral sclerosis and parkinsonism-dementia that occurred several decades ago among the Chamorros of Guam.

Efficacy and clinical relevance of cognition enhancers. Herrmann WM; Stephan K. *Alzheimer Disease and Associated Disorders*, 1991, 5 Suppl 1:S7-12.

The cognition-enhancers piracetam, acetyl-L-carnitine, and nimodipine are more effective than placebos in improving the mental functioning of patients suffering from Alzheimer's and other age-related dementias.

Neurochemical hypothesis: participation by aluminum in producing critical mass of colocalized errors in brain leads to neurological disease. Joshi JG. *Comparative Biochemistry and Physiology. C:Comparative Pharmacology*, 1991, 100(1-2): 103-5.

Aluminum interferes with metabolism of glucose and of iron, as well as other functions. Metabolic errors induced by aluminum in specific areas of the brain to which the metal can be transported may lead to neurological disorders.

Neuropsychiatric aspects of trace elements. Linter CM. *British Journal of Hospital Medicine*, 1985 Dec, 34(6):361-5.

Trace elements may be causative or therapeutic factors in a wide range of illnesses. Knowledge of trace element metabolism has increased dramatically in the past decade.

Neuropsychiatric disorders caused by cobalamin deficiency in the absence of anemia or macrocytosis. Lindenbaum J; Healton EB; Savage DG; Brust JC; Garrett TJ; Podell ER; Marcell PD; Stabler SP; Allen RH. *New England Journal of Medicine*, 1988 Jun 30, 318(26):1720-8.

Neuropsychiatric disorders due to cobalamin deficiency occur commonly in the absence of anemia.

Cobalamin therapy is helpful in reducing neuropsychiatric abnormalities in these cases.

Pathological brain ageing: evaluation of the efficacy of a pharmacological aid. Guarnaschelli C; Fugazza G; Pistarini C. *Drugs under Experimental and Clinical Research*, 1988, 14(11):715-8.

L-acetylcarnitine given to aged patients was shown to be effective in enhancing cognitive ability, motor activity, and self-sufficiency, and in relieving depression.

Pernicious anemia in the demented patient without anemia or macrocytosis. A case for early recognition. Gross JS; Weintraub NT; Neufeld RR; Libow LS. *Journal of the American Geriatrics Society*, 1986 Aug, 34(8):612-4.

Pernicious anemia in elderly patients suffering from dementia can occur in the absence of anemia. Treatment with vitamin B12 has a therapeutic effect.

Pharmaco-electroencephalographic and clinical effects of the cholinergic substance-acetyl-L-carnitine-in patients with organic brain syndrome. Hermann WM; Dietrich B; Hiersemenzel R. *International Journal of Clinical Pharmacology Research*, 1990, 10(1-2):81-4.

Acetyl-L-carnitine is promising as a treatment for elderly patients with impaired brain function, as shown in two double-blind, placebo-controlled studies. Side effects were not generally seen.

Pyridoxine, ascorbic acid and thiamine in Alzheimer and comparison subjects. Agbayewa MO; Bruce VM; Siemens V. *Canadian Journal of Psychiatry. Revue Canadienne de Psychiatrie*, 1992 Nov, 37(9):661-2.

A group of patients with Alzheimer's disease showed lower functional levels of vitamin B1 than those of a group of normal subjects.

Reduced gastrointestinal absorption of calcium in dementia. Ferrier IN; Leake A; Taylor GA; McKeith IG; Fairbairn AF; Robinson CJ; Francis RM; Edwardson JA. *Age and Ageing*, 1990 Nov, 19(6):368-75.

Patients suffering from Alzheimer-type dementia and multi-infarct dementia showed reduced ability to absorb calcium intestinally.

Relationship of normal serum vitamin B12 and folate levels to cognitive test performance in subtypes of geriatric major depression. Bell IR; Edman JS; Miller J; Hebben N; Linn RT; Ray D; Kayne HL. *Journal of Geriatric Psychiatry and Neurology*, 1990 Apr-Jun, 3(2):98-105.

Elderly patients with psychotic depression were assessed for vitamin B12 and folate levels. Those with higher B12 levels tended to do better on measures of cognitive ability. Metabolic factors, including B12, may play specific roles in psychiatric disorders of the elderly.

Panic Disorder

Double-blind, Placebo-controlled, Crossover Trial of Inositol Treatment for Panic Disorder. Benjamin J; et al. *American Journal of Psychiatry*, 1995 July, 152(7):1084-6.

In this double-blind, placebo-controlled study, panic disorder patients with or without agoraphobia received 12 g of inositol per day. Results showed a significant decline in the frequency and severity of panic attacks and agoraphobia relative to controls.

Premenstrual Syndrome

Assessment of magnesium status. Elin RJ. *Clinical Chemistry*, 1987 Nov, 33(11):1965-70.

Assessing the magnesium status of an individual is difficult: Most data are taken from blood tests, yet most of the magnesium in the body is in bone and soft tissues. A better understanding of magnesium transport and metabolism is needed, as changes in magnesium status have been implicated in a number of conditions, including heart conditions, high blood pressure, and premenstrual syndrome.

Calcium supplementation in premenstrual syndrome: a randomized crossover trial. Thys-Jacobs S; Ceccarelli S; Bierman A; Weisman H; Cohen MA; Alvir J. *Journal of General Internal Medicine*, 1989 May-Jun, 4(3):183-9.

In a double-blind study, daily calcium supplementation was given to women suffering from premenstrual syndrome. The calcium was shown to be an effective treatment for premenstrual symptoms, including water retention and pain. It also alleviated menstrual pain.

Clinical and biochemical effects of nutritional supplementation on the premenstrual syndrome. Stewart A. *Journal of Reproductive Medicine*, 1987 Jun, 32(6):435-41.

A study of women with premenstrual syndrome showed frequent nutritional deficiencies, particularly of vitamin B6 and magnesium. A multivitamin and mineral supplement corrected some of the deficiencies and improved the symptoms of premenstrual tension.

Controlled trial of pyridoxine in the premenstrual syndrome. Williams MJ; Harris RI; Dean BC. *Journal of*

International Medical Research,
1985, 13(3):174-9.

Pyridoxine, compared with a
placebo, was effective in alleviating
premenstrual symptoms.

Effect of a nutritional supplement on
premenstrual symptomatology in
women with premenstrual syndrome:
a double-blind longitudinal study.
London RS; Bradley L; Chiamori NY.
*Journal of the American College of
Nutrition*, 1991 Oct, 10(5):494-9.

Nutritional supplements proved
more effective than a placebo in
relieving premenstrual syndrome.

Efficacy of alpha-tocopherol in the
treatment of the premenstrual
syndrome. London RS; Murphy L;
Kitlowski KE; Reynolds MA.
Journal of Reproductive Medicine,
1987 Jun, 32(6):400-4.

Daily alpha-tocopherol supplements
were shown to be effective in reducing
premenstrual symptoms in a double-
blind, placebo-controlled study.

Magnesium and the premenstrual
syndrome. Sherwood RA; Rocks BF;
Stewart A; Saxton RS. *Annals of
Clinical Biochemistry*, 1986 Nov, 23
(Pt 6):667-70.

Women with premenstrual syndrome
had significantly lower than normal
levels of magnesium in their red
blood cells.

Oral magnesium successfully
relieves premenstrual mood changes.
Facchinetti F; Borella P; Sances G;
Fioroni L; Nappi RE; Genazzani AR.
Obstetrics and Gynecology, 1991
Aug, 78(2):177-81.

Magnesium supplementation, when
compared with a placebo, was
effective in relieving premenstrual
mood changes.

Premenstrual and menstrual
symptom clusters and response to
calcium treatment. Alvir JM; Thys-
Jacobs S. *Psychopharmacology
Bulletin*, 1991, 27(2):145-8.

Calcium supplementation was shown
to alleviate three premenstrual
symptoms-mood changes, water
retention, and pain-and to relieve
menstrual pain.

Premenstrual syndrome. Tactics for
intervention. Havens C.
Postgraduate Medicine, 1985 May
15, 77(7):32-7.

Nutritional supplements are
sometimes appropriate in the
treatment of premenstrual syndrome,
along with dietary changes, regular
exercise, and, at times, diuretics and
other drugs. Vitamin B6, and
possibly vitamin E or zinc sulfate,
may be used.

Pyridoxine (vitamin B6) and the
premenstrual syndrome: a
randomized crossover trial. Doll H;

Brown S; Thurston A; Vessey M. *Journal of the Royal College of General Practitioners*, 1989 Sep, 39(326):364-8.

In a double-blind, placebo-controlled study, vitamin B6 supplementation was shown to be effective in alleviating emotional symptoms of premenstrual syndrome. Depression, irritability, and tiredness were reduced in women taking B6.

Pyridoxine in the treatment of premenstrual syndrome: a retrospective survey in 630 patients. Brush MG; Bennett T; Hansen K. *British Journal of Clinical Practice*, 1988 Nov, 42(11):448-52.

Vitamin B6 supplements seemed to be beneficial in alleviating premenstrual symptoms, according to a retrospective study. No side effects of the treatment were reported.

[Value of Standardized Ginkgo Biloba Extract (Egb 761) in the Management of Congestive Symptoms of Premenstrual Syndrome.] Tamborini A; Taurelle R. *Rev Fr Gynecol Obstet*, 1993 July-September, 88(7-9):447-57.

This double-blind, placebo-controlled study examined the effects of Ginkgo biloba extract on congestive symptoms of PMS in a group of 165 women. Results showed that the extract proved to be effective in relieving symptoms, particularly those associated with the breasts.

Schizophrenia

Acetazolamide and thiamine: an ancillary therapy for chronic mental illness. Sacks W; Esser AH; Feitel B; Abbott K. *Psychiatry Research*, 1989 Jun, 28(3):279-88.

Treatment of chronic schizophrenic patients with the drug acetazolamide, plus thiamine, was shown to be effective on a number of assessment scales. No untoward effects were seen for this therapy.

Enhancement of recovery from psychiatric illness by methylfolate. Godfrey PS; Toone BK; Carney MW; Flynn TG; Bottiglieri T; Laundy M. Chanarin I; Reynolds EH. *Lancet*, 1990 Aug 18, 336(8712):392-5.

One third of a group of psychiatric patients with either major depression or schizophrenia showed signs of folate deficiency, and took part in a double-blind, placebo-controlled study of methylfolate supplementation (in addition to standard treatment). Both depressed and schizophrenic patients showed significantly improved clinical and social recovery with the supplements, and the differences between the outcomes of the methylfolate- and placebo-receiving groups increased over time. These findings add to the evidence that disturbances of methylation in the nervous system may be a factor in some forms of mental illness.

Plasma levels and urinary vitamin C excretion in schizophrenic patients. Suboticanec K; Folnegovic-Smalc V; Turcin R; Mestrovic B; Buzina R. Human Nutrition. *Clinical Nutrition*, 1986 Nov, 40(6):421-8.

Schizophrenia may be associated with impaired ascorbic acid metabolism. Schizophrenic patients were shown to have lower vitamin C levels than those of a nonschizophrenic group of psychiatric patients that had been on the same hospital diet as the schizophrenics for at least two months. Even when the schizo-phrenics were given vitamin C supplements to raise their levels to those of the other group, they excreted less of the vitamin in their urine.

Pyridoxine improves drug-induced parkinsonism and psychosis in a schizophrenic patient. Sandyk R; Pardeshi R. *International Journal of Neuroscience*, 1990 Jun, 52(3-4):225-32.

Pyridoxine supplementation should be considered in psychiatric patients with drug-induced movement disorders, such as Parkinsonism and tardive dyskinesia. An underlying pyridoxine deficiency in these patients may increase the risk of

these drug-induced disorders, as well as worsen psychotic behavior. The effects of pyridoxine on movement disorders, and on psychosis, seem related to its enhancing serotonin and melatonin functions.

Subacute combined degeneration of the spinal cord due to folate defiency in association with a psychotic illness. Donnelly S; Callaghan N. *Irish Medical Journal*, 1990 Jun, 83(2):73-4.

A dietary deficiency of folic acid in a psychotic patient caused spinal cord degeneration. Treatment with folic acid relieved this problem significantly, and may have contributed to an improvement in the patient's psychiatric illness.

The biology of folate in depression: implications for nutritional hypotheses of the psychoses. Abou-Saleh MT; Coppen A. *Journal of Psychiatric Research*, 1986, 20(2):91-101.

Folate deficiency is common in psychiatric disorders, particularly in depressive illness. Alcoholic, lithium-treated, and anorexic patients are often folate-deficient. Folate deficiency-with or without deficiencies of other nutritional factors-may predispose people to psychiatric disturbances, or aggravate existing disturbances.

Unification of the findings in schizophrenia by reference to the effects of gestational zinc deficiency. Andrews RC. *Medical Hypotheses*, 1990 Feb, 31(2):141-53.

It is hypothesized that schizophrenia is caused by the action of gestational zinc deficiency-which may or may not be caused by diet-on genetically susceptible fetuses. A nongenetic but nevertheless transmissible immune defect may play a role in this disorder.

Vitamin C in the Treatment of Schizophrenia. Sandyk R; Kanofsky JD. *International Journal of Neuroscience*, 1993 Jan, 68(1-2): 67-71.

This paper reports on a single case of 37-year-old schizophrenic who was observed to have benefited from ascorbic acid supplementation to his ongoing neuropleptic medication.

Amelioration of Negative Symptoms in Schizophrenia by Glycine. Javitt DC; et al. *American Journal of Psychiatry*, 1994 August, 151(8):1234-6.

Results of this double-blind, placebo-controlled study involving 14 chronic schizophrenics on medication found that the administration of glycine led to significant improvements in symptoms associated with the disease.

Sleep Disorders/Insomnia

Correction of Non-24-hour Sleep/Wake Cycle by Melatonin in a Blind Retarded Boy. Palm L; et al. *Ann Neurol*, 1991 March, 29(3): 336-339.

This article reports on the case of a severely mentally retarded 9-year-old boy with chronic sleep/wake disturbance. Melatonin given at 6:00 P.M. normalized the sleep/wake pattern and entrained the endogenous rhythm to a normalized 24-hour chronological day.

Sleep-inducing Effects of Low Doses of Melatonin Ingested in the Evening. Zhdanova IV; et al. *Clin. Pharmacol Therapy*, 1995, 57(5):552-8.

In this double-blind, placebo-controlled study, healthy volunteers received either 0.3 or 1.0 mg of melatonin at 6, 8, or 9 P.M. Results showed that either doses given at either time reduced sleep onset latency.

Delayed Sleep Phase Syndrome Response to Melatonin. Dahlitz M; et al. *Lancet*, 1991 May 11, 337(8750):1121-4.

This double-blind, placebo-controlled study examined the effcts of 5 mg of melatonin for four weeks on the sleep/wake cycle in 8 patients with a delayed sleep phase syndrome. Results showed significantly earlier sleep onset time and wake time relative to controls.

Improvement of Sleep Quality in Elderly People by Controlled-release Melatonin. Garfinkel D; et al. *Lancet*, 1995 August 26, 346(8974):541-4.

Results of this double-blind, placebo-controlled study showed that 2 mg per night of controlled-release melatonin for 3 weeks significantly improved sleep quality in elderly subjects.

Melatonin Replacement Corrects Sleep Disturbances in a Child with Pineal Tumor. Etzioni A; et al. *Neurology*, 1996 January, 46(1): 261-3.

This article reports on the case of a child with a germ cell tumor involving the pineal region experiencing a melatonin secretion suppression associated with severe insomnia. Supplementation with 3 mg per night for 2 weeks normalized sleep.

The Effects of Exogenous Melatonin on the Total Sleep Time and Daytime Alertness of Chronic Insomniacs: A Preliminary Study. MacFarlane JG; et al. *Biological Psychiatry*, 1991 August 15, 30(4):371-6.

This double-blind, placebo-controlled study examined the effects of 75 mg per os of melatonin administered nightly at 10 P.M. on total sleep time and daytime alertness of chronic insomniacs. Results showed a significant increase in the subjective assessment of total sleep time and daytime alertness relative to controls.

Can Melatonin Improve Shift Workers' Tolerance of the Night Shift? Some Preliminary Findings. Folkard S; et al. *Chronobiol Int.*, 1993 October, 10(5):315-320.

Results of this double-blind, placebo-controlled study showed that 5 mg per night of melatonin had positive effects with respect to sleep and alertness on police officers working successive night shifts.

The Treatment of Sleep Disorders with Melatonin. Jan JE; et al. *Neurobiol*, 1994 February, 36(2): 97-107.

In this study, 15 disabled children with severe, chronic sleep disorders received 2 to 10 mg of oral melatonin. Results showed significant positive effects.

Sleep Laboratory Investigations on Hypnotic Properties of Melatonin. Waldhauser F; et al. *Psychopharmacology*, 1990, 100(2):222-6.

In this double-blind, placebo-controlled study, 20 healthy volunteers underwent artificially induced insomnia and were treated with melatonin. Results showed that the administration of melatonin at bedtime reduced the time the subjects were awake before sleep onset, sleep latency, and the number of awakenings during the total sleep period.

Melatonin Possesses Time-Dependent Hypnotic Effects. Tzischinsky O; Lavie P. *Sleep*, 1994 October, 17(7):638-45.

This double-blind, placebo-controlled study examined the hypnotic effects of 5 mg of melatonin in healthy, young adults. Results showed that melatonin significantly increased sleep propensity, the spectral power in the theta, delta, and spindles bands, and subjective sleepiness while significantly reducing the power in the alpha and beta bands and oral temperature.

Melatonin Replacement Therapy of Elderly Insomniacs. Haimov I; et al. *Sleep*, 1995 September, 18(7): 598-603.

This double-blind, placebo-controlled study examined the effects of melatonin replacement therapy on melatonin-deficient elderly insomniacs. Subject received 2 mg tablets of melatonin for 7 consecutive days, 2 hours prior to going to bed. During another phase of the study, subjects received 1 mg of sustainde-release melatonin each night for 2 months. Results shoed that 1-week treatment with 2 mg sustained-release melatonin was effective for sleep maintenance, while sleep initiation was improved by the fast-release melatonin. Such effects were increased following the 2-month 1-mg sustained-release melatonin treatment.

Aqueous Extract of Valerian Root Improves Sleep Quality in Man. Leatherwood PD; et al. 1982 July, 17(1):65-71.

This double-blind, placebo-controlled study examined the effects of valerian root on sleep measure in 128 subjects. Results showed that valerian led to significant reduction in subjectively evaluated sleep latency scores and significantly enhanced the quality of sleep.

Effect of Valerian on Human Sleep. Balderer G; Borbely AA. *Psychopharmacology*, 1985, 87(4):406-9.

This study examined the effect of an aqueous extract of valerian root on sleep in healthy, young subjects. Results showed that doses of both 450 mg and 900 mg of valerian extract reduced perceived sleep latency and wake time after sleep onset under home conditions.

Treatment of Severe Chronic Insomnia with Lptryptophan and Varying Sleeping Times. Demisch K; et al. *Pharmacopsychiatry*, 1987 November, 20(6):245-8.

Results of this study showed that the administration of 2 g of L-tryptophan over a period of 4 weeks significantly improved sleeping patterns and mood in patients suffering from chronic insomnia.

Evaluation of L-tryptophan for Treatment of Insomnia: A Review. Schneider-Helmer D; Spinweber CL. *Psychopharmacology*, 1986, 89(1): 1-7.

This review article notes that studies have shown doses of L-tryptophan ranging from 1 to 15 g to be effective in reducing sleep onset time in patients suffering from insomnia.

L-dopa-responsive Dystonia: 2 Familial Cases of Adult Onset with Sleep Disorders. El Alaoui-Faris M; et al. *Rev Neurol*, 1995 May, 151(5):347-9.

This article reports on the cases of a woman and her son with progressive dystonia and chronic insomnia. Treatment with low dose L-Dopa had significantly beneficial effects over a period of five years with respect to dystonia and insomnia without dyskinesia.

Double blind study of a valerian preparation. Lindahl O; Lindwall L. *Pharmacology, Biochemistry and Behavior*, 1989 Apr, 32(4):1065-6.

A valerian root preparation was compared with a placebo in a double-blind test of its sedative effects. It showed significant effectiveness in improving sleep, and no side effects were observed.

Neuropsychopharmacologic properties of a Schumanniophyton problematicum root extract. Amadi E; Offiah NV; Akah PA. *Journal of Ethnopharmacology*, 1991 May-Jun, 33(1-2):73-7.

An extract of Schumanniophyton problematicum, a plant popular among Nigerian native healers for the treatment of psychosis, was given to mice. The extract, which appears to depress the central and autonomic nervous systems, can inhibit hyperactivity caused by amphetamines, induce passivity, and prolong sleeping time induced by the tranquilizer pentobarbital.

Neurotropic action of the hydroalcoholic extract of Melissa officinalis in the mouse. Soulimani R; Fleurentin J; Mortier F; Misslin R; Derrieu G; Pelt JM. *Planta Medica*, 1991 Apr, 57(2):105-9.

An extract of Melissa officinalis was tested in mice and shown to have sedative properties at low doses, and pain-relieving and sleep-inducing properties at higher doses.

Panax ginseng extract modulates sleep in unrestrained rats. Rhee YH; Lee SP; Honda K; Inoue S. *Psychopharmacology*, 1990, 101(4):486-8.

Panax ginseng extract was found to enhance the amount of slow-wave sleep in rats.

Parasomnias (non-epileptic nocturnal episodic manifestations) in patients with magnesium deficiency. Popoviciu L; Delast-Popoviciu D; Delast-Popoviciu R; Bagathai I; Bicher G; Buksa C; Covaciu S; Szalay E. *Romanian Journal of Neurology and Psychiatry*, 1990 Jan-Mar, 28(1):19-24.

Severe sleep disorders, such as night terrors, may be linked to brain damage caused by magnesium deficiency.

Pharmacological investigations on Achyrocline satureioides (LAM.) DC., Compositae. Simoes CM; Schenkel EP; Bauer L; Langeloh A. *Journal of Ethnopharmacology*, 1988 Apr, 22(3):281-93.

Among the therapeutic properties of Achyrocline satureioides (Lam.) DC. is its sleep-enhancing effect, which was shown in mice.

Potassium affects actigraph-identified sleep. Drennan MD;

Kripke DF; Klemfuss HA; Moore JD. *Sleep*, 1991 Aug, 14(4):357-60.

A double-blind, placebo-controlled study with normal young males on a low-potassium diet showed that potassium supplements may increase sleep efficiency, lessening the frequency of wakefulness immediately after the onset of sleep.

Preliminary psychopharmacological evaluation of Ocimum sanctum leaf extract. Sakina MR; Dandiya PC; Hamdard ME; Hameed A. *Journal of Ethnopharmacology*, 1990 Feb, 28(2):143-50.

An extract of the leaves of Ocimum sanctum was shown in mice to have a sedative effect.

Psychotropic effects of Japanese valerian root extract. Sakamoto T; Mitani Y; Nakajima K. *Chemical and Pharmaceutical Bulletin*, 1992 Mar, 40(3):758-61.

Valerian extract, which acts on the central nervous system, was shown to prolong drug-induced sleep in mice. The extract may also be an antidepressant.

Treatment of persistent sleep-wake schedule disorders in adolescents with methylcobalamin (vitamin B12). Ohta T; Ando K; Iwata T; Ozaki N; Kayukawa Y; Terashima M; Okada T; Kasahara Y. *Sleep*, 1991 Oct, 14(5):414-8.

Two adolescents suffering from persistent sleep-wake rhythm disorders were helped by treatment with vitamin B12, although neither had shown evidence of B12 deficiency, or of hypothyroidism, which can cause deficiency.

Vitamin B12 treatment for sleep-wake rhythm disorders. Okawa M; Mishima K; Nanami T; Shimizu T; Ijima S; Hishikawa Y; Takahashi K. *Sleep*, 1990 Feb, 13(1):15-23.

Patients with sleep-wake schedule disorders were helped by daily administration of vitamin B12. (Blood levels of the vitamin were within the normal range before treatment.)

Neuro-depressive properties of essential oil of lavender. (in French) Delaveau P; Guillemain J; Narcisse G; Rousseau A. *Comptes Rendus des Seances de la Societe de Biologie et de Sesfiliales*, 1989, 183(4):342-8.

Essential oil of lavender given to mice relieves anxiety and prolongs drug-induced sleeping time, although only for the first five days it is administered.

Neurodepressive effects of the essential oil of Lavandula angustifolia Mill. (In French) Guillemain J; Rousseau A; Delaveau P. *Annales Pharmaceutiques Francaises*, 1989, 47(6):337-43.

Oil of lavender given to mice produced a sedative effect.

Quality of Schisandra incarnata Stapf. (in Chinese) Song W. Chung-Kuo Chung; Yao Tsa Chih. *China Journal of Chinese Materiamedica*, 1991 Apr, 16(4):204-6, 253.

The medicinal plant Schisandra incarnata has sleep-enhancing properties.

Smoking

Deficiency of Vitamin E in the Alveolar Fluid of Cigarette Smokers' Influence on Alveolar Macrophage Cytotoxicity. Pacht ER; et al. *Journal of Clinical Investigations*, 1986 March, 77(3):789-96.

Results of this study found that vitamin E may be a key antioxidant for the lower respiratory tract and that young smokers deficient in vitamin E may be predisposed to an enhanced oxidant attack on their lung parenchymal cells.

Vitamin E Suppresses Increased Lipid Peroxidation in Cigarette Smokers. Hoshino E; et al. *JPEN Journal of Parenter Enteral Nutr*, 1990 May-June, 14(3):300-5.

This study examined the effects of vitamin E on lipid preoxidation in healthy smokers. Results found that supplementation with 800 mg per day of vitamin E for two weeks decreased BPO in smokers. Tryptophan and High-carbohydrate Diets as Adjuncts to Smoking Cessation Therapy. Bowen DJ; et al. *Journal of Behav Med*, 1991 April, 14(2):97-110.

Results of this study indicated that the administration of tryptophan to patients trying to quit smoking led to a reduction in total number of daily cigarettes and in symptoms of withdrawal and anxiety relative to controls.

Stress

Stress-induced 5-HT1A Receptor Desensitization: Protective Effects of Ginkgo Biloba Extract (EGB 761). Bolanos-Jimenez F; et al. *Fundam Clin Pharmacol*, 1995, 9(2):169-74.

This study examined the effects of sub-chronic cold stress on hippocampal 5-HT1A receptors functioning and potential protective effects of Ginkgo biloba extract in old isolated rats. Results showed that the extract prevented the stress-induced desensitization of 5-HT1A.

Treatment with Tyrosine, a Neurotransmitter Precursor, Reduces Environmental Stress in Humans. Banderet LE; Lieberman HR. *Brain Res Bull*, 1989 April, 22(4):759-62.

Results of this study showed that 100 mg/kg of tyrosine significantly reduced stress symptoms associated

with 4.5 hours of exposure to cold and hypoxia in human subjects.

Blunting by Chronic Phosphatidylserine Administration of the Stress-induced Activation of the Hypothalamo-pituitary-adrenal Axis in Healthy Men. Monteleone P; et al. *European Journal of Clinical Pharmacology*, 1992, 42(4):385-8.

This double-blind, placebo-controlled study examined the effects of the administration of 800 mg per day of phosphatidylserine for 10 days on neuroendocrine responses to physical stress in healthy males. Results showed that treatment counteracted activation of the hypothalamo-pituitary-adrenal axis induced by stress.

Tardive Dyskinesia

Choline and Lecithin in the Treatment of Tardive Dyskinesia: Preliminary Results from a Pilot Study. Gelenberg AJ; et al. *American Journal of Psychiatry*, 1979 June, 136(6):772-6.

Results of this study found the oral administration of choline and licethin to 5 male tardive dyskinesia led to improvements in all of them.

Treatment of Chronic Dyskinesia with CDP-choline. Arranz A; Ganoza G. *Arzneimittelforschung*, 1983, 33(7A):1071-3.

Results of this study showed that daily doses of 500-1200 mg of CDP-choline administered to elderly patients with tardive dyskinesia produced significant decreases in symptoms associated with the condition.

Variable Clinical Response to Choline in Tardive Dyskinesia. Nasrallah HA; et al. 1984 August, 14(3):697-700.

Results of this double-blind, crossover study showed that the administration of choline chloride to tardive dyskinesia produced improvements in 7 of the 11 patients treated.

Treatment of Tardive Dyskinesia with Vitamin E. Egan MF; et al. *American Journal of Psychiatry*, 1992 June, 149(6):773-7.

In this double-blind, placebo-controlled study, tardive dyskinesia patients were given up to 1600 IU per day of vitamin E for 6 weeks. In nine patients with tardive dyskinesia for five years or fewer, results found AIMS scores to be significantly lower than controls.

Vitamin E in the Treatment of Tardive Dyskinesia. Elkashef AM; et al. *American Journal of Psychiatry*, 1990 April, 147(4):505-6.

Results of this double-blind, placebo-controlled study found that AIMS scores were significantly reduced following vitamin E supplementation in 8 tardive dyskinesia patients relative to controls.

Effectiveness of Vitamin E for Treatment for Long-term Tardive Dyskinesia. Dabiri LM; et al. *American Journal of Psychiatry*, 1994 June, 151(6):925-6.

Results of this double-blind, placebo-controlled study showed a significant reduction of AIMS scores in 11 patients with tardive dyskinesia who received supplementation with vitamin E for 12 weeks relative to controls.

Vitamin E Treatment of Tardive Dyskinesia. Adler LA; et al. *American Journal of Psychiatry*, 1993 Sept, 150(9):1405-7.

In this double-blind, placebo-controlled study, tardive dyskinesia patients received 1600 IU per day of vitamin E for 8 to 12 weeks. Results showed a significant reduction in AIMS scores relative to controls.

Vitamin E Attenuates the Development of Haloperidol-induced Dopaminergic Hypersensitivity in Rats: Possible Implications for Tardive Dyskinesia. Gattaz WF; et al. *Journal of Neural Transm Gen Sect*, 1993, 92(2-3):197-201.

Results of this study found that vitamin E administration to chronic

Haloperidol treatment in rats prevented the development of behavioral supersensitivity to apomorphine, prompting the authors to argue that the concomitant administration of vitamin E to neuroleptics in humans may serve to prevent the development of tardive dyskinesia.

Vitamin E in Extrapyramidal Disorders. Bischot L; et al. *Pharm World Science*, 1993 August 20, 15(4):146-50.

This article reviewed the effects of vitamin E on tardive dyskinesia and Parkinson's disease. Double-blind, placebo-controlled studies have shown doses of up to 1600 IU per day improved symptoms in patients with tardive dyskinesia. With respect to Parkinson's disease, studies have found that 2000 IU per day of vitamin effectively slowed disease progression while not being able to entirely prevent it.

Vitamin E in Tardive Dyskinesia: Time Course of Effect after Placebo Substitution. Adler LA; et al. *Psychopharmacol Bulletin*, 1993, 29(3):371-4.

Results of this placebo-controlled study showed that vitamin E supplementation significantly improved the symptoms associated with tardive dyskinesia over a 36-week period.

Vitamin E in the Treatment of Tardive Dyskinesia: The Possible Involvement of Free Radical Mechanisms. Lohr JB; et al. *Schizophrenia Bulletin*, 1988, 14(2):291-6.

Results of this placebo-controlled study found a significant reduction in AIMS scores in patients with persistent tardive dyskinesia receiving vitamin E supplementation relative to controls.

Effect of Selenium and Vitamin E on Iminodipropionitrile Induced Dyskinesia in Rats. Tariq M; et al. *International Journal of Neuroscience*, 1994 October, 78(3-4):185-92.

This study examined the effects of selenium and vitamin E on experimentally induced dyskinesia in rats. Results showed that treatment with both nutrients individually reduced IDPN–induced dyskinesia and the combination of both together produce a near-total absence of symptoms.

L-tryptophan in Neuroleptic-induced Tardive Dyskinesia. Sandyk R; et al. *Int Journal Neurosci*, 1988 September, 42(1-2):127-30.

This article reports on the case of a patient with neuroleptic-induced tardive dyekinesia who experienced a major improvement following supplemental L-tryptophan.

Environmental Causes of Mental Disease—
A Bibliography

Aschengau, A.; Ziegler, S. and Cohen, A. "Quality of Community Drinking Water and the Occurrence of Late Adverse Pregnancy Outcomes." *Archives of Environmental Health* 48 (1993): 105-113.

Aschner, M. and Kimelberg, M., eds. *The Role of Glia in Neurotoxicity*. Boca Raton: CRC Press, 1996.

Bailey, A.J.; Sargent, J.D.; Goodman, D.C.; Freeman, J. and Brown, M.J. "Poisoned Landscapes: The Epidemiology of Environmental Lead Exposure in Massachusetts Children 1990-1991." *Social Science Medicine* 39 (1994): 757-776.

Bellinger D. et al. "Pre- and Postnatal Lead Exposure and Behavior Problems in School-Aged Children." *Environmental Research* 66, no. 1 (July 1994): 12-30.

Brockel, Becky A. and Cory-Slechta, Deborah A. "Lead, Attention, and Impulsive Behavior: Changes in a Fixed-Ratio Waiting-for-Reward Paradigm." *Pharmacology Biochemistry and Behavior* 60, no. 2 (June 1998): 545-552.

Bryce-Smith, D. "Environmental Chemical Influences on Behaviour and Mentation." *Chemical Sciety Review* 15 (1986): 93-123.

Cook, E. H., Jr., et al. "Association of Attention Deficit disorder and the dopamine Transporter gene." *American Journal of Human Genetics* 56 (1995).

Gazzaniga, Michael, Ivry, Richard B. and Mangun, George R. *Cognitive Neuroscience*. New York: W. W. Norton, 1998.

Kahn, CA., Kelly, PC., Walker, WO. 1995. "Lead screening in children with attention deficit hyperactivity disorder and developmental delay." *Clinical Pediatrics* 34, no.9 (Sept 1995): 498-501.

Minder, Barbara; Das-Smaal, Edith A.; Brand, Eddy F. J. M. and Orlebeke, Jacob F. "Exposure to Lead and Specific Attentional Problems in Schoolchildren." *Journal of Learning Disabilities* 27, no. 6 (June/July 1994): 393-398.

Levitt, Miriam. "Toxic Metals, Preconception, and Early Childhood Development." *Social Science Information* 38 (1999): 179-201.

Manuzza, S., et al. "Hyperactive Boys Almost Grown Up." *Archives of General Psychiatry* 46 (1989): 1073-1079.

Manuzza, S., et al. "Adult Psychiatric Status of Hyperactive Boys Grown Up." *American Journal Of Psychiatry* 155 (1998): 493-498.

Masters, Roger D. and Coplan, Myron. J. "Water Treatment with Silicofluorides and Lead Toxicity." *International Journal of Environmental Studies* 56 (1999a): 435-449.

Masters, Roger D. and Coplan, Myron J. "A Dynamic, Multifactorial Model of Alcohol, Drug Abuse, and Crime: Linking Neuroscience and Behavior to Toxicology." *Social Science Information* (1999b) In press.

Masters, Roger D.; Coplan, Myron J. and Hone, Brian T. "Silicofluoride Usage, Tooth Decay, and Children's Blood Lead." Poster Presentation, Environmantal Influences on Children: Brain, Development, and Behavior, Conference at New York Academy of Medicine, New York, NY, May 24-25, 1999.

Masters, Roger D.; Coplan, Myron J. and Hone, Brian T. "Heavy Metal Toxicity, Development, and Behavior." Poster Presentation, 17th International Neurotoxicology Conference, Doubletree Hotel, Little Rock, AR, October 17-20, 1999.

Masters, Roger D.; Hone, Brian T. and Doshi, Anil. "Environmental Pollution, Neurotoxicity, and Criminal Violence." J. Rose, ed. *Environmental Toxicology*. London: Gordon and Breach, 1998. 13-48.

Mendelsohn, Alan L.; Dreyer, Benard P.; Fierman, Arthur H.; Rosen, Carolyn M.; Legano, Lori A.; Kruger, Hillary A.; Limß, Sylvia W. and Courtlandt, Cheryl D. 1998. "Low-Level Lead Exposure and Behavior in Early Childhood." *Pediatrics* 101, No. 3 (March 1998): e10.

Mielke, H. "Lead in the Inner Cities." *American Scientist* 87 (1998): 62-73.

Needleman, Herbert L., ed. *Human Lead Exposure*. Boca Raton: CRC Press, 1991.

Needleman, Herbert L., et al. "Bone Lead Levels and Delinquent Behavior." *JAMA* 275 (1996): 363-69.

Needleman, Herbert L. "Environmental Neurotoxins and Attention Deficit Disorder." Presentation at Conference on Environmental Neurotoxins and Developmental Disability, Academy of Medicine, New York (May 24-25, 1999).

Tuthill, R. W. "Head Lead Levels Related to Children's Classrooom Attention-Deficit Behavior." *Archives of Environmental Health* 51 (1996): 214-20.

Useful Books

Richard Ash, *DHEA: Unlocking the Secrets to the Fountain of Youth* (contributor), Detroit Lakes: BL Publications, 1997.

Sidney M. Baker, *The Circadian Prescription* (with Karen Baar), New York: Penguin Putnam, 2000.
Detoxification and Healing: The Key to Optimal Health, New Canaan: Keats, 1997.
Child Behavior: The Classic Childcare Manual from the Gesell Institute of Human Development (contributor), New York: Harper Perennial, 1992.

Syd Baumel, *Natural Antidepressants*, Los Angeles: Keats Publishing, 1998.
Dealing with Depression Naturally, Los Angeles: Keats Publishing, 1995.

Dr. Mary Ann Block, *No More Antibiotics: Preventing and Treating Ear and Respiratory Infections the Natural Way*, Kensington Publishing Corp., 2000.
No More Ritalin: Treating ADHD Without Drugs, New York: Kensington Publishing Corp., 1996.

Peter Breggin, *The War Against Children of Color: Psychiatry Target Inner-City Youth* (with Ginger Ross Breggin), Monroe: Common Courage Press, 1998.

Talking Back to Ritalin: What Doctors Aren't Telling You About Stimulants for Children, Monroe: Common Courage Press, 1998.
Talking Back to Prozac: What Doctors Aren't Telling You About Today's Most Controversial Drug, New York: Tor Books, 1994.

Paula Caplan, *They Say You're Crazy: How the World's Most Powerful Psychiatrists Decide Who's Normal*, Reading: Addison-Wesley Publishing Co., 1995.
You're Smarter Than They Make You Feel: How the Experts Intimidate Us and What We Can Do About, New York: The Free Press, 1994.

Catharine Carrigan, *Healing Depression: A Holistic Guide*, New York: Marlowe & Co., 1999.

Dr. H. Richard Casdorph and Dr. Morton Walker, *Toxic Metal Syndrome*, Wayne: Avery Publishing, 1995.

Dr. Hyla Cass, *All About St. John's Wort*, Wayne: Avery Publishing, 1999.
Kava: Nature's Answer to Stress, Anxiety & Insomnia, Rocklin: Prima Communications, Inc., 1998.
St. John's Wort: Nature's Blues Buster, Wayne: Avery Publishing, 1998.

Ty Colbert, *Broken Brains or Wounded Hearts: What Causes Mental Illness*, Santa Ana: Kevco, 1996.

Depression & Mania : Friends or Foes, Santa Ana: Kevco, 1995.

Dr. William Crook, *Healing Depression: A Holistic Guide*, New York: Marlowe and Company, 1999.

Help For The Hyperactive Child: a Practical Guide Offering Parents of Attention Deficit Disorder Alternatives to Ritalin, New York: Professional Books, 1991.

Dr. Gabriel Cousens, *Depression-Free for Life: An All-Natural 5 Step Plan to Reclaim Your Zest for Living*, New York: William Morrow & Co., 2000.

Conscious Eating, Santa Rosa: Vision Books, 1998.

Dr. Helen A. Derosis, *Women and Anxiety: A Step by Step Program for Managing Anxiety and Depression*, New York: Hatherleigh Co., Ltd., 1998.

Jerry Dorsman, *How to Quit Drugs for Good*, New York: Prima Communications, 1999.

How to Quit Drinking Without AA, Rocklin: Prima Communications, 1997.

Dr. Samuel Dunkell, *Goodbye Insomnia, Hello Sleep*, New York: Dell Publishing Co., Inc., 1996.

Dr. John Eades, *The Seventh Floor Ain't Too High For Angels To Fly*, Deerfield Beach: Health Communications, Inc., 1995.

Eva Edelman, *Natural Healing for Schizophrenia and Other Common Mental Disorders*, Eugene: Borage Books, 1998.

Norman Ford, *Sleep RX, 75 Proven Ways to Get a Good Night's Sleep*, Saddle River: Prentice Hall, 1994.

Dr. Lynne Freeman, *Panic Free: Eliminate Anxiety and Panic Attacks Without Drugs and Take Control of Your Life*, Denver: Arden Books, 1999.

Dr. James Gordon, *Manifesto For A New Medicine: Your Guide to Healing Partnerships and the Wise Use of Alternative Therapies*, Reading: Addison Wesley Longman, Inc., 1996.

Letha Hadady, *Asian Health Secrets: The Complete Guide to Asian Herbal Medicine*, New York: Crown Publishing Group, 1996.

Dr. Abram Hoffer and Dr. Morton Walker, *Smart Nutrients: A Guide to Nutrients That Can Prevent and Reverse Senility*, Wayne: Avery Publishing, 1994.

Dharma Singh Khalsa, *Brain Longevity: The Breakthrough Medical Program That Improves Your Mind and Memory*, New York: Warner Books, 1997.

Michael Lapchick, *The Label Reader's Pocket Dictionary of Food Additives: A Comprehensive Quick Reference Guide to More Than 250 of Today's Most Common Food Additives*, New York: John Wiley & Sons, 1993.

Jay Lombard, *The Brain Wellness Plan: Breakthrough Medical, Nutritional and Immune-Boosting Therapies*, New York: Kensington Publishing Corp., 1998.

Joan Matthews-Larson et al, *Seven Weeks to Emotional Healing: Proven Natural Formulas for Eliminating Anxiety, Depression, Anger, and Fatigue from Your Life*, New York: Ballantine Publishing Group, 1999.
Seven Weeks to Sobriety, New York: Ballantine, 1992.

Michael Norden, *Beyond Prozac: Brain-Toxic Lifestyles, Natural Antidotes & New Generation Antidepressants*, New York: Regan Books, 1995.

James Pearl, *Sleep Right in Five Nights*, New York: Quill, 1996.

Dr. Alan Pressman, *Integrative Medicine: The Patient's Essential Guide to Conventional and Complementary Treatments for More Than 300 Common Disorders*, New York: St. Martin's Press, 2000.
Ginkgo: Nature's Brain Booster. New York: Avon, 1999.
ed., *The Complete Idiot's Guide to Alternative Medicine*, New York: Alpha Books, 1999.
Glutathione: The Ultimate Antioxidant, New York: St. Martin's Press, 1998.
The GSH Phenomenon: Nature's Most Powerful Antioxidant and Healing Agent, New York: St. Martin's Press, 1997.

Peggy Ramunda, *You Mean I'm Not Lazy, Stupid or Crazy?!: A Self-Help Book for Adults With Attention Deficit Disorder*, New York: Scribner, 1995.

Valerie Davis Raskin, *When Words Are Not Enough: The Woman's Prescription for Depression and Anxiety*, New York: Broadway Books, 1997.

Dr. Judythe Reichenberg-Ullman, *Prozac-Free : Homeopathic Medicine for Depression, Anxiety, and Other Mental and Emotional Problems*, Rocklin: Prima Pub, 1999.
Ritalin Free Kids: Safe and Effective Homeopathic Medicine for ADD and Other Behavioral and Learning Problems (with Robert

Ullman and Edward Chapman), Rocklin: Prima, 1996.

Joel Robertson, *Natural Prozac: Learning to Release your Body's Own Anti-Depressants*, New York: Harper Collins, 1997.

Sherry Rogers, *Depression: Cured at Last!*, Sarasota: SK Publishing, 1997.

Ethan Russo, ed., *Handbook of Psychotropic Herbs : A Scientific Analysis of Herbal Remedies for Psychiatric Conditions, with Case Studies*, Binghamton: Haworth Herbal Press, 2000.

Dr. Judith Sachs, *Break the Stress Cycle!: 10 Steps to Reducing Stress for Women*, Holbrook: Adams Media, 1998.
 Nature's Prozac: Natural Therapies and Techniques to Rid Yourself of Anxiety, Depression, Panic and Stress, Englewood Cliffs: Prentice Hall, 1997.

Ray Sahelian, *New Memory Boosters: Natural Supplements That Enhance Mind, Memory and Mood*, Thomas Dunne Books, 2000.
 5-HTP: Nature's Serotonin Solution, Garden City Park: Avery, 1998.
 Kava: The Miracle Anti-Anxiety Herb, New York: St. Martin's, 1998.
 Pregnenolone: Nature's Feel Good Hormone, Garden City Park: Avery, 1997.
 DHEA: A Practical Guide, Garden City Park: Avery, 1996.

Alexander Schauss, *Anorexia and Bulimia: A Natural Approach to the Deadly Eating Disorders*, New Canaan: Keats, 1997.

Karyn Seroussi and Bernard Rimland, Ph.D., *Unraveling the Mystery of Autism and Pervasive Developmental Disorder: A Mother's Story of Research and Recovery*, New York: Simon and Schuster, 2000.

Dr. Lendon Smith, *Feed Your Body Right*, New York: M. Evans & Co., 1995.
 Feed Yourself Right, New York: McGraw-Hill, c1983.
 Feed Your Kids Right, New York: McGraw-Hill, c1979.

James & Nancy Strohecker, eds. *Natural Healing For Depression: Solutions From the World's Great Health Traditions and Practitioners*, New York: Perigee Books, 1999.

Dr. Jacob Teitelbaum, *From Fatigued To Fantastic*, New York: Avery Pub., 1996.

Dr. Lynda Toth, *Why Can't I Remember?: Reversing Normal Memory Loss*, New York: Avery Pub., 1999.

Dr. Melvyn R. Werbach, *Nutritional Influences on Illness: A Sourcebook of Clinical Research*, 2nd ed., Tarzana: Third Line Press, 1993.

Bruce Wiseman, *Psychiatry: The Ultimate Betrayal*, Los Angeles: Freedom Pub., 1995.

Dr. Jonathan Zeuss, *The Wisdom of Depression: A Guide to Understanding and Curing Depression Using Natural Medicine*, New York: Harmony Books, 1998.

The Natural Prozac Program: How to Use St. John's Wort, the Antidepressant Herb, New York: Three Rivers Press, 1997.

Marcia Zimmerman, *The ADD Nutrition Solution: A Drug-Free Thirty-Day Plan*, New York: Holt, 1999.

Websites

www.garynull.com (news, reports, documents, activism, resources)

www.thenutritionreporter.com

www.intacad.com (Academy of Nutrition- International Clinical Nutrition Review)

www.orthodmed.org/jom (Journal of Orthomolecular Medicine)

www.healthy.net/library/journals

erf@rachel.org (Rachel's Environment and Health Weekly, a publication of the Environmental Research Foundation. To subscribe: listserv@rachel.org)

www.healthfinder.com (government portal)

www.noaw.com (Living with Schizophrenia)

www.naturopathic.org

pi@orst.edu (linus pauling institute)

www.orthomed.org

www.ceri.com (Cognitive Enhancement Research Institute— includes resources and referrals)

www.latitudes.org

www.holisticmed.com (information, chats, Q&As, etc. listed by disorders. Especially good discussion group on ADD: www.holisticmed.com/add/)

www.futurehealth.org

www.newmedicinenet.com

www.holisticdepression.net (Holistic Depression Network)

www.somethingfishy.org (Eating Disorders Shared Awareness)

www.alternate_health.com

www.healthyideas.com

www.obgyn.net (women's health)

www.aanp.org (American Academy of Nurse Practitioners)

B

THE
*D*ANGERS
OF PROZAC

Gary Null, Ph.D. and
Martin Feldman, M.D.

Nearly a decade has passed since Prozac, the antidepressant drug, was introduced to the market and quickly achieved the label of a "wonder drug." During that time, Prozac has indeed helped many people who suffer from severe depression. But the early claims that Prozac would alleviate depression without causing harmful side effects have not been realized.

Indeed, just the opposite has proven to be true. Prozac has produced serious side effects in some users, prompting a host of lawsuits against Eli Lilly & Co., the drug's manufacturer.[1] These adverse effects include akathisia (a condition in which a person feels compelled to move about), permanent neurological damage, and suicidal obsession and acts of violence.

In 1990, the Citizens Commission on Human Rights (CCHR), a Scientology organization that investigates psychiatric violations of human rights, wrote a letter to the House of Representatives in which it stated, "The wide use of Prozac has been largely generated by Lilly's false claim that Prozac has fewer side effects than other antidepressant drugs. This is a serious misrepresentation to the public which is destroying lives."[2]

The letter notes that Eli Lilly changed its advertisements to remove the statement that Prozac causes "fewer side effects." In one ad, for example, the manufacturer said instead that the drug produces "fewer tricyclic-like side effects." However, the CCHR believes Prozac should be recalled. The letter concludes, "...the drug should be immediately recalled as a serious health hazard, and kept off the market until the manufacturer can guarantee that the drug will not kill more people."

A 1990 article in Trial, published by the Association of Trial Lawyers of America, also points to the "dark side" of Prozac, noting that it not only produces troubling side effects but also can be harmful and even deadly when combined with certain other drugs. "Prozac has greatly benefited many severely depressed patients. Others, however, have suffered serious side effects," states the report. "Eli Lilly & Co.'s failure to adequately warn physicians of side effects and of the danger of drug interactions has doubtless resulted in injuries that could otherwise have been avoided. Now that the dangers are better known, doctors should inform patients of these risks."[3]

The Side Effects of Prozac

The CCHR letter notes that the Food and Drug Administration (FDA) received almost twice as many adverse reaction reports on Prozac in two years than it did on Elavil, another antidepressant, in 20 years. Even Valium, a widely used prescription drug, accumulated fewer adverse reaction reports in 20 years than Prozac did in two years, says the CCHR.[4]

Prozac relieves depression by affecting the level of serotonin, a neurotransmitter that connects receptor sites and fires nerve cells. The CCHR letter states that the drug's chemical structure, which is unlike that of other medications, makes it "an utter wild card" in predicting what effects it may have.[5] And yet, doctors not only prescribe Prozac for depression, its approved use, but also for smoking cessation, weight loss and other problems.

The adverse effects of Prozac can be traced to the drug's effect on brain chemistry. As Peter R. Breggin, M.D., explains in Talking Back to Prozac: What Doctors Aren't Telling You About Today's Most Controversial Drug, Prozac acts as a stimulant to the nervous system.[6] Therefore, it can produce side effects that mimic those of amphetamines and are exaggerations of the desired effects of Prozac in relieving depression.

According to Dr. Breggin, the FDA psychiatrist who wrote the agency's safety review of Prozac stated that the drug's effects—including nausea, insomnia and nervousness—resembled the profile of a stimulant drug, rather than a sedative.[7] Dr. Breggin adds that nearly all of the side effects of Prozac listed in the Physician's Desk Reference "fit into the stimulant profile." Among others, these stimulant symptoms include headaches, nervousness, insomnia, anxiety, agitation, tremors, weight loss, nausea, diarrhea, mouth dryness, anorexia and excessive sweating.[8]

In short, a drug that acts as a stimulant also can overstimulate the body systems. In his book, Dr. Breggin offers the example of a person who takes Prozac to relieve depression (the beneficial effect) and suffers from agitation and insomnia (the negative effects). These adverse effects "are inherent in the stimulant effect that produces feelings of energy and well-being," Dr. Breggin writes. "In this sense, the difference between 'therapeutic effects' and 'toxic effects' are merely steps along a continuum from mild to extreme toxicity."[9]

With that in mind, what follows is a discussion of some of the side effects that have been associated with Prozac:

Akathisia. As noted, people may suffer from a variety of side effects when the central nervous system is overstimulated. Studies show that two effects of overstimulation—akathisia and agitation—are experienced by some people who take fluoxetine (the chemical name for Prozac).

Simply put, akathisia is a need to move about. The person feels anxious or irritable and is compelled to stand up, pace, shuffle his or her feet and the like. The inner sense of anxiety, says Dr. Breggin, is "like chalk going down a chalkboard, only it's your spine."[10] Prozac also can cause extreme agitation, and this condition often is associated with akathisia.

Eli Lilly states in Prozac's information sheet that the drug can cause akathisia. However, Eli Lilly has said that less than 1 percent of Prozac users experience this side effect, while a 1989 report in the Journal of Clinical Psychiatry estimates that the actual share of Prozac users who suffer from akathisia is between 10 percent and 25 percent.[11] Other reports on the link between Prozac and akathisia have appeared in psychiatric journals.[12, 13, 14]

Akathisia is related to a breakdown in the ability to control impulses. Thus, it has been associated with violent and suicidal acts in a number of studies and reports. A two-year study published in Psychopharmacology Bulletin in 1990 found a higher akathisia rating among people involved in violent acts than those who observed the incidents.[15] Another double-blind clinical study established a link between akathisia and suicidal or homicidal thoughts, according to a report in the Journal of Clinical Psychopharmacology.[16]

Akathisia was associated with acts of extreme violence in an article in the American Journal of Forensic Psychiatry, which described three patients who attacked other people or committed murder.[17] Other researchers have noted that patients who take Prozac and develop akathisia may, in turn, become preoccupied with thoughts of suicide.[18, 19] A 1991 article in the Journal of Clinical Psychiatry, for example, reports on three patients who attempted suicide during fluoxetine treatment and were then reexposed to the drug. The second time around, all three developed severe akathisia and said the condition made them feel suicidal; they also attributed their previous suicide attempts to akathisia.[20]

Psychosis. A person's nervousness may reach a psychotic level when the overstimulation of the nervous system is severe. People can become paranoid, extremely depressed, suicidal and dangerous to others around them. They may behave in bizarre ways, perhaps by spending all their money or directing traffic naked. The mental effects of fluoxetine treatment have been discussed in several psychiatric reports.[21, 22]

More specifically, Prozac's ability to induce mania in patients has been documented in a number of medical journals.[23, 24, 25, 26, 27, 28, 29, 30] This adverse effect supports Dr. Breggin's position, as stated earlier, that a drug's therapeutic effects and its toxic effects are simply a matter of degree in the same continuum. As he writes in his book, "Many patients who swear by Prozac are probably experiencing imperceptible or barely perceptible degrees of mania."[31]

Suicide. Beyond the link between akathisia and acts of violence, some users of Prozac have said that the drug caused them to develop suicidal thoughts and obsessions. In some cases, the use of Prozac allegedly has prompted people to commit murder. This aspect of the drug has generated controversy and led to discussions in both medical publications and the general media about the connection between Prozac and acts of violence.[32, 33, 34, 35, 36, 37, 38, 39, 40, 41, 42, 43, 44, 45, 46]

It should be noted that in several studies, the findings suggested that Prozac did not lead to suicidal preoccupation or found that the drug was not associated with an increased risk of suicidal acts. Other reports on clinical experiences with Prozac and its effects following an overdose support the safety of the drug.[47, 48, 49, 50, 51, 52, 53, 54]

However, other research supports the contention that Prozac leads some users to become suicidal or violent. In his book, Dr. Breggin says that it is the drug's ability to cause a variety of psychological and neurological disorders that underlies such destructive behavior. Five of these disorders—agitation, panic, anxiety, mania and akathisia—can prompt suicidal or violent acts, says Breggin. Four other conditions caused by Prozac—depression, paranoia, obsessive-compulsive thoughts and behavior, and insomnia—may precipitate the irrational fears, suicidal thoughts and despair that lead to violent thoughts or actions.[55]

What follows is a summary of some of the research on the link between Prozac and suicidal thoughts and behavior:

➤A study published in the American Journal of Psychiatry in 1990 reported on the "surprising possibility that fluoxetine [Prozac] may induce suicidal ideation in some patients." This study, conducted by Dr. Martin Teicher and colleagues at Harvard Medical School, concerned six patients who were depressed but not suicidal before they started taking Prozac. Within weeks of taking the drug, said the researchers, the patients experienced "intense, violent suicidal preoccupation."[56]

➤ In an analysis of 1,017 patients treated with antidepressant drugs by 27 psychiatrists, researchers found that 3.5 percent of those who took fluoxetine alone and 6.5 percent of those who took fluoxetine and tricyclics became suicidal only after their treatments began. The researchers concluded that the incidence of suicidal ideation was not significantly different between patients taking Prozac alone and those taking other drugs.[57] However, Dr. Teicher and his associates at Harvard Medical School have noted the results of this analysis support their suggestion that fluoxetine may precipitate suicidal ideation.[58]

➤Researchers at the State University of New York in Syracuse reported on "two patients in whom suicidal ideation and fluoxetine treatment were strongly associated" in the New England Journal of Medicine in 1991.[59]

➤A Prozac study involving children aged 10 to 17, conducted at the Yale University School of Medicine, found that "suicidal ideation of self-injurious behavior persisted for up to one month after the fluoxetine was discontinued," according to the researchers' report in the Journal of the American Academy of Child and Adolescent Psychiatry.[60]

➤Psychiatrist William Wirshing and associates reported in the Archives of General Psychiatry on five patients who developed akathisia when they took Prozac. They noted that the condition may have accounted for suicidal ideation in the patients.[61]

➤In a 1990 letter to the American Journal of Psychiatry, a doctor described a patient who "developed depression and suicidal ideation approximately 30 days after beginning fluoxetine, [and] had had no previous suicidal ideation or attempts."[62]

➤In a report on antidepressants and suicidal tendencies, Dr. Teicher and his colleagues say that such medications may "redistribute" the risk of suicide, reducing the risk for some patients while possibly increasing it for others. They state, "Although antidepressants diminish suicidal behavior in many patients, about as many patients experience a worsening suicidal ideation on active medication as they do on placebo. Furthermore, at least as many patients attempted suicide on fluoxetine and tricyclic antidepressants as on placebo..."[63]

The stories of individual patients also illuminates the effects of Prozac on some users. Perhaps the most notorious of these individuals is Joseph Wesbecker, who committed mass murder and then killed himself while he was taking Prozac. Wesbecker's rampage received national media attention after he went to his former place of employment in 1989 and shot 20 people, eight of them fatally, before killing himself.[64]

Other Prozac users claim the drug made them hostile and suicidal. Janet Sims, for example, received Prozac for her "low mood" when she and her husband attended marriage counseling. She attacked her husband and became obsessed with suicide. Sims eventually underwent electric shock treatments.[65] Sharyn DiGeronimo became hostile, self-destructive and obsessed with suicide when she took Prozac because she was feeling down.[66]

Depression. People who are overstimulated may end up suffering from depression as well. Eli Lilly knew that Prozac caused depression and reported the relationship to the FDA, according to Dr. Breggin. "Lilly admitted on paper, in its final statement about the drug's side effects, that it commonly caused patients to get depressed. Then it got scratched out at the FDA... It just disappeared from the label."[67]

The result is that a drug intended to relieve depression may have the opposite effect. As Dr. Breggin states, "[People] start taking the drug and in the beginning they feel better... Maybe the drug gives them a burst of energy. Stimulants will do that. They make people feel energized. Then they get more depressed. They may get suicidal feelings. They don't know that Eli Lilly once listed depression as an effect of the drug. And so they end up thinking they need more Prozac, and their doctor agrees."[68]

In a related area, doctors at Johns Hopkins University School of Medicine have reported that five patients developed apathy, indifference, and loss of initiative when they took fluoxetine or fluvoxamine, another antidepressant. The doctors noted that the mechanisms producing these side effects bore a clinical resemblance to "those of frontal lobe dysfunction," in which patients may "display apathy, flatness of affect and lack of emotional concern, childishness and euphoria, socially inappropriate behavior, and difficulty in foreseeing the outcome of an action."[69]

Sexual dysfunction. Prozac can induce sexual dysfunction because it affects the level of serotonin, a neurotransmitter that connects receptor sites and fires nerves. Men who take the drug may not be able to get an erection or to ejaculate, and women may have difficulty obtaining an orgasm.

In one study, 45 of 60 men who took Prozac experienced retarded ejaculation or ejaculatory incompetence, suggesting that "such sexual dysfunction is a more common side effect of fluoxetine than is reported in the Physician's Desk Reference."[70] Another study found that 8.3 percent of Prozac users had problems achieving orgasm.[71] Other reports document cases of prolonged erection and loss of ejaculation or sexual stimulation as a side effect of Prozac.[72, 73] Cases of sexual dysfunction may subside when the drug is discontinued.[74]

Dr. Breggin adds, "Again, when Lilly studied this matter for the FDA, they found only a small amount of people were having sexual dysfunction. Then after the drug was approved, they found out that they were wrong and that a very large percentage of people were having this particular problem."[75]

Tardive dystonia and tardive dyskinesia. Some Prozac users have charged that the drug causes tardive dystonia or tardive dyskinesia (TD), two forms of neurological damage in which the muscles tense up or move involuntarily. These disorders can produce bizarre-looking postures and movements. Consequently, people who are taking Prozac to relieve mental illness may in fact appear to be mentally ill. What's more, the symptoms may continue after they stop taking the drug; in some cases the condition may be permanent.

Doctors have reported a variety of neurological symptoms in people taking Prozac. These symptoms including acute dystonia and reversible dystonia.[76, 77, 78] In two cases, patients developed complex movement disorders while they were taking fluoxetine. This disorder was marked by rhythmic palatal movements, myoclonus and possibly dystonia in one patient, and myoclonic jerking and rapid, sterotypic movements of the toes in the other.[79] Another report says that four patients with idiopathic Parkinson's disease experienced an increased amount of motor disability when they took Prozac.[80] However, a review of 23 patients with Parkinson's disease who took Prozac found that 20 of them did not experience a worsening of their condition. The researchers concluded that fluoxetine in doses of up to 40 mg per day does not appear to be linked to an increase in the signs and symptoms of Parkinson's disease.[81]

Many psychiatric drugs, such as Haldol and Thorazine, have been found to cause tardive dyskinesia in about 20 percent of long-term users. The manufacturers' prescription information for these drugs includes appropriate warnings. But that is not the case with Prozac's package insert, which warns that users have developed dystonia and dyskinesia but not that the drug may cause permanent damage to the nervous system.

Generally, when psychiatric drugs cause permanent disorders such as TD, it is after patients have used the medication for a year or longer. With Prozac, however, the condition appears to set in much more rapidly. One woman in Texas who sued Eli Lilly claims she experienced permanent damage within two days of taking two Prozac capsules a day. Another user began to experience severe muscle spasms in her arms after she took Prozac for eight days; she still had TD and a diminished ability to function two years later.

The FDA has received reports linking Prozac to tardive dystonia and tardive dyskinesia. Ironically, however, the agency seems to have taken the position that the symptoms occur too soon in Prozac users, and therefore are not "tardive" (which means "late developing") disorders. In explaining why it has not acknowledged that Prozac may cause TD, the FDA also has said that some reports did not contain sufficient information and that some claimants were using other drugs as well.

Prozac's Clinical Trials

How did a drug with such potentially dangerous side effects make it into the marketplace? One reason is that the clinical trials for Prozac were flawed, according to documents released under the Freedom of Information Act. Consider:

➤Eli Lilly told physicians involved in the trials to record a variety of adverse reactions, including suicidal ideation, morbid thoughts, agitation, sadness and insomnia, as "symptoms of depression," rather than as separate effects. In a review of Prozac, FDA Efficacy Reviewer J. Hillary Lee stated, "Note: the exhortation [by Lilly] to exclude experiences caused by depression may have altered the relative frequencies of many adverse experiences. Each investigator would have had his own idea of what depressive experiences might comprise resulting in a lack of generality from one investigator to the next. Not surprisingly, many antidepressants and ansiolytic agents do produce adverse reactions which are known to be symptoms of depressions (e.g., insomnia, nausea, anxiety, tension, restlessness) leading to a possible underrepresentation of these effects."

➤Tony DiCicco, an FDA Consumer Safety Officer, said the studies conducted by Eli Lilly to demonstrate Prozac's efficacy and safety were badly flawed. He stated, "This agency has discovered a flaw in the experimental design and execution of the fluoxetine studies. In the main efficacy trials, patients who were not doing well could be dropped out at the end of the second week and switched to fluoxetine (after breaking the blind and determining if the patient was on imipramine or placebo)... This led to the situation where an end point analysis would compare patients' scores after six weeks of treatment...leading to a biased comparison."

Meanwhile, the FDA's original efficacy review of Prozac found that the drug was no more effective than a placebo. The FDA, for reasons that are not clear, told Eli Lilly to reevaluate the drug based on fewer variables. The manufacturer did so, reducing the number of variables by two-thirds, and issued a new evaluation of Prozac's effectiveness. The FDA approved this new evaluation.

In fact, the FDA appears to have looked the other way in regard to several problems before Prozac's release. The FDA discovered in 1986 that Eli Lilly had withheld information about the onset of psychotic episodes on at least 52 patients during the drug's clinical trials. Yet no actions were taken against the manufacturer or Prozac. Documents also show that Eli Lilly and the FDA knew of 15 suicides that occurred during the drug's clinical trials, even though the Prozac label said that three people died during the trials.

Dr. Breggin, for his part, believes strongly that Prozac should not have been approved by the FDA for a variety of reasons.[82] Among them:

➤Eli Lilly hand-picked doctors to conduct studies of Prozac, and these doctors ignored evidence of its stimulant properties. Patients who became agitated received sedatives such as Klonopin, Ativan, Xanax and Valium, a procedure that Dr. Breggin says invalidates the studies. After all, the use of sedatives means that any effects on the patients were not caused by Prozac alone. As Dr. Breggin argues, "Basically, the FDA should have said, 'We're approving Prozac in combination with addictive sedatives.'"

➤The number of people tested during Prozac's clinical trials is far fewer than the manufacturer claims. Eli Lilly has stated that 11,000 people took part in the clinical trials for the drug, including about 6,000 who took Prozac. But Dr. Breggin shows in his book that a mere 286 people completed the four- to six-week-long trials on which Prozac's approval was based.[83] Eli Lilly has never challenged this information. "They've had me under oath in court, and they haven't contested a single word I've written in the book," Dr. Breggin says.

➤The tests excluded people who were suicidal, psychotic or suffering from other mental and emotional disorders. These, of course, are the very types of people who would later be prescribed Prozac. Although Eli Lilly has not studied how many Prozac users have attempted suicide or committed suicide, adds Dr. Breggin, it could easily do so even today.

"One of the easiest things to study is whether your patients are alive or not. It's much easier to study that than whether they've gotten over their depression. That's a hard thing to judge. How do you know if somebody is feeling better or not feeling better? It's very complicated."

Evidence presented in the trial of Joseph Wesbecker also indicates that Eli Lilly knew that Prozac users had a much higher rate of attempted suicide than did patients taking placebos or other drugs. Dr. Breggin has testified as a medical expert in the trial of Wesbecker, who killed eight people, wounded a dozen others and then killed himself while he was taking Prozac.

Would a manufacturer sell an unsafe drug, and would the FDA approve it? Dr. Breggin says the answer is "yes" because psychiatry is a part of the medical industrial complex, which looks to market its products and services just like any other industry.

The fact is, hundreds of approved drugs later have major new warnings added to their labels or are withdrawn from the market. About 16 other drugs got the green light during the time that Prozac was approved, and nine of these have since had major changes to their labels. The FDA informs doctors, but not the public, that the approval of a drug does not mean it is safe.

Meanwhile, a drug's dangerous side effects may not be recognized during the testing stage because the FDA's individual studies usually consist of small groups of patients. For example, if 40 groups of 100 patients are tested (for a total of 4,000), the scientists may not notice a reaction in one patient.

The FDA Panel

Another problem is that FDA doctors may have close affiliations with drug companies. Dr. Breggin points out that Paul Leber, who approves psychopharmacological drugs at the FDA, is "a friend to Prozac." A statement in some of Eli Lilly's material even noted the relationship. Also, one doctor who voted in favor of the drug received payment from Eli Lilly to makes speeches about the drug's benefits and safety. "Dozens of doctors are getting paid by Lilly and doing clinical research for them. Nonetheless, they think they can sit fairly in judgment about whether Prozac is harmful or not," says Dr. Breggin.[84]

Furthermore, when the FDA convened a panel in late 1991 to review concerns about Prozac and violence, eight of the 10 panel members were psychiatrists. The livelihood of these professionals depends, in part, on the prescription of antidepressants such as Prozac, which raises questions about their objectivity in reviewing the safety of prescription drugs.

In fact, the FDA disclosed before the panel hearing that a number of the members had financial conflicts of interest because they had received grants from various manufacturers of antidepressants. One member even had grants pending from Eli Lilly; the CCHR also discovered that this member did not disclose his engagement to speak at seminars funded by Eli Lilly or two pending grants from antidepressant manufacturers. He had received some $4 million worth of research grants from such manufacturers in the eight years preceding the Prozac hearing.

In the end, nearly all of the panel members either had conflicts of interest or belonged to the psychiatric profession. The panel voted 10 to zero that there was no evidence proving that antidepressants were linked to violent or suicidal thoughts and behaviors.

According to the critics, the FDA panel did not acknowledge the importance of the "rechallenging" process in its review of Prozac. With rechallenging, patients who have experienced side effects which subside when they stop taking a drug begin taking it again to see if the same negative effects reoccur. If they do, the side effects in question can be closely linked to the drug.

Dr. Martin Teicher, the Harvard researcher, told the FDA panel of at least eight patients who had been rechallenged with Prozac and experienced violent, suicidal thoughts, establishing a connection between the drug and these effects. Dr. Teicher said that rechallenging could provide more definitive data about a drug, and more quickly, than do clinical trials, but the panel was not interested in the findings. What's more, when Dr. Teicher asked to present slides correlating Prozac with violent, suicidal thoughts, the panel refused to see them. It did, however, allow slide presentations that defended Prozac.

References

1. Arizona inmate files $200 million suit, claims drug caused aggressive behavior, 18(37) Product Safety & Liability Reporter, September 14, 1990, p. 1025-26.
2. Citizens Commission on Human Rights (CCHR), International Office, Los Angeles. Letter to The Honorable John D. Dingell, Chairman, Energy and Commerce Committee, House of Representatives, July 24, 1990.
3. Lewis J, Prozac: Dark side of a wonder drug, Trial, August 1990, p. 62-4.
4. CCHR, op cit.
5. Ibid.
6. Breggin PR and Breggin GR, Talking back to Prozac: What doctors aren't telling you about today's most controversial drug. New York, St. Martin's Press, 1994, p. 121
7. Breggin, Talking Back to Prozac, p. 75.
8. Ibid, p. 78.
9. Ibid, p. 105.
10. Breggin PR, in interview with Gary Null. November 1994.
11. Lipinski JF, Mallya G, Zimmerman P, Pope HG, Fluoxetine-induced akathisia: clinical and theoretical implications, 59(9) Journal of Clinical Psychiatry, September 1989, p. 339-42.
12. Wirshing WC, Van Putten T, Rosenberg J, Fluoxetine, akathisia and suicidality: Is there a causal connection?, 49(7) Archives of General Psychiatry, July 1992, p. 580-81.
13. Sabaawi M, Holmes, TF, Fragala MR, Drug-induced akathisia: Subjective

experience and objective findings, 159(4) Military Medicine, April 1994, p. 286-91.

14. Kalda R, Media- or fluoxetine-induced akathisia, 150(3) American Journal of Psychiatry, March 1993, p. 531-32.

15. Crowner ML, Douyon R, Convit A, Gaztanaga P, Volavka J, Bakall R, Akathisia and violence, 26(1) Psychopharmacology Bulletin, 1990, p. 115-17.

16. Shear KM, Frances A, Weiden P, Suicide associated with akathisia and depot fluphenazine treatment, Journal of Clinical Psychopharmacology, August 1983, p. 235-36.

17. Schufte JL, Homicide and suicide associated with akathisia and haloperidol, American Journal of Forensic Psychiatry, Vol. VI, No. 2, 1985, p. 3.

18. Power AC, Cowen, PJ, Fluoxetine and suicidal behavior: Some clinical and theoretical aspects of a controversy, 161(12) British Journal of Psychiatry, December 1992, p. 735-41.

19. Hamilton MS, Opler LA, Akathisia, suicidality, and fluoxetine, 53(11) Journal of Clinical Psychiatry, November 1992, p. 401-6.

20. Rothschild, AJ, Locke CA, Reexposure to fluoxetine after serious suicide attempts by three patients: The role of akathisia, 52(12) Journal of Clinical Psychiatry, December 1991, p. 491-3.

21. Hersh CB, Sokol MS, Pfeffer CR, Transient psychosis with fluoxetine, 30(9) Journal of the Academy of Child and Adolescent Psychiatry, September 1991, p. 851.

22. Mandalos GE, Szarek BL, Dose-related paranoid reaction associated with fluoxetine, Journal of Nervous and Mental Disease, 1990, 178:57-8.

23. Nakra BR, Szwabo P, Grossberg GT, Mania induced by fluoxetine, 146(11) American Journal of Psychiatry, November 1989, p. 1515-16.

24. Sholomskas AJ, Mania in a panic disorder patient treated with fluoxetine, 147(8) American Journal of Psychiatry, August 1990, p. 1090-91.

25. Venkataraman S, Naylor MW, King CA, Mania associated with fluoxetine treatment in adolescents, 31(2) Journal of the Academy of Child and Adolescent Psychiatry, March 1992, p. 276-81.

26. Piredda SG, Rubinstein SL, Hypomania induced by fluoxetine?, 32(1) Biological Psychiatry, July 1992, p. 107.

27. Hon D, Preskorn SH, Mania during fluoxetine treatment for recurrent depression, 146(12) American Journal of Psychiatry, December 1989, p. 1638-39.

28. Lebegue B, Mania precipitated by fluoxetine, 144(12) American Journal of Psychiatry, December 1987, p. 1620.

29. Chouinard G, Steiner W, A case of mania induced by high-dose fluoxetine treatment, American Journal of Psychiatry, May 1986, p. 686.

30. Turner SM, Rolf JG, Beidel DC, Griffin S, A second case of mania associated with fluoxetine, 142(2) American Journal of Psychiatry, February 1985, p. 274-75.

31. Breggin, Talking Back to Prozac, p. 103.

32. Angier N, Suicidal behavior tied again to drug, New York Times, February 7, 1991, p. B15.

33. Associated Press, Third lawsuit against Ely Lilly Antidepressant Drug, Chicago Tribune, August 8, 1990.

34. Belli A, Family Takes on Drug Firm: Prozac blamed on man's suicide, The Dallas Morning News, June 23, 1991.

35. Blodgett N, Eli Lilly drug targeted, ABA Journal, November 1990, p. 24.

36. Cassada ME, Prozac noted by Massey's attorney, Danville Register & Bee, September 17, 1991.

37. Charles H, Woman who took Prozac, killed husband gets probation, Press-Telegram, April 20, 1991.

38. The Economist (London), Prozac and suicide: Open verdict, January 19, 1991, p. 76.

39. Dewan MJ, Prakash M, Prozac and suicide, Journal of Family Practice, 1991, 33:312.

40. Drake RE, Ehrlich J, Suicide attempts associated with akathisia, American Journal of Psychiatry, April 1985, p. 499-501.

41. Fetner H, Watts H, Geller B, Fluoxetine and preoccupation with suicide, 148(9) American Journal of Psychiatry, September 1991, p. 258.

42. Hoover CE, Additional cases of suicidal ideation associated with fluoxetine, 147(11) American Journal of Psychiatry, November 1990, p. 1570-71.

43. Tollefson GD, Fluoxetine and suicidal ideation, 147(12) American Journal of Psychiatry, December 1990, p. 1691-92.

44. Breggin P, A case of fluoxetine-induced stimulant side effects with suicidal ideation associated with a possible withdrawal reaction ('crashing'), International Journal of Risk and Safety in Medicine, 1992, 3:325-28.

45. Breggin P, News and Views on Psychiatry: Prozac, suicide and violence: An analysis with reports from the Prozac Survivors Support Group, Inc., The Rights Tenet, Winter/Spring 1991. p. 4-6.

46. Brewerton TD, Fluoxetine-induced suicidality, serotonin, and seasonality, Biological Psychiatry, 1991, 30:190-96.

47. Ashleigh AE, Fesler AF, Fluoxetine and suicidal preoccupation, 149(12) American Journal of Psychiatry, December 1992, p. 1750.

48. Beal DM, Harris D, Bartos M, Korsak C, Safety and efficacy of fluoxetine, 148(12) American Journal of Psychiatry, December 1991, p. 1751.

49. Warshaw MG, Keller MB, The relationship between fluoxetine use and suicidal behavior in 654 subjects with anxiety disorders, 57(4) Journal of Clinical Psychiatry, April 1996, p. 158-66.

50. Beasley CM Jr., Dornseif BE, Bosomworth JC, Sayler ME, Rampey AH Jr., Heiligenstein JH, Thompson VL, Murphy DJ, Masica DN, Fluoxetine and suicide: A meta-analysis of controlled trials of treatment for depression, BMJ, September 21, 1991, 303:6804, p. 685-92.

51. Miller RA, Discussion of fluoxetine and suicidal tendencies, 147(11), American Journal of Psychiatry, November 1990, p. 1571.
52. Berkley RB, Discussion of fluoxetine and suicidal tendencies, 147(11), American Journal of Psychiatry, November 1990, p. 1572.
53. Henry JA, Toxicity of antidepressants: Comparisons with fluoxetine, Int Clin Psychopharmacol, June 1992 (6 Suppl), p. 22-7.
54. Borys DJ, Setzer SC, Ling LJ, Reisdorf JJ, Day LC, Krenzelok EP, Acute fluoxetine overdose: A report of 234 cases, 10(2) Am J Emerg Med, March 1992, p. 115-20.
55. Breggin, Talking Back to Prozac, p. 176-77.
56. Teicher MH, Glod C and Cole JO, Emergence of Intense Suicidal Preoccupation during fluoxetine treatment, 147(2) American Journal of Psychiatry, February 1990, p. 207-10.
57. Fava M, Rosenbaum JF, Suicidality and fluoxetine: Is there a relationship?, 52(3) Journal of Clinical Psychiatry, March 1991, p. 108-11.
58. Teicher MH, Glod CA, Cole JO, Dr. Teicher and associates reply [to Tollefson], 147(12) American Journal of Psychiatry, December 1990, p. 1692-93.
59. Masand P, Gupta S and Dewan M, Suicidal ideation related to fluoxetine treatment, letter in 324(6) New England Journal of Medicine, 324: February 7, 1991, p. 420.
60. King RA, Riddle MA, Chappell PB, Hardin MT, Anderson GM, Lombroso P and Scahill L, Emergence of self-destructive phenomena in children and adolescents during fluoxetine treatment, 30(2) Journal of the American Academy of Child and Adolescent Psychiatry, March 1991, p. 179.
61. Wirshing, op cit.
62. Dasgupta K, Additional cases of suicidal ideation associated with fluoxetine, 147(11) American Journal of Psychiatry, November 1990, p. 1570.
63. Teicher MH, Glod CA, Cole JO, Antidepressant drugs and the emergence of suicidal tendencies, 8(3) Drug Safety, March 1993, p. 186-212.
64. Geoffrey C, A prozac backlash, Newsweek, April 1, 1991, p. 64.
65. Angier N, Eli Lilly facing million-dollar suits on its antidepressant drug Prozac, The New York Times, 117: August 16, 1990, p. B13.
66. Talan J, Worries over an antidepressant, Newsday, July 3, 1990, Part III, p. 1.
67. Breggin interview, op cit.
68. Ibid.
69. Hoehn-Saric R, Lipsey JR, McLeod DR, Apathy and indifference in patients on fluvoxamine and fluoxetine, 10(5) Journal of Clinical Psychopharmacology, October 1990, p. 343-45.
70. Patterson WM, Fluoxetine-induced sexual dysfunction, 54(2) Journal of Clinical Psychiatry, February 1993, p. 71.
71. Herman JB, Brotman AW, Pollack MH, Falk WE, Biederman J, Rosenbaum JF, Fluoxetine-induced sexual dysfunction, 51(1) Journal of Clinical Psychiatry, January 1990, p. 25-7.

72. Murray MJ, Hooberman D, Fluoxetine and prolonged erection, 150(1) American Journal of Psychiatry, January 1993, p. 167-68.

73. Morris PL, Fluoxetine and orgasmic sexual experiences, 21(4) Int J Psychiatry Med, 1991, p. 379-82.

74. Walker PW, Cole JO, Gardner EA, Hughes AR, Johnson A, Batey SR, Lineberry CG, Improvement in fluoxetine-associated sexual dysfunction in patients switched to buproprion, 54(12) Journal of Clinical Psychiatry, December 1993, p. 459-65.

75. Breggin interview, op cit.

76. Mahendra D, Fluoxetine-associated dystonia, American Journal of Psychiatry, January 1994, p. 149.

77. Black B, Uhde TW, Acute dystonia and fluoxetine, 53(9) Journal of Clinical Psychiatry, September 1992, p. 327.

78. Reccoppa L, Welch WA, Ware MR, Acute dystonia and fluoxtine, 51(11) Journal of Clinical Psychiatry, November 1990, p. 487.

79. Bharucha KJ, Sethi KD, Complex movement disorders induced by fluoxetine, Mov Disord, 11: May 1996, p. 324-26.

80. Steur EN, Increase of Parkinson disability after fluoxetine treatment, 43(1) Neurology, January 1993, p. 211-13.

81. Caley CF, Friedman JH, Does fluoxetine exacerbate Parkinson's disease?, 53(8) Journal of Clinical Psychiatry, August 1992, p. 278-82.

82. Breggin interview, op cit.

83. Breggin, Talking Back to Prozac, p. 45-6.

84. Breggin interview, op cit.

AUTISM: IS THERE A VACCINE CONNECTION?

F. E. Yazbak

The routine administration of a live virus vaccine booster, during the postpartum period to previously vaccinated women who have remained rubella-susceptible should be reconsidered.

It is likely that continued rubella susceptibility in these women is not due to a problem with the vaccine, but with the woman herself, and therefore it seems reasonable not to attempt to correct it by the administration of more boosters.

Some re-vaccinated mothers are developing unusual problems, and many remain rubella-susceptible. Their children also appear to have an inordinate number of difficulties of their own. Twenty out of twenty five families (80%) in this study have children with autism.

Large-scale independent investigations on the possible link between live virus vaccines, MMR, and autism should be undertaken.

An epidemic increase in the incidence of autism nationwide has been noted in the last few years and was described in "Autism 99, A National Emergency."[1] This increase is still ongoing and indeed accelerating.

Many parents have suspected that such an increased incidence may be due to the administration of certain vaccines, a view vehemently denied by the vaccine authorities. Mothers who themselves were re-vaccinated in adulthood with live virus vaccines have also wondered if by receiving such vaccines, they could have in any way compromised their children's immune system, and predisposed them to adversely react to their own vaccinations.

Andrew Wakefield in an impressive study[2] published in *The Lancet* last year, reported remarkable and original findings, in a series of twelve cases at the Royal Free Hospital, London. He made it clear that his findings only raised questions, and that more studies on the possible relationship between Mumps-Measles-Rubella (MMR) vaccination and autism were needed. His research was immediately criticized, and the vaccine "establishment" viciously attacked him personally.

Brent Taylor and associates,[3] also from the Royal Free Hospital, published their own study this past June in *The Lancet* and reported no increase in autism in the UK after the introduction of the MMR vaccine in 1988.

Their research, which was financed by The Public Health Laboratory and the Medicines Control Agency, was hailed by the vaccine authorities, world wide, as the absolute proof, and the final word, that indeed there was no MMR/Autism link. However, parents of children with autism were not convinced, and many researchers rejected Taylor's methodology and conclusions. No large-scale independent studies have been carried out in the United States.

A study was therefore initiated to examine any connections between the administration of the MMR vaccine or any of its components to a woman in the childbearing age and the development of autism in her children.

Methodology

Members of vaccine and parent groups were contacted via e-mail, and notices were included in newsletters in the UK, Australia, and U.S.

The study outline and questionnaire were also posted in a well-known web site.[4]

Over 280 replies were received in 120 days. Of these, 240 were complete and accepted.

The discovery of unexpected and alarming findings in twenty five families where the mothers received a live virus vaccine shortly after delivery, prompted the release of this information at this time, because of its serious implications.

Review of present recommendations

The following are statements of the vaccine manufacturer and the Centers For Disease Control and Prevention, relative to the administration of live virus vaccines after delivery (the postpartum period):

➤"It has been found convenient in many instances to vaccinate rubella-susceptible women in the immediate postpartum period."[5]

➤"Recent studies have shown that lactating postpartum women immunized with (rubella) live attenuated vaccine may secrete the virus in breast milk and transmit it to breast fed infants.

In the infants with serological evidence with rubella infection, none exhibited severe disease; however, one exhibited mild clinical illness typical of acquired rubella. Caution should be exercised when Meruvax II is administered to a nursing mother."[6]

➤"It is not known whether measles or mumps vaccine virus is secreted in human milk. Recent studies have shown that lactating postpartum women immunized with live attenuated Rubella vaccine may secrete the virus in breast milk and transmit it to breast-fed infants.

In the infants with serological evidence of rubella infection, none exhibited severe disease: however, one exhibited mild clinical illness typical of acquired rubella. Caution should be exercised when MMR-II is administered to a nursing woman."[7]

➤"Excretion of small amounts of the live attenuated rubella virus from the nose or throat has occurred in the majority of susceptible individuals 7-28 days after vaccination. There is no confirmed evidence to indicate that such virus is transmitted to susceptible persons who are in contact with the vaccinated individuals. Consequently, transmission through close personal contact, while accepted as a theoretical possibility is not regarded as a significant risk. However, transmission of the vaccine virus to infants via breast milk has been documented. There are no reports of transmission of live attenuated measles or mumps viruses from vaccinees to susceptible contacts."[7]

➤"Although vaccine virus may be isolated from the pharynx, vaccinees do not transmit rubella to others, except occasionally in the case of the vaccinated breast feeding woman. In this situation, the infant may be infected, presumably through breast milk, and may develop a mild rash illness, but serious effects have not been reported.

Infants infected through breast-feeding have been shown to respond normally to rubella vaccination at 12–15 months of age. Breast feeding is not a contraindication to rubella vaccination and does not alter rubella vaccination recommendations."[8]

➤"Rubella vaccine recommendation: Prenatal screen with postpartum vaccination."[9]

Descriptions of cases

All mothers received postpartum boosters because they were rubella-susceptible.

Case 1: Mother received MMR in 1994, few hours postpartum. She had no miscarriages prior to 1994 and has had three since. The child, a boy, was normal till he received his MMR vaccine at age 13 months. Autistic symptoms were noted 1-2 months later. A maternal aunt has also remained rubella-susceptible in spite of multiple vaccinations.

Case 2: Mother who was fully immunized received MMR boosters in 1983 and 1991. She was again given another MMR in 1993, 4 hours postpartum. The child, a boy, was breast-fed and was well until age 15 months when he received an MMR vaccine. He developed autistic symptoms within the month, and also has gastro-intestinal (GI) problems.[2]

Case 3: Mother had measles and mumps as a child. She received rubella vaccine in 1985, two days postpartum. She did not breast feed because the child had a harelip and cleft palate. The child, a boy, received an MMR at age 15 months. He had gradual onset of autistic symptoms, and is now severely affected. He has received a course of IVIG infusions, and has elevated measles and rubella titers. He is also positive for Myelin Basic Protein Antibody (MBP). A younger sister is normal and immunized.

Case 4: Mother was fully immunized and received two MMR boosters. She was given a rubella vaccine in the immediate postpartum period. She has developed asthma and "immune problems" lately. The child, a boy 18 months of age is still breast-feeding, has allergies, and recurrent ear infections, but no evidence of autism to date.

Case 5: Mother, who was fully immunized, received an MMR vaccine in 1989 shortly after the birth of her 3rd child. This child, a girl, is not autistic, but has had frequently recurring ear infections and required a T&A. Two older brothers born in 1981 and 1987 are normal. So are the younger two sisters born in 1991 and 1997. The mother has had two miscarriages, one at 12 weeks in December 1996 and the other at 14 weeks in January 1999. Family history is positive for immune disease.

Case 6: Mother, who previously had been fully immunized, received an MMR booster 24 hours after she had a normal uncomplicated delivery. The child, a boy is now 13 years old. He had an uneventful newborn period, and breast-fed well. He remained fine till age 4 months when he received his second DPT, after which he developed a high fever and screamed for a long while. He then became extremely listless and difficult to arouse, breast-fed poorly, and started with gastro-esophageal reflux (which progressed and eventually required fundoplication). The boy went on to develop athetoid movements, and was later diagnosed with cerebral palsy. He is severely affected, has serious problems with interpersonal communication and at times "tunes out the world, and does not respond." His first MMR vaccination was delayed because of his neurological impairment. A younger brother is well and immunized.

Case 7: Mother, who had been previously immunized, received a rubella vaccine immediately after the birth of her first son in November 1989. She remained rubella susceptible, and was given another rubella vaccine three days after the birth of her second son. She is still rubella susceptible.

The oldest boy, born 11/6/1989, was breast-fed for a very short period. He was routinely immunized, and seems to be normal.

The second son, born 5/31/1991, was breast fed for one month, and received all his immunizations on schedule. At age 2 he started exhibiting autistic symptoms. He was diagnosed as PDD-NOS at Stanford at age 3. He was re-evaluated at UCSF a year later, and a diagnosis of autism was made. He seems to have autistic entero-colitis[2] and complains of itching, earaches and headaches. The third child, a girl, has verbal apraxia.

Case 8: Mother received rubella vaccine booster 8 weeks postpartum in 1983. That child, a boy, breast fed for one month, was immunized and seems intact. The second child, a boy was born in 1991. Mother reports that her delivery was difficult and that the baby was treated for meconium aspiration.

This boy received his first MMR vaccine at age 14 months, started exhibiting autistic symptoms around age 3, and was diagnosed as Asperger's Syndrome.

Case 9: Mother had a severe reaction to the measles vaccine at age 5. She was given an MMR booster on 9/11/1993, a few days after she delivered a daughter. That daughter, born September 6, 1993, was breast-fed for five months. She was routinely immunized in the first year of life. She "was sociable, but was not talking and had some OT issues" at 16 months, when she received her first MMR vaccine. She developed autistic symptoms "within days" of the vaccine, and was diagnosed with autism. She also had symptoms of autistic entero-colitis.[2]

A younger daughter born 11/20/1997 was nursed for sixteen months.

According to her mother: "She has some autistic symptoms but not all: she has a sensory integration disorder, and severe speech and language problems.

"She has the same digestive difficulties as her sister, and has been on casein and gluten-free diet since birth. She has not been vaccinated."

Case 10: Mother received rubella vaccine two months after the delivery of her first child, a girl who was born on 5/20/1992 and is well and immunized. The following child, a boy, born 1/14/1994 was breast-fed for six months. He received his first MMR around age 15 months in April 1995.

He started exhibiting autistic symptoms in July of that year, and lost more skills as time went by. He is positive for MBP, and has high measles titers.

The third child, a boy, age 2, is normal.

Case 11: Mother received rubella vaccine in 1991, immediately after the birth of her second child, a boy, whom she nursed for seven months.

Mother states: "My health problems began after his birth." The boy "was happy and talking until his MMR at 15 months. He has leaky gut symptoms,[2] digestive difficulties and candida." This boy was diagnosed with autism and has received 12 monthly infusions of IVIG, with good clinical results reportedly. His rubella titers were elevated initially, but came down towards normal after the infusions.

The oldest boy, born in 1990, is in good health and has been immunized.

Case 12: Mother received rubella vaccine postpartum "while in the hospital." She is now "starting with arthritis." Her only child, a boy, born May 1996, was breast fed for 13 months. He has severe reactions to most foods, and needed a rotation diet. He has not been immunized and shows no signs of autism.

Case 13: Mother received rubella vaccine in 1993, at the six-week postpartum check-up, while she was breast-feeding. She is now 35, and claims to be "extremely arthritic in my legs, have been since the vaccine."

The child, a girl, born May 1993, has received all her immunizations and does not appear to be autistic.

However, she has been diagnosed with Mc Cune Albright Syndrome and presented with precocious puberty, hyperthyroidism and a cystic ovarian tumor. Her right ovary and tube were surgically removed.

A second daughter, born 6/94 was diagnosed with Kawasaki Syndrome, three weeks after her 15 months immunizations. She was treated with IVIG infusions but went on to develop an aneurysm of her left descending coronary artery. She has "slow motor skills" and attends a special early childhood program.

Case 14: Mother received an MMR booster on 12/18/1991, two days after the birth of her first child, a girl, whom she only breast fed for 3 to 4 days.

Thirteen months later, she became pregnant with her second child. This boy was breast fed for two days only, and was routinely immunized. He received his first MMR at age 12 months, started with symptoms between 16 and 20 months, and was later diagnosed with autism. He is due for his second MMR vaccine. The mother claims that she has developed an immune disorder, and that she has a positive ANA. The older girl is well and has been immunized.

Case 15: Mother had MMR vaccine in 1993. She failed to develop adequate rubella titers, and was given another MMR booster in 1997, shortly after she delivered her second child, a daughter, who has been immunized and seems normal to date.

The oldest child, a boy born 12/7/1993, received one hepatitis B vaccination, and all his scheduled HIB, DPT and polio vaccines, as recommended, and without apparent immediate reaction. He received his first MMR at age 15 months. Mother reports that he started developing symptoms suggesting autism at the age of 18 months, and that his symptoms progressed, and became more marked, till the diagnosis of autism was confirmed. He has not received a second MMR.

Case 16: Mother received a rubella vaccine booster three days after the birth of her first child, a girl born 2/22/1992, who is well. The subsequent child, a boy, was not breast fed. He received his first MMR vaccine at 14 months of age, and his second at age 4 years. He has autism and his symptoms reportedly started at age 22 months.

Case 17: Mother was given a rubella vaccine booster shortly after the delivery of her first child who was born April 5, 1993. This girl has been immunized and is well. The following child, a boy, born 10/19/1994, was not breast-fed. He was routinely immunized and seemed well. At age 18 months, he received his first MMR vaccine. Parents noted unusual symptoms starting age 20 months, and the child has now been diagnosed as PDD/NOS. The third child, a daughter, born 7/28/1997, is well and has been immunized.

Case 18: Mother received a rubella vaccine booster shortly after delivering a son. This young man born 2/18/1986 has been diagnosed as having Asperger's Syndrome (AS).

Case 19: Mother received an MMR vaccine on 1/6/1991, two days after the birth of her first son who is healthy, has no developmental problems and has been routinely vaccinated. A second son, born 9/2/1992 was normal until the age of 18 months when he received his first MMR. He reportedly started with autistic symptoms within two months and the diagnosis of autism was later confirmed.

Case 20: Mother received an MMR booster in 1982 when she resumed her college education. In 1991, she was still rubella-susceptible and was given another MMR booster in January 1991, after the birth of her first child a boy who is being treated for Attention Deficit Disorder but who according to the mother has some autistic traits. Her second boy born in December 1992 received his first MMR vaccine at the age of 18 months, and was diagnosed with autism around the age of 33 months. A younger sister is developmentally normal but has allergies and eczema. The mother was found to be immune to rubella in 1992 but was told she was again rubella-susceptible in 1994.

Case 21: Mother, who is a physician, received a rubella vaccine immediately after the birth of her first child in 1989. She acquired rubella immunity and the boy seems developmentally normal.

A second son born in 1993 was diagnosed with autism at the age of three.

Case 22: Mother received an MMR vaccine shortly after she delivered her first child, a girl who is in good health and seems neurologically intact. The next child also a girl, who was conceived eight months after the mother's vaccination, exhibited autistic symptoms before her first birthday, and has been diagnosed with autism.

Case 23: Mother had a rubella titer of 9.2 during her first pregnancy. She delivered prematurely on October 1, 1993, and because her titer was below 10, she was given an MMR vaccine on October 3, 1993. The child, a girl, stayed in the nursery for 34 days but has developed normally and is doing well.

A second daughter was born 3 to 5 weeks prematurely on 1/15/1996. She was breast-fed for 6 months. She uttered a few words before her first birthday. On January 20, 1997, she received the MMR, HIB and Varicella vaccines. Her speech was noted to be quite delayed by the age of 18 months, and she soon thereafter developed severe behavioral difficulties. A diagnosis of autism was confirmed in October 1998.

The mother's rubella titer in July 1995 was 12.[3]

Case 24: Mother, who had been previously vaccinated, received a rubella vaccine booster on 8/15/1989, less than 24 hours after the birth of her first child. This boy was not breast-fed. He had G-E reflux, needed several formula changes and was constipated, but he appeared to be developing normally in the first year of life. He received his first MMR on 11/16/1990. According to the mother he appeared to interact much less with his surroundings by the time he was eighteen months old. His speech decreased and he was diagnosed with autism.

The second child a girl is 8 years old and is sensitive to gluten and Casein. She has several educational issues and is being evaluated for ADD.

Case 25: Mother received a rubella vaccine in 1979.

She delivered her first child in 1986 and received a second rubella vaccine.

In 1992, she delivered a second child and was given yet another rubella vaccine. This last child was noted to have speech and other problems and was diagnosed as having Asperger's Syndrome.

Discussion

Methodology

A prospective study of the general population is not feasible, and credible retrospective studies would have to compare matched groups:

➤With and without autism
➤With and without maternal re-vaccination
➤With and without children's vaccinations
➤And any variations thereof.

Identifying, selecting, and contacting such large groups would require a huge organization without any assurance of a large-scale response. The methodology used was the only one possible under the circumstances. In any case, the findings are impressively meaningful by themselves and in spite of any possible statistical bias.

General Discussion

In a very short time, and with limited research, twenty five families were identified, where the mothers were vaccinated in the postpartum period. Fourteen mothers received the rubella vaccine and eleven the MMR vaccine. Twenty cases were from the United States, four from the United Kingdom and one from Australia.

Twenty of the twenty five families (80%) report having children with autism, AS or PDD. One of these families, (Case 9), has two affected children, and the younger child, who is less affected, has not received the MMR vaccine. In another family (Case 20) there is one diagnosed and one suspected child with autism.

In nine cases, the child born immediately before the mother's booster developed autism. In ten others, that particular child was spared but the following child was diagnosed with the disease and in one case it was a previous child who was affected.

If there was a mother to child vaccine virus transmission in cases 3 & 24, it was not through breast milk, and it could have been through direct contact.

In two instances (Cases 16 & 17) where the mother did not breast-feed, the child born just before the maternal booster was normal. However the following child has autism.

In five families (Cases 4, 5, 6, 12, and 13) the children who were not diagnosed with autism report unusual problems, and in one (Case 6), the child seems to have autistic tendencies. In another (Case 12), the intact and only child has not received any MMR vaccine.

The first girl in case 9 who was born just before mother's vaccination was much more affected with the disease, than her younger sister born four years later.

Several mothers did not develop rubella antibodies in spite of repeated vaccinations.

Symptoms of immune diseases have been reported in many families.

Gender distribution[10]

Of the children born just before mother's vaccination and who developed autism seven were males, one was a female and in one case, the sex of the child was not listed.

Among the ten cases where it was the subsequent child who developed autism, there were eight males and two females.

Cases 5, 10, 13, 14, 15, 16, 17, 22, 23 represent situations where the children, all girls, whose births immediately preceded a maternal live virus vaccine booster, did not exhibit symptoms of autistic spectrum disorders. However some of them have developed immune, educational or unusual problems.

In cases 10, 14, 16, and 17 the subsequent male child was diagnosed with autism.

In cases 5 and 13, the girls who followed did not develop autism, while in cases 22 & 23, they did.

In case 15, it was the preceding child, a boy, who had the syndrome.

Conclusions

In spite of its statistical imperfections, this small study reveals new findings, which can not and should not be all blamed on coincidence and /or sample bias. It is hoped that it will prompt the vaccine manufacturers and the regulatory agencies to review this situation and their present recommendations with an open mind.

The routine administration of a live virus vaccine booster during the postpartum period to women who have previously been vaccinated, and yet have remained rubella-susceptible, should be seriously reconsidered.

It seems that women, who do not develop protective titers to rubella, after their initial vaccination and booster, have some immune difficulty of their own, which they may transmit to their children. It is most likely that their continued rubella susceptibility is not due to a problem with the vaccine, and therefore it seems reasonable not to attempt to correct it by the administration of more boosters.

In this study, re-vaccinated mothers seem to be developing unusual problems, and many have remained rubella-susceptible.

Their children also seem to have an inordinate number of difficulties.

Twenty out of the twenty five families have at least one child with autism.

Autistic symptoms often started shortly after the children were vaccinated.

Health providers should clearly explain to mothers that at least the rubella vaccine virus would be excreted in their nose, throat and breast milk, when obtaining "informed consent."

Serious research on whether measles vaccine virus is passed from mother to infant through breast milk should be undertaken.

The postpartum vaccination of women with live virus vaccines should be promptly and thoroughly reviewed.

Independent research looking into all possible causes of autism is imperative.

A second study, Part II on Intrapartum Vaccination with attenuated live virus vaccines is also being published at this time.[11]

References

1. Yazbak, F.E. : http://www.garynull.com/Documents/autism_99.htm
2. Wakefield AJ, Murch SH, Anthony A, et al: Ileal-lymphoid hyperplasia, non-specific colitis, and pervasive developmental disorder in children. Lancet 1998:351:637-41
3. Brent Taylor, Elizabeth Miller, C Paddy Farrington, Maria-Christina Petropoulos, Isabelle Favot-Mayaud, Jun Li, Pauline A Waight : Autism and

measles, mumps, and rubella vaccine: no epidemiological evidence for a causal association. Lancet 1998:353 # 9169

4. http://www.garynull.com/issues/MMRstudy.htm
5. PDR 1999, p. 1833
6. PDR 1999, p. 1834
7. PDR 1999, p. 1820
8. Epidemiology and Prevention of Vaccine-Preventable Diseases, (CDC) 5th edition, January 1999, p. 185
9. Epidemiology and Prevention of Vaccine-Preventable Diseases, (CDC) 5th edition, January 1999, p 187
10. Lang-Radosh, K.L., pers. comm. A review of male susceptibility to autism spectral disorders (in progress).
11. Yazbak, F.E. : Autism, Is there a vaccine connection? Part II. Vaccination during pregnancy.

Some of the above statements may not represent the views of organizations to which I belong.

This study is dedicated to all the wonderful mothers of children with autism. FEY.

E-mail: TLAutStudy@aol.com

Autism: Is There a Vaccine Connection? Part II

By F. E. Yazbak

The Centers for Disease Control and Prevention[1,2,3,4] and the vaccine manufacturers[5,6,7] have always warned against the administration of live virus vaccines during pregnancy, and shortly prior to conception.

This report describes six mothers who received live virus vaccines and one who received a Hepatitis B vaccine during pregnancy[8] after having received an MMR booster five months prior to conception.

All the children who resulted from these pregnancies have had developmental problems, six out seven (85%) were diagnosed with autism, and the seventh seems to exhibit symptoms often associated with autistic spectrum disorders.

A remarkable study from California released in March 1999, showed a 273% increase in autism in that state in the last ten years.[9]

Shortly thereafter "Autism 99, A National Emergency," a study based on the yearly reports of The U.S. Department of Education to Congress, described similarly impressive nationwide increases.[10]

Parents of children with autism are looking for answers to questions such as:

➤What could be causing such an increase in autism in this generation of children, when autism was so rare in the past ?

➤What environmental factors could be implicated?

➤Could something that happened to the mothers somehow predispose their children to autism?

Many parents have reported that their children's autistic symptoms had started shortly after they received their MMR vaccination. Was it possible the vaccine somehow reacted with antibodies which the child had received from his or her mother? And, if so, could that reaction start a chain of immune events which eventually would lead to autism?

A study was devised to investigate whether there is any association between vaccination with live virus vaccine and autism.

It was decided to target mothers who had received a live virus vaccine after the age of 16, whether or not they had an autistic child. If maternal antibodies were in any way a factor in the children's illness, then it would be reasonable to presume that the higher the maternal titers the more likely they are to precipitate the suspected immune reactions. Late re-vaccinations were the most liable to result in higher titers.

Women in the target group are usually re-vaccinated for two reasons:

➤They need to fulfill requirements for higher education or employment.

➤They fail to develop protective antibodies in response to prior live virus vaccinations.

This second group of mothers is particularly interesting, because their inability to produce protective antibody titers may not have been due to problems with the vaccine but rather to some immune dysfunction in the mothers themselves which could be passed to their children.

Neither a prospective study of the general population nor credible retrospective studies are presently available and therefore members of vaccine groups and parents of children with autism were contacted via e-mail, newsletters and the internet, and asked to identify friends and relatives.

Over 280 replies were received in 120 days. Of these, about 240 entries were complete and accepted. They will be included in the main study, due to be published soon.

Seven situations where a mother was vaccinated during pregnancy are reported.

Case Reports

Case 1: Mother who had been fully immunized received an MMR booster in College in 1985 and another during her postgraduate training in 1988.

In 1992, she applied for employment in a hospital and was found to be measles susceptible Because she was pregnant and was afraid of the rubella vaccine component of the MMR, she requested and was given the single measles vaccine. She was carrying twins, and one died in utero at about term. A few days later, the mother was induced (pitocin) and delivered.

The second twin, a boy, seemed healthy at birth. He is now described by the mother as "a high-need child... vaccine affected...

and nervous system oriented." Mother does not believe he is autistic yet describes several social and sensory constellations of symptoms which could be associated with autistic spectrum disorders. Mother has remained measles susceptible but has declined further vaccines

Case 2: Mother received a rubella vaccine while pregnant with her first child. This boy has autism and according to the mother, "he seemed to lose some of the delayed skills that he already had" after he was given the MMR vaccine.

The mother also states: "My other two sons have a lot of traits."

Case 3: Mother had all three live virus vaccines as a child and a booster as a teenager. In 1984, she was given a measles vaccine to fulfill college requirements. When she found out that she was pregnant she immediately contacted the health office at the college and her own HMO physicians, who were not concerned.

Mother delivered a boy who reportedly had poor eye contact and was less responsive than expected. He was given his first MMR at age 16 months and according to the mother seemed to deteriorate after that.

By age two, he was "visibly autistic," and the diagnosis was made at 26 months.

Case 4: Mother received an MMR booster in June 1994 five months prior to conception. She was also given a dose of hepatitis B vaccine on 9/1/94 and another on 10/6/94. Her third and last hepatitis B vaccine was administered on 4/6/95, while she was pregnant.

She delivered a boy on 8/4/95 and breast-fed him for 8 months. The child was "normal in the first year of life except for some digestive problems." He received his hepatitis B vaccines on 9/1/95, 10/2/95, and 6/6/96, and his first MMR at 16 months of age. He started exhibiting autistic symptoms at the age of 18 months and lost all language by the time he was 23 months old.

He has been diagnosed with autism, has tested positive for Myelin Basic Protein Antibody, and has elevated measles antibody titers. He is often severely constipated and in need of stool softeners.

A younger brother is developing normally and has been immunized routinely.

Case 5: Mother returned to college and was given an MMR vaccine in March 1990. A few days later she realized she was pregnant at the time of the vaccination. She delivered a boy in November whom she breast fed for six months and who started exhibiting autistic symptoms at the age of 10 months.

The diagnosis of autism was subsequently confirmed.

This boy received his first MMR on 12/18/91, his second on 8/18/95 and his hepatitis B series in 1998. The second child, a girl, born May 1992 is in good health and has been routinely vaccinated.

Case 6: This mother who was born 7/18/1965 was fully immunized as a child. She delivered her first child after a 5-month gestation on December 18, 1985. The baby weighed 2 lbs. and lived one month.

On 10/8/1987 she delivered a daughter who reportedly has an anxiety disorder.

In April 1992, the mother who was 13 weeks pregnant, was admitted to a hospital to undergo cervical banding. While in the hospital she was given a rubella vaccine booster because she was rubella-susceptible.

She delivered thirteen weeks prematurely on July 5, 1992. The baby, a girl, weighed 1lb 11oz and remained in the Neonatal Intensive Care Unit for 115 days. She developed and was treated for sepsis, broncho-pulmonary dysplasia, and apnea. She was also given her routine immunizations.

On October 19, 1992, the baby had an alarming hypotonic-hyporesponsive episode following her second set of DPT, Polio and HIB vaccines.

She was discharged from the hospital on October 28, with oxygen and an apnea monitor. Growth and development were reported delayed during the first year of life. The baby was given her MMR vaccine in October 1993, and according to the parents she started with head banging and self abusing behavior shortly thereafter. She also developed severe constipation.

A diagnosis of autism was confirmed at age 40 months.

Case 7: This Canadian mother received a rubella vaccine in 1981 when she was only a few days pregnant. She delivered a girl who appeared to be developmentally delayed starting at the age of two to three months and was mostly breast-fed for the first six months. The child received her first MMR on 7/14/1983, shortly after her first birthday and has been diagnosed with autism.

Discussion

The Centers for Disease Control and Prevention (CDC) and the vaccine manufacturer have long advised against the administration of live virus vaccines to women during and immediately before delivery.

Seven cases of women vaccinated during pregnancy are described in this report.

Three mothers received the rubella vaccine, two the measles vaccine, and one the MMR vaccine. The seventh mother (case 4) received the recombinant Hepatitis B vaccine, but had received an MMR vaccine five months prior to conception.

Problems with either the pregnancy or the child are reported in every instance. If these problems are indeed related to the vaccination, then the recommendation not to vaccinate during pregnancy is justified and should be enforced.

Six out of the seven children (85%) who resulted from these pregnancies were diagnosed with autism, and the seventh, (case 1) whose mother received a measles vaccine, exhibits symptoms which suggest autistic spectrum. This child's twin brother was stillborn.

One mother (case 2) may have more than one child with autism.

A mother vaccinated with the rubella vaccine in the thirteenth week of pregnancy (case 6) gave birth to a very small premature infant who had a stormy neonatal period.

The problems with two children (cases 1 and 6) were apparent at delivery.[3]

It is impossible to know in case 4 whether the hepatitis B vaccine given during pregnancy, or the MMR vaccine administered five months prior to conception, played any role whatsoever in the development of the child's autism.

If the MMR vaccine did, then it could conceivably affect mothers vaccinated some ten, twenty or more months prior to conception and in some way contribute to the development of autism in their children.

Selection bias alone can not explain all the reported findings.

Another study on vaccination after delivery[11] is reported separately.

The results of the main research on the effects of maternal vaccination with live virus vaccines after age 16 will be published in March 2000.

Conclusions

Seven mothers who were vaccinated during pregnancy have reported problems with the pregnancy or the resulting children.

These problems may not have happened if the mothers had not been vaccinated, and therefore the recommendation not to administer live virus vaccines during early pregnancy and shortly before conception should be enforced more stridently.

Consideration should be given to re-instate the Vaccine in Pregnancy Registry and to follow up the children born to mothers vaccinated during pregnancy for an extended period of time, as it is obvious that not all problems with the children were readily apparent at birth.[3]

Six out of the seven children born to mothers vaccinated during pregnancy have been diagnosed with autism. If live virus vaccination during early pregnancy or several months prior to conception is in any way a factor in the development of autism, then a similar relationship between autism and live virus vaccination in general should be seriously investigated by independent longitudinal large scale studies.

Susceptible adult females do not necessarily develop protective antibodies after receiving live virus vaccine boosters.

The administration of Hepatitis B vaccine during pregnancy should be reviewed.

The logic of ongoing research to develop new vaccines which can be administered to pregnant women in an effort to "vaccinate two for the price of one" should be very critically questioned.

References

1. CDC: Epidemiology and Prevention of Vaccine-Preventable Diseases, 5th Ed. page152: "Women known to be pregnant should not receive measles vaccine. Pregnancy should be avoided for 1 month following receipt of measles vaccine and 3 months following MMR vaccine."
2. CDC: Epidemiology and Prevention of Vaccine-Preventable Diseases, 5th Ed. page184: "Women known to be pregnant or attempting to become pregnant should not receive rubella vaccine. Although there is no evidence that

rubella vaccine virus causes fetal damage (see below), pregnancy should be avoided for 3 months after rubella or MMR vaccination."

3. CDC: Epidemiology and Prevention of Vaccine-PreventableDiseases, 5th Ed. page 186: "From 1971 to 1989 the Centers for Disease Control and prevention (CDC) maintained a registry of women vaccinated during pregnancy to determine whether congenital rubella congenital syndrome would occur in infants of such mothers. Sub-clinical fetal infection has been detected serologically in approximately 1% to 2% of infants born to susceptible vaccinees regardless of the vaccine strain. However, based on data collected by the CDC in the vaccine in pregnancy (VIP) registry (1971-1989) no evidence of CRS has occurred in offspring of the 321 susceptible women who received rubella vaccine and who continued pregnancy to term. The observed risk of vaccine induced malformations is now 0% ...As of April 30, 1989, CDC discontinued the VIP registry."

4. CDC: Epidemiology and Prevention of Vaccine-PreventableDiseases, 5th Ed. page 242: "Pregnant women who are otherwise eligible can be given hepatitis B vaccine"

5. PDR 1999, page 1737: "Do not give Attenuvax to pregnant females; the possible effects of the vaccine on fetal development are unknown at this time. If vaccination of postpubertal females is undertaken, pregnancy should be avoided for three months following vaccination."

6. PDR 1999, page 1833 : "Do not give Meruvax to pregnant females; possible effects of the vaccine on fetal development are unknown at this time. If vaccination of postpubertal females is undertaken, pregnancy should be avoided for three months following vaccination".

7. PDR 1999, page 1834 : "It is also not known whether Meruvax can cause fetal harm.
In a ten year survey involving over 700 pregnant women who received rubella vaccine within three months before or after conception none of the newborns had abnormalities compatible with rubella congenital syndrome."

8. PDR 1999, p. 1884 : "The (Hepatitis B) vaccine should be given to a pregnant woman only if clearly needed."

9. Changes in the population of persons with Autism and Pervasive Developmental Disorders in California's Developmental Services system : 1987 through 1998. A report to the legislature.
http://www.dds.ca.gov/autismreport.cfm

10. Yazbak, F.E. :Autism 99 A National Emergency

11. Yazbak, F.E. : Autism, Is there a vaccine connection? Part I: Vaccination after delivery.

The above may not represent the opinions of organizations to which I belong.

Dedicated to all the people of good will who are helping children and adults with autism. FEY.
E-mail: TLAutStudy@aol.com

Autism: Is There a Vaccine Connection? Part III

By F. E. Yazbak

Two studies, published in late December 1999, described the very high incidence of autism in children whose mothers had received live virus vaccines in the postpartum period,[1] prior to conception and during pregnancy.[2]

In the following weeks, twenty two more mothers reported having been vaccinated in those same periods. Every one of them (100%) subsequently had at least one child who developed Autism/PDD.

All three studies clearly demonstrate that the administration of a live virus vaccine booster to a mother, around conception, pregnancy, or delivery, may carry certain risks and merits immediate review.

There is crucial need for large-scale independent investigations of a vaccine–autism connection.

The Autism Pandemic

A substantial increase in the incidence of autism has been noted for sometime.

The current Diagnostic and Statistical Manual Fourth Edition (DSM IV) has for years clearly defined the criteria required to make a diagnosis of autism and other autistic spectrum disorders.

In 1999, two works "The Autism Report to the California Legislature" and "Autism 99, A National Emergency"[3, 4] clearly demonstrated an impressive and accelerating increase in Autistic Syndromes (DSM IV) in the last few years.

More recently, it was reported that in California alone, 1,944 new cases of autism (DSM IV) were added to the system between January 1999 and January 2000, a 19% increase in one year, or 6 new cases a day, seven days a week![5]

Excluded from these statistics are PDD, PDD-NOS and Asperger's Syndrome. Also excluded are the 15,000 plus children in the Early Start Program who are younger than three years of age. (Using the conservative estimate by the California DDS that each new child with autism added to the system will cost taxpayers $2 million over a lifetime of care, the 1,944 new children added in 1999 alone are projected to cost taxpayers $3.8 billion.)

Accelerating increases in autism have also been documented in other states. The argument that these increases are solely due to better detection is not valid because standardized diagnostic criteria have remained unchanged for years.

Denying this true increase in the incidence of autism is therefore callous.

Believing that a parent would accept such a label lightly, or that a school authority would include an unconfirmed case in its program is preposterous.

This autism explosion clearly indicates that research should cease to be limited to genetic causes. It would be wiser and more reasonable to direct funds and efforts to investigate all environmental and antigenic insults that could compound a familial predisposition to immune disease.

This very affected generation of children is unquestionably the most vaccinated yet, and as a group, their parents have also certainly been more extensively vaccinated than any previous parents' group.

The role of vaccines in precipitating autism should therefore become the focus of extensive and unbiased research.

Parents continue to report that gastro-intestinal symptoms[6] promptly follow the administration of the MMR vaccine to children, and that acquired speech and social skills stagnate and then regress after such vaccination.

To investigate what could be predisposing certain children to develop autism around the time of their MMR vaccination, a study was devised to examine the role of their mothers' re-vaccination with live virus vaccines.

The stipulation was that women who failed to develop protective titers to rubella did not do so because the vaccine was defective, but because they themselves had some immune problem, which they transmitted to their children.

As mentioned, two studies were released earlier because of their clinical and medico-legal implications.

The first: "Autism: Is there a vaccine connection? Part I" described mothers who were vaccinated in the postpartum period. Twenty out of twenty five of these mothers (80%) reported having at least one child with autism.[1]

The second study: "Autism: Is there a vaccine connection? Part II" reviewed seven situations where the mothers were vaccinated immediately before or during early pregnancy. Six out of those seven mothers (85%) reported having children with autism, and the seventh described in her child many suggestive symptoms of the autistic syndrome.[2]

In the present study, unfortunate outcomes are documented in each case.

Every mother who has received a live virus vaccine has had at least one child develop autism, in connection with or following such a vaccination.

Case Presentations

Case 1: This mother who was born in 1953 delivered her first child in November 1984 and was given a rubella vaccine shortly thereafter. This girl who was not breastfed is normal.

The mother then had three miscarriages before conceiving her second child, a boy who was born 9/8/1987. Again the mother was given a rubella vaccine shortly after delivery, and this time she breastfed her baby for four months.

This boy "was a happy healthy infant and he began walking around 12 months."

He received his first MMR at the age of 29 months. "He was approaching three when I became concerned with his inability to produce understandable verbal language." A long list of medical and educational diagnoses was exhausted before the diagnosis of autism was confirmed. "I have always felt there was a strong connection."

The third child, a daughter was born on 11/28/1988. Mother was given yet a third postpartum rubella booster and also breastfed this child who now has severe dyslexia, ADHD and learning disabilities.

Case 2: Mother born in 1965 reports that she had been fully immunized and boosted. On 7/30/1992, she delivered a boy and was given an MMR booster within 24 hours.

The child was breastfed and "developed normally until we saw a slow deterioration after his MMR vaccine at 16 months. He was diagnosed with autism at age 2."

He was vaccinated against Hepatitis B in July 1994, October 1994 and June 1996.

A younger brother born 9/19/98 is normal: "I feel the risk of vaccinating my second child outweigh the benefits. He has not and will not receive any vaccines."

Case 3: Mother born 1/24/61 was given a rubella vaccine booster on 4/5/1992 one day after her son was born. This boy was breastfed for eight months.

He received the Hepatitis B vaccine on 4/4/92, 5/7/92, and 10/12/92.

Mother felt that he started exhibiting autistic symptoms early, but that his first MMR vaccine "definitely worsened his symptoms". "He was different from other babies, never cried and slept all the time. Wet diapers, heat, cold, even shots didn't seem to phase him. His senses seemed to have shut down. His immune system is also really weak, he gets sick all the time, and is very thin and pale looking. He was exposed to "strept" a year and a half ago and now has Tourette's syndrome too."

"I believe my rubella vaccine postpartum and nursing contributed to his autism. I wish I could go back in time and refuse to take that rubella vaccine on April 5, 1992."

Case 4: This mother who was born in 1960, received a measles vaccine on 3/20/69, and a rubella vaccine on 7/16/1970. In March 1980, she was given a rubella vaccine booster shortly after the birth of her first child, a boy, whom she breastfed for nine months, and who is normal.

The second child a girl born on 8/10/1982 is also normal. Both children have not received hepatitis B vaccinations and did not react to any vaccines.

The mother who is a nurse was given her first dose of Hepatitis B vaccine in May and her second in June 1990. On 7/18/91 she received the third dose plus an MMR booster.

She became pregnant in the fall of 1991, and delivered a boy on 5/4/1992 whom she breastfed for 8 weeks. He did not receive the hepatitis B series.

He cried constantly for five months, and according to his mother developed autistic symptoms very early. He received his first MMR vaccine at 18 months.

"I believe that my son's autism worsened due to the MMR."

Case 5: This mother who was born in 1965, received an MMR booster in 1980. Her first daughter born 12/17/81 is normal and has been vaccinated routinely.

A second daughter was born on 10/24/91 and the mother received an MMR booster in the delivery room. The mother had a respiratory infection with some mucus and did not nurse this child, who was routinely vaccinated.

She was "a very happy baby, she said 'I love mommy' and 'Bye Bye,' she was pointing, knew her colors and some names of animals."

At the age of 17 months the girl was given DPT, Polio, HIB and MMR vaccines.

"We started noticing a difference in her speech and hand flapping just two months after her last round of shots. That is a lot of shots on one day."

This girl now has autism.

Case 6: This mother who was born in 1975 received one hepatitis B vaccine in 1996. On 3/18/1998, she delivered her first child, a boy who was given a hepatitis B vaccine in the nursery (without her knowledge). He received his second and third dose in May and November of 1998.

On 3/19/1998 the mother received a rubella vaccine. She nursed her baby for four months, but he had difficulties with breast milk and later with several formulas. "He had gastro-intestinal symptoms all through the first year of life. Very early he also had no eye contact and disliked being held. His behavioral difficulties became dramatically worse after his MMR vaccine," which he received with the DTaP and HIB boosters on 4/22/1999.

The child was evaluated and the diagnosis of autism was suggested.

The parents promptly initiated a strict gluten free/casein free (GF/CF) diet and started him on anti-fungal therapy with good results.

Case 7: This mother received an MMR booster in November 1991, 2 days after the birth of her second child, a daughter. She became pregnant again in February of 1992 and went on to deliver a daughter who developed autism.

"Though all of my children have disabilities, the youngest is the most severe."

Case 8: This mother had a normal and healthy first son. While traveling in Thailand, she was bitten by a dog. She was given a tetanus toxoid booster, and started on the rabies vaccine series.

When she discovered that she was pregnant, she decided to stop the rabies vaccines in spite of her doctor's assurance that they were safe.

Her second child, also a boy, was born in the US and received his first hepatitis B vaccine shortly after birth. He has experienced problems early and has autistic tendencies, some developmental delay and several other medical issues.

Case 9: Mother age 39, received an MMR booster because she was going back to college where there was an outbreak of measles.

She believes that one week later her middle child, was conceived. This boy was born on 9/29/91 without difficulty after a 38 weeks gestation.

The mother started nursing him but developed mastitis 10 days after delivery and was treated with antibiotics. This boy has had developmental difficulties all along. He has an abnormal EEG (Landau Klefner pattern) and has been taking Depakote. He has received all his immunizations on schedule except for the hepatitis B series. He did not seem to have a reaction to the MMR vaccine, and reportedly does not have GI symptoms. He has had recurrent yeast infections.

An older boy, now ten years of age, has ADHD.

A younger sister, age 6, is fine.

Case 10: This mother born in February 1959 has a family history of immune disease. She was routinely vaccinated but "needed" and received a rubella booster shortly after she delivered her first child, a girl, on 11/5/1987.

This girl is developmentally normal and has been routinely vaccinated, including the hepatitis B series at the age of 9.

The mother then had a miscarriage. She subsequently became pregnant and delivered a boy in December 1989. This child has significant speech difficulties and was classified as service eligible by the school special education committee.

He has been routinely vaccinated except for the hepatitis B series.

After a second miscarriage the mother became pregnant again and delivered a boy on September 7, 1992, whom she nursed for 18 months. This boy received a series of hepatitis B vaccines in the first year of life, an MMR at 12 months and a single measles at 61 months. He had severe constipation in infancy. The few words and eye contact he acquired in the first year of life were lost between 12 and 15 months. The diagnosis of autism was later confirmed.

Case 11: This mother delivered her first child, a girl, on 1/25/1992.

Two days later she was given an MMR vaccine booster "in case you have more kids."

The girl who was breastfed, had a reaction to her second DPT with prolonged high pitch cry and fever, but reportedly has developed normally.

In 1995 mother had a miscarriage.

In 1996 she became pregnant again. She had a viral illness in the end of her third month of gestation and felt there was "something different with the pregnancy after that." On August 3, 1997 she delivered a boy who is still breastfeeding.

He was "hypertonic" at birth and developed several allergies and food sensitivities later. He also had several bouts of ear infections as an infant. At the age of 11 months, he had a very severe case of chicken pox after which he lost language and eye contact. He has been diagnosed with autism. He has shown improvement on a Gluten-free and Casein-free diet.

He has not received any vaccines.

Case 12: This mother's first pregnancy resulted in a daughter who is now 22 years old.

She is in good health and goes to college.

Her second child, a boy, died at the age of three months of SIDS.

Her next child a boy was born on 9/21/1979. The following day, the mother received an MMR vaccine. The boy was breastfed for six months and received his first MMR vaccine at 15 months.

By the age of eighteen months, he stopped talking. "He became withdrawn, refused to be held, and reacted to any change with severe temper tantrums."

Simultaneously, he also started with prolonged diarrhea.

He has been diagnosed with autism. His chromosomal analysis is normal.

The subsequent children in the family were:

A girl, 19, and a boy, 17, both with serious learning disabilities.

A boy, 15, with Tourette's syndrome, PDD and an IQ of about 100.

A boy, 11, with PDD and an IQ of 70.

A boy, 10, with PDD and an IQ of 50.

Lastly a girl who was born in 1991 at 32 weeks gestation.

She weighed 3 lbs, had hypo-plastic left heart syndrome, and only one kidney.

She lived two days.

Family history on both sides was negative for autism and the mother's chromosomal studies were normal.

Case 13: This mother was born in 1966. On 2/15/1997, she delivered a boy and was given an MMR vaccine the following day. The baby received his first hepatitis B vaccine on 2/17/1997 and his second and third on 3/25 and 11/17, 1997. The baby was breastfed for three months. He had severe G-E reflux and constipation. He was switched to Nutramigen and had an endoscopy, and a barium enema. He walked alone before he was one, and was saying a few words. Reportedly, he was developing normally until he received his first MMR at the age of 15 months. Autistic symptoms started between 15 and 18 months. He lost the speech he had acquired, and his behavior and eating habits changed drastically.

Case 14: This mother born in 1963 had measles and mumps as a child.

In 1985, she was given an MMR vaccine because there were cases of rubella in college. On November 24, 1993, she delivered her first child, a normal girl, whom she breastfed.

The following day, she was given a rubella vaccine because her titers were low and "they wouldn't discharge me without giving me the shot."

The mother became pregnant again within seven months of the booster, and delivered a boy on 3/24/1995, who was also breastfed (for eight months). He cooed and smiled earlier but appeared to have problems by the time he was nine months old. He has had very poor expressive language and was diagnosed with autism. Family history on both sides is totally negative for autism.

Case 15: This mother delivered her first son on 2/6/1990. The following day, she received a rubella vaccine. This boy reportedly has an attention deficit disorder.

Her second child a girl is normal.

The mother reports that there were family problems and that she was depressed during her third pregnancy. She experienced some "indigestion" around the third week of gestation that she could relieve by drinking one ounce of beer (a day). This apparently lasted 4 weeks.

She also had an ear infection and was treated with Erythromycin.

At term, she was induced with pitocin. On 4/19/1993 she delivered a boy who was breastfed for a year. He was always severely constipated. He reportedly developed clear autistic symptoms by the age of 18 months before his MMR vaccine.

Case 16: This mother who was born in 1954 received a rubella vaccine in 1985.

Her oldest child, a girl who was born on 3/27/1986, has developed normally and has been immunized.

The mother delivered her second daughter on 2/25/1990. There was "some delay in taking her first breath due to meconium" according to the mother.

On 2/26/1990, the mother who was nursing received a rubella vaccine.

On 3/21/90 the mother consulted her physician because "she was coughing, had red spots all over and itchy arms and hands."

The girl has had developmental difficulties all along and has been diagnosed as PDD-NOS.

Case 17: This mother born in 1967 had two uncomplicated pregnancies and two beautiful normal children. During her second pregnancy, her rubella titers were found to be low. Somehow no one noted the results and no booster was administered postpartum.

Two years later, the doctor gave her an MMR vaccine because her earlier shot "didn't take" and urged her not to become pregnant for three months.

She conceived 4 months later. The pregnancy was "plagued with several colds... I had a tachycardia throughout which was not treated with medications."

The delivery was uncomplicated but "it took the baby a minute before crying."

The child, a boy, was routinely vaccinated. He always had strong smelling stools and recurrent fungal infections in the first year of life. He received his first MMR at 15 months of age and lost the few words he had acquired.

His autistic symptoms became more evident and he has now been diagnosed with PDD-NOS.

Case 18: This mother, born in 1964, was vaccinated routinely as a child but still came down with all three diseases: measles, rubella and mumps. She was evaluated at the time and found to have some immune problem for which she received injections of gamma globulin.

In 1983, she received an MMR vaccine because there was an outbreak of measles at college. In 1991, 1992 and 1997, she was found to be immune to measles.

She was immune to rubella in January 1991, when she was pregnant with her first boy, who is fine. In October 1992, when she became pregnant with her second boy, she was found to be rubella-susceptible. She delivered on 5/5/1993 and her doctor gave her yet another MMR that same day "against my will. For what little I knew, if I couldn't have it while I was pregnant, I didn't want it if I was going to be nursing. My MD would not discharge me from the hospital without the vaccine first—I was bullied and lost. This guilt I will always carry."

This second boy has been diagnosed with autism. On the 4th day of life, "he curled up into a ball and screamed for 24 hours straight" (this event may represent the beginning of his GI insult).

The child became severely constipated through the first year of life and has had severe diarrhea since then.

His body temperature has always been below normal, and he actually has had a ruptured appendix and generalized peritonitis without a fever.

A third child, a girl, is normal.

The mother has several markers for Lupus. She received the hepatitis B vaccine series on 9/98, 10/98, and 3/99.

Case 19: This mother, born in 1971 was routinely vaccinated as a child.

She had a miscarriage on 1/6/1993 at 28 weeks gestation.

Four weeks later, she was given an MMR booster because she was rubella-susceptible.

On 3/10/1994, she delivered a boy four weeks prematurely. This boy reportedly has ADHD, motor dyspraxia and sensory integration dysfunction.

Her second boy was born on 7/8/1995. He has been diagnosed with "autistic spectrum disorder." His symptoms started before he was one.

The last boy was born on 12/22/1996. Like his oldest brother he has been diagnosed with sensory integration dysfunction and dyspraxia, both motor and verbal.

All three boys were breastfed and routinely immunized.

Case 20: This mother who was born in 1963 and who is a juvenile diabetic delivered a boy on 1/6/1998 and breastfed him for a month. On 1/9/1998 she was given an MMR booster.

This boy was in good health in the first year of life. He seemed to develop normally and reportedly had no problems. He was given his MMR vaccine at the age of 15 months.

Autistic symptoms appeared between 15 and 18 months of age, and a diagnosis of autism was confirmed at the age of two.

Three months after her own MMR booster, the mother developed significant swelling and pain in her joints. These symptoms have been recurring regularly.

In the spring of 1999 she had a miscarriage.

Case 21: This mother who delivered her first child, a normal girl, on 9/20/1989 received an MMR vaccine booster the following day.

On 2/8/1995, her second child, a boy, was born. Unlike his older sister, he was given a hepatitis B vaccine in the nursery. He was breastfed for one year, and developed normally till he received his first MMR vaccine at the age of fifteen months. Autistic symptoms appeared very shortly thereafter, and have been clearly documented by videos. The diagnosis of autism was later confirmed.

This boy's measles and rubella titers remain very elevated. "Most doctors do not believe this and feel it is just a coincidence, but they did not see their child disappear before their eyes.... I truly believe he was predisposed and the MMR set it off."

Case 22: This mother who was born in 1957 suffers from scleroderma.

She reports having been routinely vaccinated as a child.

On 2/19/1997, she delivered her first son at full term and she breastfed him.

She was given an MMR booster prior to discharge, and developed a fever and a rash.

The boy appeared bright, verbal and sociable during the first year of life.

At the age of 15 months, he was given his first MMR, and reacted promptly with fever, irritability and loose stools. Shortly thereafter he also lost the speech he had acquired and seemed to withdraw. He now has eczema, persistent diarrhea and sleep difficulties.

He has been diagnosed with "autistic spectrum."

A maternal aunt has social difficulties that suggest Asperger's Syndrome.

Discussion

The clinical cases of 22 mothers are reported.

➤ They all received a live virus vaccine around a pregnancy.

➤Every one of them has at least one child with autism.

Several mothers who were in good health and had normal children, report that after they were re-vaccinated with MMR or rubella vaccines:

➤They experienced health problems.

➤They had miscarriages or delivered prematurely.

➤They still remained rubella-susceptible.

➤Their children developed autism and other disabilities.

Seven mothers received a rubella vaccine in the postpartum period.

In five cases, the child born just before that vaccination developed autism.

In the other two cases, a subsequent child did.

Eleven mothers received the MMR vaccine after delivery. In seven cases, the child whose birth immediately preceded the vaccination developed autism.

In the four other cases, it was a subsequent child who was affected.

In one situation, the boy born just before maternal MMR vaccination and three younger brothers have all been diagnosed with either autism or PDD.

Three mothers received an MMR vaccine from one week to four months prior to conception. In every case the infant developed autistic symptoms early during the first year of life.

One mother received several doses of rabies vaccines just before and after conception. The boy she delivered had early onset autism.

In many instances, the children's autistic manifestations reportedly started or worsened after they received their first MMR vaccine.

In one case, clinical autism started at the age of eleven months after chickenpox.

No mother seems to have been fully informed about the risks of the vaccine she was receiving and several seem to have been badgered into accepting it.

Whether Hepatitis B vaccination in the newborn period is an antigenic insult which increases the risk of developing autism should be thoroughly examined.

All reporting mothers live in the United States.

Conclusions

The administration of live virus vaccines to a mother just before or during early pregnancy is inappropriate.

Postpartum vaccination with MMR or rubella vaccines may not be safe or wise:

➤Possible risks to both mother and child have been demonstrated.

➤Alleged benefits seem to pale in the face of resulting problems.

➤Maternal immunity is not assured.

An antigenic insult from a live virus vaccine may be a factor in the development of the autistic syndromes.

The vaccine authorities should carefully reconsider their former positions that:

➤There is absolutely no autism-vaccine connection.

➤The onset of autism around MMR vaccination is just a coincidence.

It is now up to them to prove that vaccines do not predispose to autism.

Independent large-scale studies should be promptly initiated.

References

1. Autism: Is there a vaccine connection? Part I. Vaccination after delivery.
   <htttp://www.garynull.com/Documents/autism99b.htm>
2. Autism: Is there a vaccine connection? Part II. Vaccination during pregnancy.
   < http://www.garynull.com/Documents/autism99b2.htm>
3. Changes in the population of persons with Autism and PDD
   California's Developmental Services System: 1987 through 1998. A report to the Legislature.
   <http://www.dds.ca.gov/autismreport.cfm>
4. Yazbak, F.E.: Autism 99, A National Emergency
   <http://www.garynull.com/Documents/autism_99.htm>
5. Rollens R.: Personal communication, January 2000
6. Wakefield AJ, Murch SH, Anthony A, et al: Ileal-lymphoid hyperplasia, non-specific colitis, and pervasive developmental disorder in children. Lancet 1998:351:637-41

Some of the above statements may not represent the views of organizations to which I belong.

This study is dedicated to my daughter Kathleen who unfortunately received two MMR boosters as an adult. She has experienced first hand how children develop spectrum diseases after immunization and has taught me a lot about autism. FEY.

E-mail: TLAutStudy@aol.com

*I*NDEX

hormone replacement therapy
for, 84–85
and hormones, 81–82
and mental activity, 85
and NADH, 78
and nutrition, 83–84
pharmaceuticals for, 84
statistics on, 78
and stress management, 85–86
treatment, 79–86
and vitamin supplements, 83–84
American Academy of Environmental
Medicine, 237–38
amino acids
and alcoholism, 67–68
analysis, 192–93
and anxiety disorders, 90–91
for depression, 125
and nutrient imbalances, 307–9
amphetamines, 70–71, 123
anacardium, 294
anorexia nervosa
and anxiety, 107–8
cognitive therapy for, 107
and heart problems, 104, 108
reflexology for, 109–11
and Ritalin, 221
and zinc deficiency, 102, 103–6
anti-aging medicine, 183
Anti-Aging Plan, The (Wolford),
78–79
anti-psychotic drugs. *see* psychiatric
drugs
antibiotics, 218–19, 231–32
and candida, 273
and chronic fatigue syndrome, 288
antidepressants, 45, 123–24
natural, 129–30
Prozac, 43, 70–71, 120–21, 200–1
St. John's Wort, 129–30
tryptophan, 120–21, 124
zinc, 105–6
antioxidants, 79–80, 81

anxiety
and alcoholism, 69
and diet, 18–19
anxiety disorders, 87–98
agoraphobia, 88
and auto-immune processes, 91
causes of, 91–92
and diet, 90, 92
and environmental allergies, 88
generalized, 88–89
homeopathic remedies, 89–90
and indigestion, 88
kava, 93–94
and mitral valve prolapse, 87–88
obsessive-compulsive disorders,
94–98
panic attacks, 87, 88
and peptides, 91–92
post traumatic stress disorder, 89
treatments for, 89–91
arsenicum album, 294
Aslan, Ana, 80
aspartame, 16
asthma, 262
Atkins, Robert
on addictions, 63
on depression, 124
on importance of nutrition, 18–19
on insomnia, 167
on obsessive-compulsive
disorders, 97–98
attention-deficit hyperactivity
disorder, 50–51, 203–23
in adults, 169–72
and alkalinity, 216–17
and allergies, 204–5
and antibiotics, 218–19
and dairy products, 214
diagnosis of, 206–7, 213–14
discipline for, 219
environmental factors, 208–9,
218–19
exercise for, 171

Breggin, Peter
  on aggression, 200–2
  on psychiatric drugs, 41–43
  on Ritalin, 221–22
  on schizophrenia, 152–53
  on tardive dyskinesia, 173–75
Brundtland, Gro Harlem, 9–10
bulimia nervosa, 108
  complications from, 100
  reflexology for, 110–11
  and zinc deficiency, 102, 103–6
Buttram, Harold
  on attention deficit disorder, 206
  on behavioral disorders, 235–39
  on environmental toxins, 195–96
  on food allergies, 246

C

caffeine, 290
  and chronic fatigue syndrome,
    286–87
  and insomnia, 163–64
Calapai, Christopher, 24–25
calcium, 127, 214, 217
candida, 19, 92, 264–65
candidiasis, 267–81
  causes of, 273–74
  and depression, 277, 281
  and diet, 274, 276, 277
  and the digestive system, 274
  and the immune system, 274,
    277–78
  and the liver, 274–75
  personal accounts of, 267–83,
    280–81
  and sugar, 276
  symptoms of, 273, 273–74, 275
  treatments for, 275–77, 280
Caplan, Paula, 47–49
cardamom, 131
Carpenter, Karen, 100, 104
Carrigan, Catherine, 114, 117–18, 122

Cass, Hyla
  on food addiction, 75
  on hypoglycemia, 263–64
  on PMS, 314–16
  on thyroid disorders, 320–22
chelation therapy, 25, 80, 82, 172
chemical imbalances, 53
chemical toxins. see environmental
  toxins
chi energy, 284
children
  and food allergies, 22, 239, 245–57
  organic diet for, 238–39
  overmedication of, 50–52
  poor eating habits of, 242–43
  vitamin supplements for, 239
children, disorders in, 195–96
  aggression, 197–202
  allergies, 245–57
  attention-deficit hyperactivity dis-
    order, 203–23
  autism, 225–32
  behavioral disorders, 233–39
chronic depression, 241–43
cholinesterase, 33, 34
chronic depression, 241–43
chronic fatigue syndrome, 283–300
  and B vitamins, 287, 290–91
  and caffeine, 286–87, 290
  causes of, 292, 297–99
  and depression, 289, 296
  and energy, 284–85
  and Epstein Barr virus, 292, 297
  and food sensitivities, 289
  and glutathione, 295–96
  herbal remedies for, 291
  homeopathy for, 292–95
  and the hypothalamus, 287–88
  and the immune system, 299–300
  and nutrition, 287, 289–91
  nutritional deficiencies, 288
  and sugar, 290
  symptoms of, 286, 296–97

digestive system
  and anxiety, 91–92
  and candidiasis, 274
  and insomnia, 164
Dumont, Matthew, 43
Dunkell, Jerry, 159–62

E

Eades, John, 71–74
eating disorders, 99–111
  causes of, 100
  reflexology for, 109–11
  and stress, 103, 105
  and zinc, 99–106
Edelman, Eva, 147–48
electro convulsive therapy, 46–47
electrolytes, 241–42
Eli Lilly, 43
Ellis, Leander
  on autism, 227
  on depression in children, 241
  on hypoglycemia, 264–65
endocrine system, 180
endorphin system, 21
endorphins, 70
energy, 284–85
environment
  influence on mental states of,
    15–19
environmental allergies. *see*
  allergies, environmental
Environmental Health Network, 325
environmental toxins, 249–51
  and attention-deficit hyperactivity
    disorder, 208–9
  and behavioral disorders, 235–38
  and children, 195–96
  formaldehyde, 36, 37, 38, 237
  and the medical community, 36–37
  and mental health problems, 32–40
  mold, 256
  organic solvents, 237

perfumes, 37
pesticides, 34–36, 237
in schools, 249–56
treatments for, 237–39
in the workplace, 256
epinephrine (adrenaline), 18, 265, 305
Epstein Barr virus, 292, 297
estrogen, 81–82, 84–85, 303–4
Everett, Sandra, 49–51
exercise
  and attention-deficit hyperactivity
    disorder, 171
  and brain health, 182, 183
  and depression, 133–136
  for fibromyalgia, 291–92
  and insomnia, 165–66
  mental, 182

F

fatigue
  and chi energy, 283–85
  and depression, 289
  levels of, 285–86
fatty acids
  analysis, 192
  and depression, 121–22
fibromyalgia, 286, 291–92
flavonoids, 66
flax seed, 17
fluoride, 209
fo-ti, 132
folic acid, 120
food addictions, 74–76
food allergies, 19–22
  and ADHD, 22, 204–5, 214–15,
    220
  and behavioral disorders, 234
  in children, 22, 239, 245–57
  dairy products, 214, 256–57
  diagnosis of, 249–51, 254–55,
    256–57
  and food addictions, 20, 74–76

Gary Null, Ph.D., is one of America's leading health and fitness writers and alternative practitioners. Trained as a nutritionist, he is the author of dozens of books and hundreds of medical articles. His one-hour health radio program airs daily on WBAI in New York City, and is carried weekly to 32 stations nationwide over the Virtual Radio Network. Null is a former faculty member of the New School for Social Research and a National TAC Master Champion Racewalker. Among his many best-selling books are *Get Healthy Now!*, *The Ultimate Anti-Aging Program*, and, with Barbara Seaman, *For Women Only!* He lives in New York City and Naples, Florida.

Louise Bernikow is a Fulbright Fellow, an award-winning magazine writer, and the author of seven books, including *Among Women* and *Alone in America*, and her memoir, *Bark if You Love Me*.